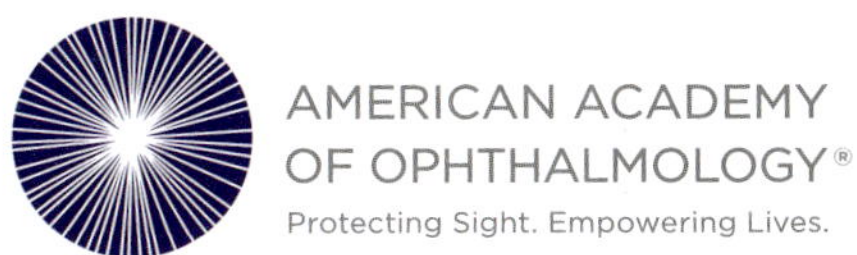

3 | Clinical Optics and Vision Rehabilitation

Last major revision 2022–2023

2024–2025

BCSC

Basic and Clinical Science Course™

EB

Published after collaborative review with the European Board of Ophthalmology subcommittee

The American Academy of Ophthalmology is accredited by the Accreditation Council for Continuing Medical Education (ACCME) to provide continuing medical education for physicians.

The American Academy of Ophthalmology designates this enduring material for a maximum of 15 *AMA PRA Category 1 Credits*™. Physicians should claim only the credit commensurate with the extent of their participation in the activity.

CME expiration date: June 1, 2025. *AMA PRA Category 1 Credits*™ may be claimed only once between June 1, 2022, and the expiration date.

To claim *AMA PRA Category 1 Credits*™ upon completion of this activity, learners must demonstrate appropriate knowledge and participation in the activity by taking the posttest for Section 3 and achieving a score of 80% or higher. For further details, please see the instructions for requesting CME credit at the back of the book.

The Academy provides this material for educational purposes only. It is not intended to represent the only or best method or procedure in every case, nor to replace a physician's own judgment or give specific advice for case management. Including all indications, contraindications, side effects, and alternative agents for each drug or treatment is beyond the scope of this material. All information and recommendations should be verified, prior to use, with current information included in the manufacturers' package inserts or other independent sources, and considered in light of the patient's condition and history. Reference to certain drugs, instruments, and other products in this course is made for illustrative purposes only and is not intended to constitute an endorsement of such. Some material may include information on applications that are not considered community standard, that reflect indications not included in approved FDA labeling, or that are approved for use only in restricted research settings. **The FDA has stated that it is the responsibility of the physician to determine the FDA status of each drug or device he or she wishes to use, and to use them with appropriate, informed patient consent in compliance with applicable law.** The Academy specifically disclaims any and all liability for injury or other damages of any kind, from negligence or otherwise, for any and all claims that may arise from the use of any recommendations or other information contained herein.

Cover image: From BCSC Section 4, *Ophthalmic Pathology and Intraocular Tumors*. Photomicrograph of focal posttraumatic choroidal granulomatous inflammation. *(Courtesy of Vivian Lee, MD.)*

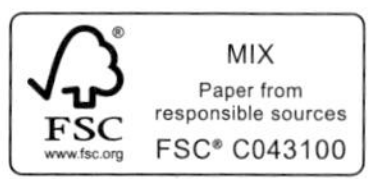

Printed in India.

Basic and Clinical Science Course

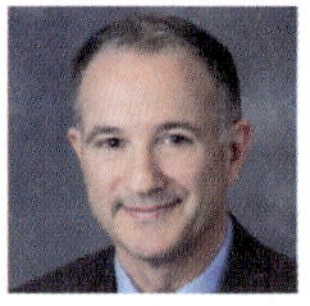

Christopher J. Rapuano, MD, Philadelphia, Pennsylvania
Senior Secretary for Clinical Education

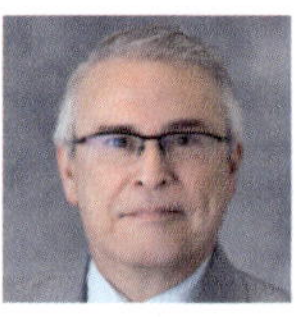

J. Timothy Stout, MD, PhD, MBA, Houston, Texas
Secretary for Lifelong Learning and Assessment

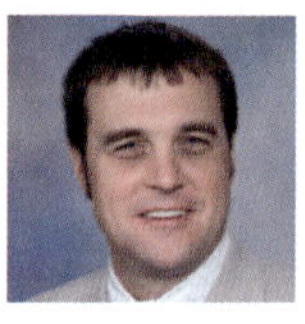

Colin A. McCannel, MD, Los Angeles, California
BCSC Course Chair

Section 3

Faculty for the Major Revision

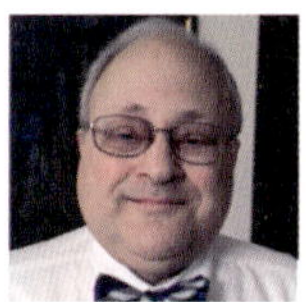

Scott E. Brodie, MD, PhD
Chair
New York, New York

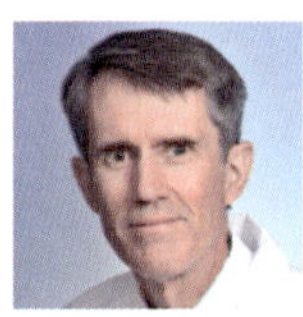

Thomas F. Mauger, MD
Morgantown, West Virginia

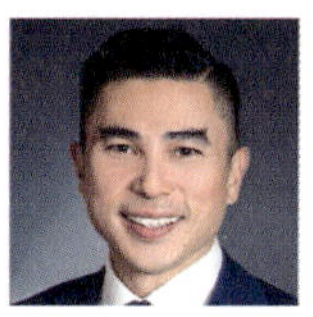

Marcus Ang, MBBS, PhD
Singapore

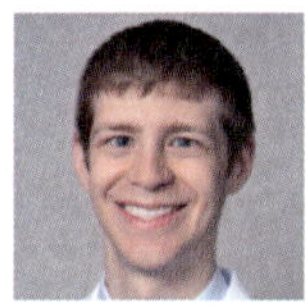

Tyler Oostra, MD
Columbus, Ohio

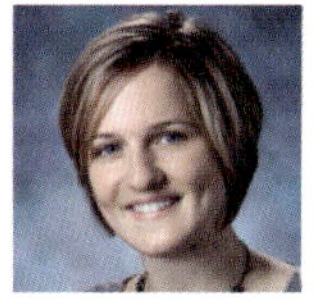

Kristina Irsch, PhD
Baltimore, Maryland
and Paris, France

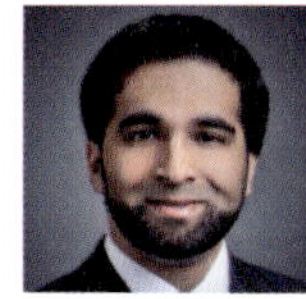

Kamran M. Riaz, MD
Oklahoma City, Oklahoma

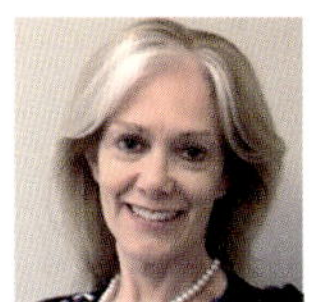

Mary Lou Jackson, MD
Vancouver, Canada

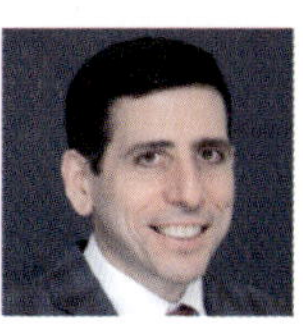

Joshua A. Young, MD
New York, New York

The Academy wishes to acknowledge the following committees for review of this edition:

Committee on Aging: Daniel C. Tu, MD, PhD, Portland, Oregon

Vision Rehabilitation Committee: Mary Lou Jackson, MD, Vancouver, Canada

BCSC Resident/Fellow Reviewers: Sharon L. Jick, MD, *Chair,* St Louis, Missouri; Jennifer Lynne Barger, MD; Tamara Lee Lenis, MD, PhD; Kenneth W. Price, MD; Brittany Simmons, MD; Heather Stiff, MD; Nandini Venkateswaran, MD; James T. Walsh, MD; Madeline W. Yung, MD

Practicing Ophthalmologists Advisory Committee for Education: Bradley D. Fouraker, MD, *Primary Reviewer*, Tampa, Florida; Cynthia S. Chiu, MD, Oakland, California; George S. Ellis Jr, MD, New Orleans, Louisiana; Philip R. Rizzuto, MD, Providence, Rhode Island; Gaurav K. Shah, MD, Town and Country, Missouri; Rosa A. Tang, MD, MPH, MBA, Houston, Texas; Troy M. Tanji, MD, Waipahu, Hawaii; Michelle S. Ying, MD, Ladson, South Carolina

The Academy also wishes to acknowledge the following committee for assistance in developing Study Questions and Answers for this BCSC Section:

Resident Self-Assessment Committee: Evan L. Waxman, MD, PhD, Chair, Pittsburgh, Pennsylvania; Robert A. Beaulieu, MD, Southfield, Michigan; Benjamin W. Botsford, MD, New York, New York; Olga M. Ceron, MD, Grafton, Massachusetts; Kevin Halenda, MD, Cleveland, Ohio; Amanda D. Henderson, MD, Baltimore, Maryland; Andrew M. Hendrick, MD, Atlanta, Georgia; Joshua Hendrix, MD, Dalton, Georgia; Matthew B. Kaufman, MD, Portland, Oregon; Zachary A. Koretz, MD, MPH, Pittsburgh, Pennsylvania; Kevin E. Lai, MD, Indianapolis, Indiana; Kenneth C. Lao, MD, Temple, Texas; Yasha S. Modi, MD, New York, New York; Mark E. Robinson, MD, MPH, Columbia, South Carolina; Jamie B. Rosenberg, MD, New York, New York; Tahira M. Scholle, MD, Houston, Texas; Ann Shue, MD, Sunnyvale, California; Jeong-Hyeon Sohn, MD, Shavano Park, Texas; Misha F. Syed, MD, League City, Texas; Parisa Taravati, MD, Seattle, Washington; Sarah Van Tassel, MD, New York, New York; Matthew S. Wieder, MD, Scarsdale, New York; Jules A. Winokur, MD, Great Neck, New York

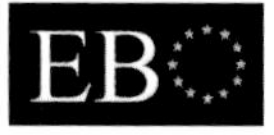

European Board of Ophthalmology: Lotte Welinder, MD, *Liaison,* Aalborg, Denmark; Roger C. Humphry, MD, MBBS, Salisbury, England

Financial Disclosures

Academy staff members who contributed to the development of this product state that within the 24 months prior to their contributions to this CME activity and for the duration of development, they have had no financial interest in or other relationship with any entity whose primary business is producing, marketing, selling, reselling, or distributing health care products used by or in patients.

The authors and reviewers state that within the 24 months prior to their contributions to this CME activity and for the duration of development, they have had the following financial relationships:*

Dr Fouraker: Addition Technology (C, L), AJL Ophthalmic, S.A. (C, L), Alcon (C, L), OASIS Medical (C, L)

Dr Jackson: Astellas Pharma (C)

Dr Lai: Twenty/Twenty Therapeutics (C)

Dr Modi: Alimera Science (C), Allergan (C), Carl Zeiss (C), Genentech (C), Novartis (C), Théa Laboratories (C)

Dr Riaz: Bausch + Lomb (L), Beaver-Visitec International (C), CorneaGen (L), ImprimisRx (S)

Dr Robinson: Horizon Therapeutics (O)

Dr Shah: Allergan (C, L, S); Bausch + Lomb (L); D.O.R.C. Dutch Ophthalmic Research Center (International) B.V. (S); Regeneron Pharmaceuticals (C, L, S)

Dr Tang: EMD Serono (L); Horizon Therapeutics (C, S); Immunovant (S); Novartis (S); Quark Pharmaceuticals (C, S); Regenera Pharma (S), Sanofi (L), ZEISS (L)

Dr Van Tassel: AbbVie (C), Aerie Pharmaceuticals (C), Allergan (C), Bausch + Lomb (C), Carl Zeiss Meditec (C), Equinox (C), New World Medical (C, L)

Dr Young: Johnson & Johnson Vision (C)

All relevant financial relationships have been mitigated.

The other authors and reviewers state that within the 24 months prior to their contributions to this CME activity and for the duration of development, they have had no financial interest in or other relationship with any entity whose primary business is producing, marketing, selling, reselling, or distributing health care products used by or in patients.

Recent Past Faculty

Pankaj C. Gupta, MD
Leon Strauss, MD, PhD
Edmond H. Thall, MD

In addition, the Academy gratefully acknowledges the contributions of numerous past faculty and advisory committee members who have played an important role in the development of previous editions of the Basic and Clinical Science Course.

* C = consultant fee, paid advisory boards, or fees for attending a meeting; E = employed by or received a W-2 from a commercial company; L = lecture fees or honoraria, travel fees or reimbursements when speaking at the invitation of a commercial company; O = equity ownership/stock options in publicly or privately traded firms, excluding mutual funds; P = patents and/or royalties for intellectual property; S = grant support or other financial support to the investigator from all sources, including research support from government agencies, foundations, device manufacturers, and/or pharmaceutical companies

American Academy of Ophthalmology
655 Beach Street
Box 7424
San Francisco, CA 94120-7424

Contents

Introduction to the BCSC

The Basic and Clinical Science Course (BCSC) is designed to meet the needs of residents and practitioners for a comprehensive yet concise curriculum of the field of ophthalmology. The BCSC has developed from its original brief outline format, which relied heavily on outside readings, to a more convenient and educationally useful self-contained text. The Academy updates and revises the course annually, with the goals of integrating the basic science and clinical practice of ophthalmology and of keeping ophthalmologists current with new developments in the various subspecialties.

The BCSC incorporates the effort and expertise of more than 100 ophthalmologists, organized into 13 Section faculties, working with Academy editorial staff. In addition, the course continues to benefit from many lasting contributions made by the faculties of previous editions. Members of the Academy Practicing Ophthalmologists Advisory Committee for Education, Committee on Aging, and Vision Rehabilitation Committee review every volume before major revisions, as does a group of select residents and fellows. Members of the European Board of Ophthalmology, organized into Section faculties, also review volumes before major revisions, focusing primarily on differences between American and European ophthalmology practice.

Organization of the Course

The Basic and Clinical Science Course comprises 13 volumes, incorporating fundamental ophthalmic knowledge, subspecialty areas, and special topics:

1 Update on General Medicine
2 Fundamentals and Principles of Ophthalmology
3 Clinical Optics and Vision Rehabilitation
4 Ophthalmic Pathology and Intraocular Tumors
5 Neuro-Ophthalmology
6 Pediatric Ophthalmology and Strabismus
7 Oculofacial Plastic and Orbital Surgery
8 External Disease and Cornea
9 Uveitis and Ocular Inflammation
10 Glaucoma
11 Lens and Cataract
12 Retina and Vitreous
13 Refractive Surgery

References

Readers who wish to explore specific topics in greater detail may consult the references cited within each chapter and listed in the Additional Materials and Resources section at the back of the book. These references are intended to be selective rather than exhaustive, chosen by the BCSC faculty as being important, current, and readily available to residents and practitioners.

Multimedia

This edition of Section 3, *Clinical Optics and Vision Rehabilitation,* includes videos and interactive content (an "activity") related to topics covered in the book. The videos and activity were developed and selected by members of the BCSC faculty and are available to readers of the print and electronic versions of Section 3 (www.aao.org/bcscvideo_section03 and www.aao.org/bcscactivity_section03). Mobile-device users can scan the QR codes below (a QR-code reader may need to be installed on the device) to access the videos and activity.

Videos

Activity

Self-Assessment and CME Credit

Each volume of the BCSC is designed as an independent study activity for ophthalmology residents and practitioners. The learning objectives for this volume are given on page 1. The text, illustrations, and references provide the information necessary to achieve the objectives; the study questions allow readers to test their understanding of the material and their mastery of the objectives. Physicians who wish to claim CME credit for this educational activity may do so by following the instructions given at the end of the book.*

Conclusion

The Basic and Clinical Science Course has expanded greatly over the years, with the addition of much new text, numerous illustrations, and video content. Recent editions have sought to place greater emphasis on clinical applicability while maintaining a solid foundation in basic science. As with any educational program, it reflects the experience of its authors. As its faculties change and medicine progresses, new viewpoints emerge on controversial subjects and techniques. Not all alternate approaches can be included in this series; as with any educational endeavor, the learner should seek additional sources, including Academy Preferred Practice Pattern Guidelines.

The BCSC faculty and staff continually strive to improve the educational usefulness of the course; you, the reader, can contribute to this ongoing process. If you have any suggestions or questions about the series, please do not hesitate to contact the faculty or the editors.

The authors, editors, and reviewers hope that your study of the BCSC will be of lasting value and that each Section will serve as a practical resource for quality patient care.

*There is no formal American Board of Ophthalmology (ABO) approval process for self-assessment activities. Any CME activity that qualifies for ABO Continuing Certification credit may also be counted as "self-assessment" as long as it provides a mechanism for individual learners to review their own performance, knowledge base, or skill set in a defined area of practice. For instance, grand rounds, medical conferences, or journal activities for CME credit that involve a form of individualized self-assessment may count as a self-assessment activity.

Introduction to Section 3

Knowledge of optics and refraction distinguishes ophthalmologists among all other physicians. Every trainee approaches this material as a novice—it is not covered in premedical studies or in the medical school curriculum. This volume represents our sincere attempt to make the learning curve as smooth and seamless as possible.

Refraction is not a spectator sport. The only way to acquire the knowledge and experience to become a skilled and efficient refractionist—to acquire the deep intuition sometimes referred to by the German term *Fingerspitzengefühl* (feeling in your fingertips)—is through practice with patients in the refracting lanes. The time spent mastering these skills early in your training will come back to you 10-fold and more over the course of your training and subsequent career.

As you work through this material, pay particular attention to the "Try It Yourself!" exercises. These are designed to give you hands-on experience with the behavior of lenses and a chance to see the refraction process through your own eyes. Do not simply skip over them.

In this edition, we have expanded and moved the material on retinoscopy to the Quick-Start Guide at the front of the book. We hope this will encourage you to experiment with the retinoscope at the beginning of your training and to acquire the skills of retinoscopy in your first few months in the clinic. If you defer working with the retinoscope until you start your neuro-ophthalmology or pediatric ophthalmology rotations, for which retinoscopy is an essential skill, you will be forced to play catch-up with your patients.

In this edition, we have also revised the title of Section 3 from *Clinical Optics* to *Clinical Optics and Vision Rehabilitation.* Discussion of vision rehabilitation has always been a part of this Section of the Basic and Clinical Science Course, but it is our intention to emphasize the importance of its role in the care of those patients whose visual disorders cannot be completely remedied.

We have deliberately included more material in this volume than the absolute minimum needed to recognize and correct refractive errors in your patients, with the awareness that this is likely the first, and often the last, text on optics and refraction that many residents will encounter. For example, the appendices may be omitted in a first reading. We hope that many of our readers will nevertheless take the opportunity to further enrich their understanding and perhaps expand upon our knowledge in the future.

Objectives

Upon completion of BCSC Section 3, *Clinical Optics and Vision Rehabilitation*, the reader should be able to

- explain the principles of light propagation and image formation
- state some of the fundamental equations that describe or measure such properties as refraction, reflection, magnification, and vergence
- explain how the principles noted above can be applied diagnostically and therapeutically
- describe the clinical application of Snell's law and the lensmaker's equation
- describe the relationship between physical optics and geometric optics
- describe the clinical and technical relevance of such optical phenomena as interference, coherence, polarization, diffraction, and scattering
- explain the basic properties of laser light and how they affect laser–tissue interaction
- identify optical models of the human eye and describe how to apply them
- describe various aspects of visual performance, including visual acuity, brightness sensitivity, color perception, and contrast sensitivity
- list the steps for performing streak retinoscopy
- identify the steps for performing a manifest refraction using a phoropter or trial lenses
- describe the use of the Jackson cross cylinder
- describe the indications for prescribing bifocal and progressive lenses as well as common difficulties encountered in their use

- identify the materials and fitting parameters of both soft and rigid contact lenses
- describe the basic methods of calculating intraocular lens (IOL) powers and the advantages and disadvantages of the different methods
- explain the conceptual basis of multifocal IOLs and how the correction of presbyopia differs between IOLs and spectacles
- explain the optical principles underlying various modalities of refractive correction: spectacles, contact lenses, IOLs, and refractive surgery
- describe the operating principles of various optical instruments in order to use them effectively
- describe the visual needs of patients with low vision and how to address these needs through use of optical and nonoptical devices and/or appropriate referrals
- state how social determinants of health can affect the low-vision patient population

QUICK-START GUIDE

Optics, Refraction, and Retinoscopy

This chapter includes related videos. Go to www.aao.org/bcscvideo_section03 or scan the QR codes in the text to access this content.

This chapter also includes a related activity. Go to www.aao.org/bcscactivity_section03 or scan the QR code in the text to access this content.

Part 1: Optics

Highlights

- A pinhole camera is the simplest imaging device.
- Lenses allow for brighter images than a simple pinhole does.
- The effect of source object location and lens power on the location of images is governed by the vergence equation.
- Refractive errors can be corrected with appropriate convex, concave, or cylindrical lenses.

Glossary

Aperture The opening in an optical system through which light travels. It may be defined by the edges of a lens or an additional diaphragm, pinhole, or slit.

Astigmatism The imagery formed by a toric lens, with power that varies according to meridian.

Axis

Optic axis A line along which there is some degree of rotational symmetry in an optical system such as a lens, a combination of lenses, or a mirror. To a first approximation, the optic axis indicates the path along which light propagates through the system.

Cylinder axis A cylindrical lens exhibits curvature in only 1 direction; in the perpendicular direction, the surface consists of straight lines. The *cylinder axis* is the orientation of these straight lines. Cylinder axis is expressed in degrees, measured counterclockwise as viewed from in front of the lens. A vertical axis lies at 90°; by convention, a horizontal axis lies at 180°.

Camera obscura A small, light-tight room or box in which a pinhole aperture forms an inverted image.

Focal length The distance between a lens and the image it forms of an object at great distance *(optical infinity).*

Hyperopia A refractive error in which distant and near objects are imaged behind the retina.

Image distance The distance from a lens to the image it forms of an object. Distances to the left of a lens are considered as negative numbers; distances to the right of a lens are considered as positive numbers. (If the object is at infinity, the image distance is the focal length of the lens.)

Meridian The orientation of a plane passing through the optic axis of a lens or of the intersection curve of such a plane with a lens surface. This orientation is usually specified in degrees, increasing counterclockwise from the horizontal as viewed from in front of the lens. The horizontal meridian is by convention designated as 180° (not 0°); the vertical meridian is at 90°.

Myopia A refractive error in which distant objects are imaged in front of the retina.

Object distance The distance from a source object to the lens, in meters. The sign conventions are the same as for image distance.

Power (of a lens) The reciprocal of the focal length. Measured in m^{-1}, referred to as *diopters (D).*

Power cross A diagrammatic representation of the action of a toric lens, showing the power and orientation of the 2 (perpendicular) principal meridians.

Principal meridian The flattest or steepest meridian of a toric lens. The principal meridians are in general perpendicular to each other *(regular astigmatism).*

Refractive index The speed of light in air or in a vacuum divided by the speed of light in a different medium. As light always travels more slowly through a material medium (sometimes referred to as a *denser* medium) than in a vacuum, the refractive index is always greater than 1.00.

Toric lens A lens with a surface resembling the outer rim of a torus, such as an automobile tire or the side of a rugby ball or an American football.

Vergence (in air) The reciprocal of the object distance *(object vergence)* or image distance *(image vergence).*

Vergence (in media other than air or a vacuum) The refractive index of the medium in which light travels divided by the object distance or image distance. Sometimes referred to as *reduced vergence*, even though it is numerically greater than the vergence in air, as refractive indices of denser media are always greater than 1.00.

Vergence equation The formula relating object vergence, lens power, and image vergence.

Introduction

The term *optics* refers to the properties and manipulation of light. In this part of the Quick-Start Guide, we introduce the basic ideas of optics—sufficient to understand the essence of clinical refraction, as presented in Part 2, Refraction. Readers already familiar with this material are welcome to go directly to Part 2.

The Camera Obscura: Pinhole Imaging

The term *camera obscura* (Latin for "dark chamber") was introduced in the 17th century to describe a device already known to the ancients: a small, light-tight room or box with a small hole on 1 side. The hole allowed the inverted image of a bright scene or bright object to be projected onto the opposite wall or side of the box, where it could be conveniently viewed or studied. The earliest known drawing of such a device is shown in Figure Q-1, where it is being used to view a solar eclipse.

Experience with such devices leads to 3 important observations:

- *The projected image is inverted.* The inverted image arises from the straight-line propagation of light rays originating from each point in the original object, with the pinhole acting as a sort of fulcrum (Fig Q-2).
- *The depth of field of the projected image is superb: objects are simultaneously in focus at all distances, from foreground objects to distant hills and even astronomical objects (Fig Q-3).* This great depth of field is due to the small aperture, which allows light rays from each object to reach only a very small region in the image plane.
- *The image is very dim.* The small aperture also greatly limits the amount of light that is available to form the image.

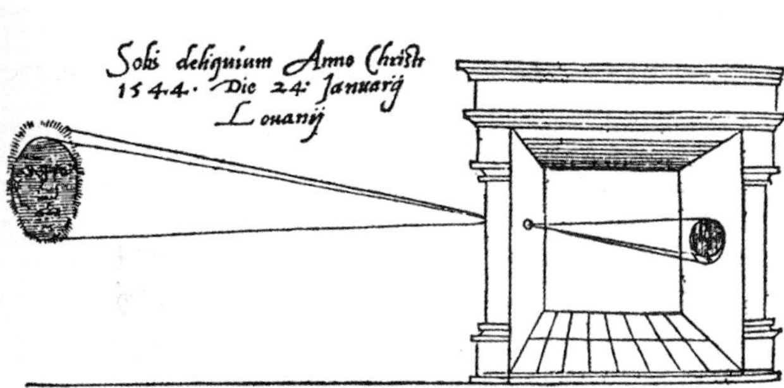

Figure Q-1 Earliest known depiction of a camera obscura. *(From* De Radio Astronomica et Geometrica; *1545.)*

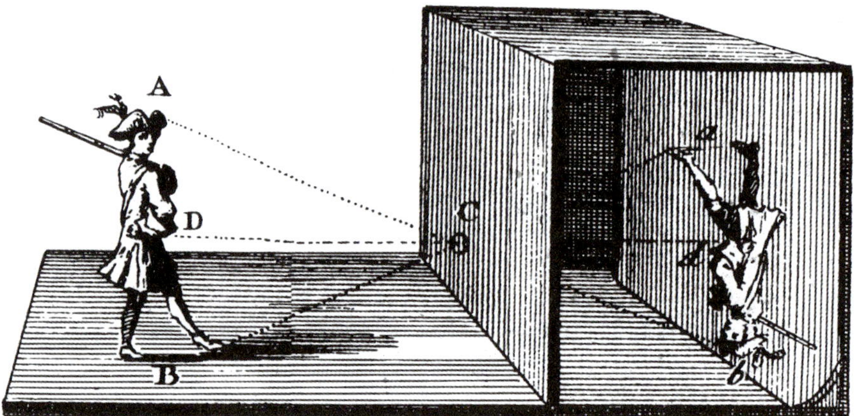

Figure Q-2 Image formation in a camera obscura. An inverted image forms when rays of light from points of the original object (eg, **A, D, B**) follow straight paths through the pinhole (**C**) to the corresponding points (eg, **b, d, a,** respectively) in the image on the far wall.

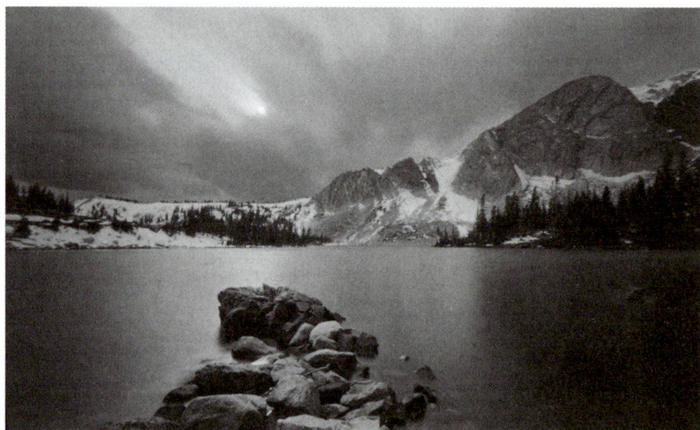

Figure Q-3 Camera obscura (pinhole camera) image. Notice the great depth of field, with both the rocks in the foreground and the mountains in the background simultaneously in sharp focus. *(Courtesy of Mark James.)*

To obtain a brighter image, capable of activating a detector (such as a photographic plate, a charge-coupled device, or the retina), the pinhole aperture must be enlarged to admit more light. Unfortunately, enlarging the aperture also allows the rays of light emanating from each point of the source object to form a cone of light, which illuminates a proportionally larger disk on the image plane (Fig Q-4). These so-called *blur circles* (or, more generally, *blur ellipses*) smear out the image, resulting in substantial blurring (Fig Q-5).

To recover a sharp image while retaining the image intensity afforded by a larger aperture, it is necessary to recombine the light rays that originate from each point of the source object so that they will converge on a single image point. This can be accomplished by placing a suitable lens in the aperture (Fig Q-6).

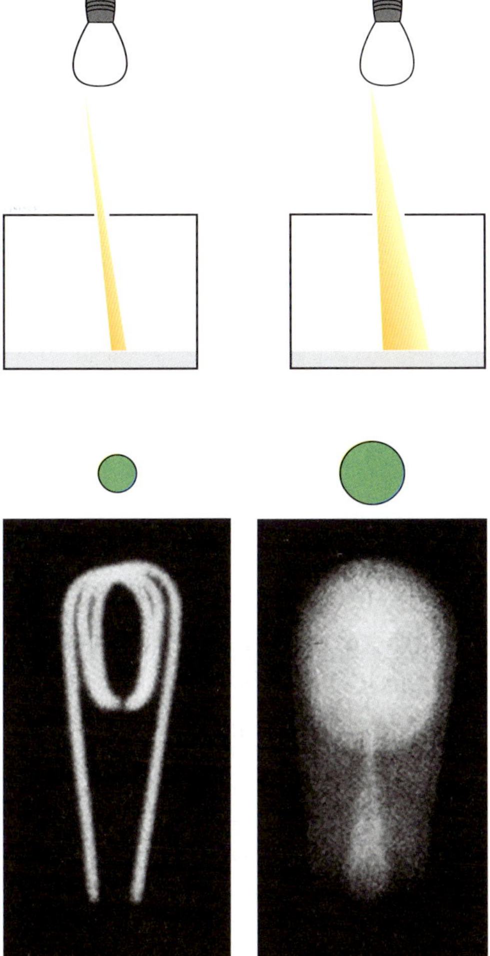

Figure Q-4 Enlarging the pinhole in a camera obscura results in larger blur-circle images of each point of the original object.

Figure Q-5 Effect of pinhole size (as indicated schematically by the green circles) on image sharpness in a camera obscura.

However, using a lens to recover the sharpness of images by enlarging the aperture necessarily sacrifices the depth of field obtained with the simple pinhole. The lens can simultaneously bring into focus rays of light from different points only for those source points at the same distance from the lens (Fig Q-7).

These observations about image formation in simple cameras essentially summarize the entire challenge of basic optics: how to form sharp images from beams of light defined by apertures of finite size while providing sufficient brightness for the application at hand. The rules for the proper selection of lenses for this purpose are discussed in the next section.

Convex Lenses

Consider a thin, spherical convex lens intended to form an image of an object at *optical infinity*—that is, at a very great distance, such as a star—located to the left of the lens. The

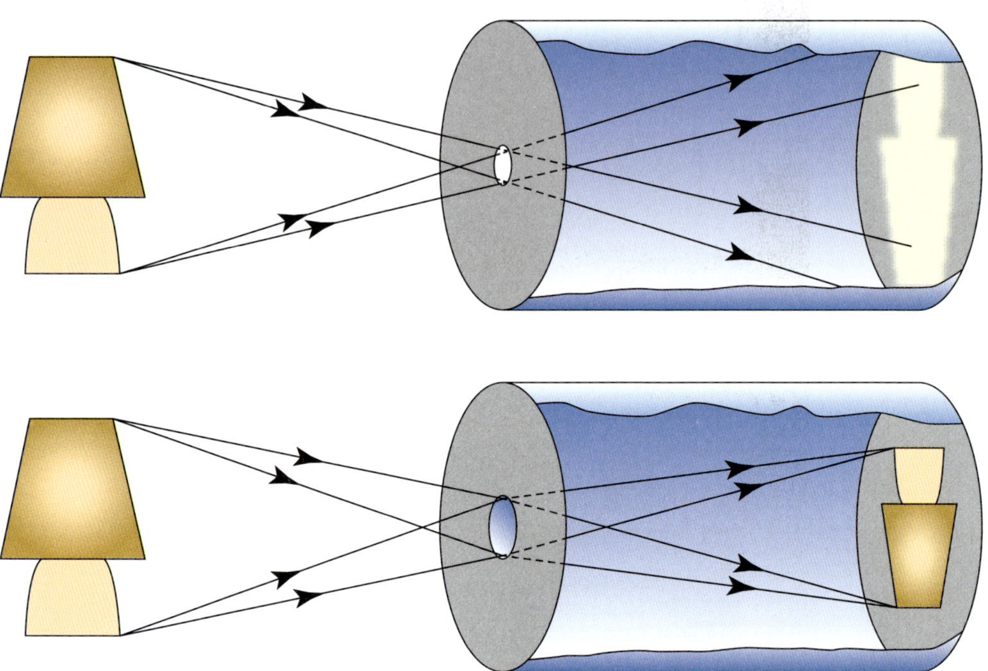

Figure Q-6 Recovering a sharp image by placing a lens in the aperture of a camera obscura after the aperture has been enlarged. The lens simultaneously recombines the rays of light from each point of the source object to land at a single point in the image plane.

image will be formed to the right of the lens at a distance *f*, measured in meters. This distance is called the *focal length* of the lens. The *power* of the lens is then $P = 1/f$, where the unit for P is reciprocal meters, which is referred to as the *diopter (D)*. For example, a lens that images starlight 0.5 m to its right has a power of $P = 1/0.5\text{ m} = 2.00\text{ D}$ (Fig Q-8).

Combining Lenses

If 2 thin lenses (with powers designated P_1 and P_2) are placed in contact with each other, and we consider them together as a single compound lens system, the power of the 2 lenses together is closely approximated by the sum of the powers of the constituent lenses: $P = P_1 + P_2$. This summation demonstrates the utility of using the reciprocal of the focal length (in diopters) to designate lens power.

EXAMPLE Q-1

If 2 convex lenses of power $P_1 = 1.00$ D and power $P_2 = 4.00$ D are combined and treated as a single unit, where does this combination lens form the image of a distant star?

$$P = P_1 + P_2 = 1.00\text{ D} + 4.00\text{ D} = 5.00\text{ D} = 1/f$$

Thus, $f = 1/P = 0.20$ m, or 20 cm, to the right of the lens, which is the location of the image of the distant star.

@ f/2
Only front battery is in focus.

@ f/16
First 2 batteries are in focus.

@ f/32
All batteries are in focus.

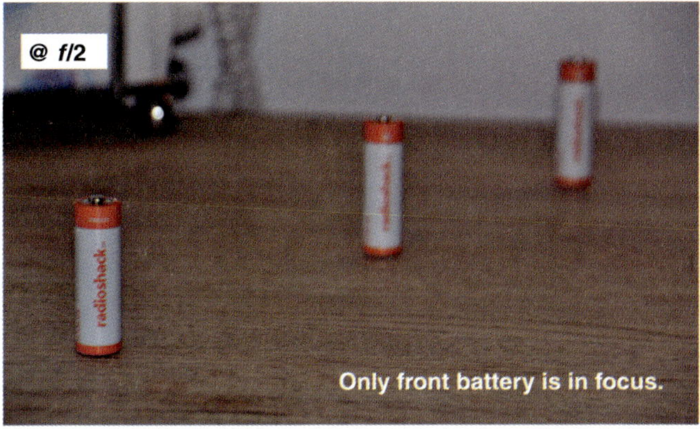

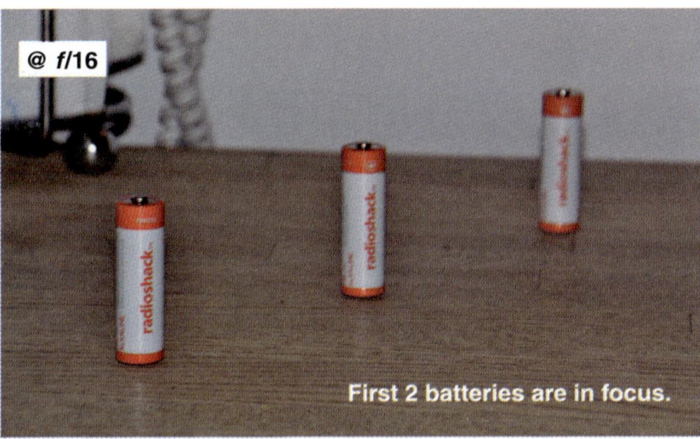

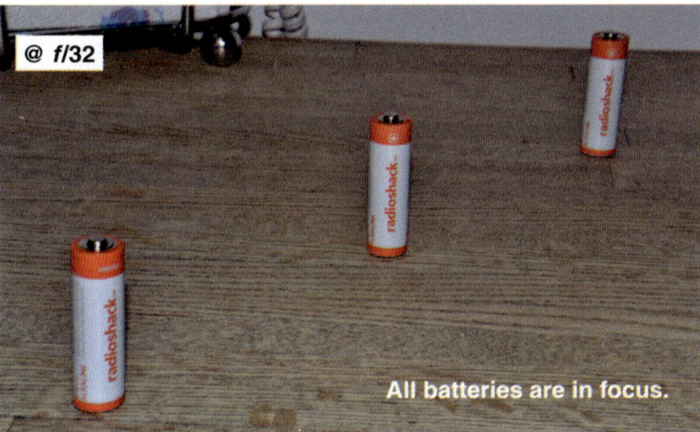

Figure Q-7 Reduced depth of field in images obtained with lenticular optics. Even in this case, smaller apertures (larger *f*/ numbers) result in greater depth of field. *(Courtesy of Scott E. Brodie, MD, PhD.)*

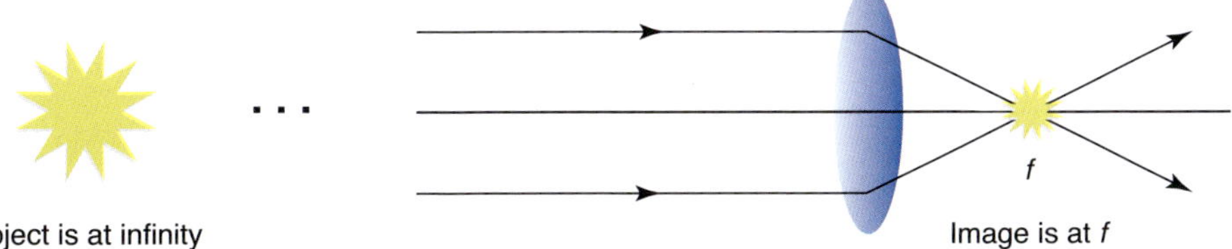

Figure Q-8 Image formation for an object at infinite distance (such as a star) by a simple convex lens. The distance from the lens to the image is f, the focal length of the lens; the power of the lens is given by $P = 1/f$, where P is given as units of diopters (D) equivalent to reciprocal meters.

EXAMPLE Q-2

Moving an image closer to the lenses: the image in Example Q-1 must be moved 2.0 cm (0.02 m) closer to the compound lens. We may do so by adding a third convex lens. Because we wish to obtain a result of $f=0.18$ m, $P=1/f=1/0.18$ m $=5.55$ D $=P_1+P_2+P_3$. Thus, $P_3=0.55$ D. This example demonstrates a general method: adding a convex lens to a system of lenses will generally shift an image that is located to the right of the lens closer to the lens system.

Imaging Nearby Objects: Vergence and the Vergence Equation

If the source object is located only a finite distance to the left of a convex lens, but at greater distance than the focal length (f), the image will be farther to the right of the lens than the image of an object that is infinitely far away, such as a star. The distance from the source object to the lens is referred to as the *object distance*; the distance from the lens to the image is known as the *image distance*. The image distance for an object at infinity is the focal length of the lens. Assuming both the source object and the image are in air, the formula for locating the image is

$$U+P=V$$

where $U=1/u$ is the *vergence* of the object at a distance u to the left of the lens, P is the power of the lens, and $V=1/v$ is the vergence of the light emerging from the lens to form the image at distance v to the right of the lens (Fig Q-9).

Note: In the *vergence equation,* distances to the *left* of the lens are treated as *negative numbers* (so, in this situation, $u<0$). The vergence, $U=1/u$, of an object to the left of a lens is likewise a *negative number*. Distances to the *right* of a lens—and, thus, in this case, the image vergence $V=1/v$—are considered *positive*. In this context, it is important to keep track of the *sign* of the power of a convex lens as a *positive number* as well. Objects infinitely far from the lens generate beams of light that reach the lens with a vergence of $V=1/\infty=0$.

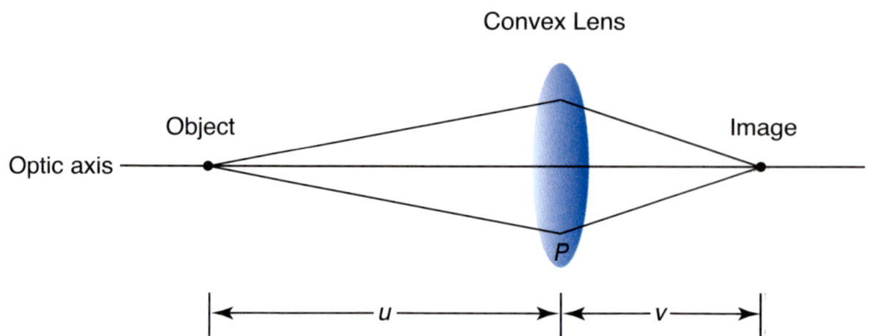

Figure Q-9 The vergence equation: the object distance is *u*, the image distance is *v*, and the power of the lens is *P*.

EXAMPLE Q-3

A lens of power $P = +3.00$ D images an object at position $u = -1.0$ m to the left of the lens as follows:

$U + P = V$: $1/(-1.0 \text{ m}) + (+3.00 \text{ D}) = +2.00 \text{ D} = V$,
so $v = 1/V = +0.50 \text{ m} = 50 \text{ cm}$,

measured to the right of the lens.

EXAMPLE Q-4

Moving the source object closer to the lens: if the object in Example Q-3 is moved closer to the lens but not closer than the focal length $f = 1/P$ (say, to a location -0.50 m to the left of the lens), then

$U + P = V$: $1/(-0.50 \text{ m}) + (+3.00 \text{ D}) = -2.00 \text{ D} + 3.00 \text{ D} = +1.00$,
so $v = 1/V = +1.0$ m.

That is, moving the source object closer to the lens shifts the image away from the lens on the other side. This, too, is a general method. What happens if you move the source object farther to the left of the lens?

Concave Lenses

Concave lenses do not by themselves form real images, but they can be used to shift an image away from (to the right of) an existing lens or lens system.

A spherical concave lens will cause light from an infinitely distant object to diverge. If these divergent rays are extended back toward the light source (eg, to the left of the lens for a source object to the left), they will intersect at a "virtual" focal point—say, at a distance f to the left of the lens (Fig Q-10). In keeping with the sign conventions above, the power of this lens is given by $P = 1/f$ (with f in meters). Here, f is a *negative* number, and the power of the concave lens is likewise a *negative* number.

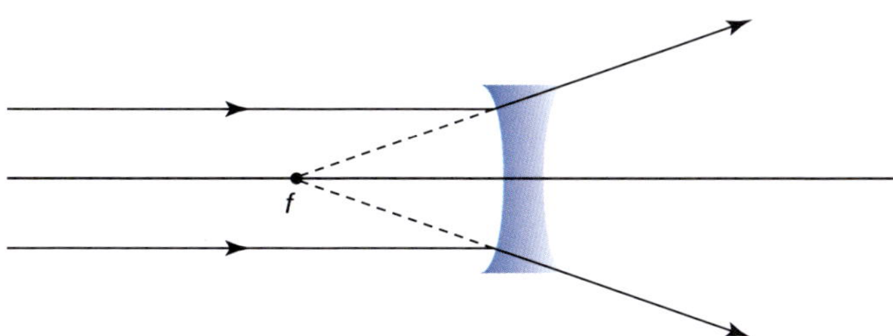

Figure Q-10 Formation of a virtual image of an object infinitely far away to the left of the lens by a concave lens. The focal point *(f)* is to the left of the lens; the focal length is a negative number, and the power of the lens $P = 1/f$ is likewise negative.

Concave lenses can be combined with other immediately adjacent lenses. The power of such a lens system follows the same simple addition formula as we introduced for convex lenses:

$$P = P_1 + P_2$$

Remember to track the algebraic signs carefully.

EXAMPLE Q-5

A lens of power $P_1 = +4.00$ D will form the image of a source object at location $u = -0.5$ m as follows: the object vergence is $U = -2.0$; the image vergence is −2.00 D + 4.00 D = +2.00 D, so the image location is $v = 1/(+2.00\ \text{D}) = +0.50$ m to the right of the lens. If a concave lens of power $P_2 = -1.00$ D is placed adjacent to the +4.00 D lens, the combination has a power of $P = +4.00\ \text{D} + (-1.00\ \text{D}) = +3.00$ D. The image vergence is then $V = -2.00\ \text{D} + 3.00\ \text{D} = +1.00$ D, so the image location is $v = 1/(+1.00\ \text{D}) = +1.0$ m. That is, adding the minus lens to the optical system has shifted the image from +0.50 m to the right of the lens to a new location, +1.0 m to the right of the lens. This example illustrates a common method: the image of a convergent optical system can be moved further away (to the right) by adding a minus lens to the system (Fig Q-11).

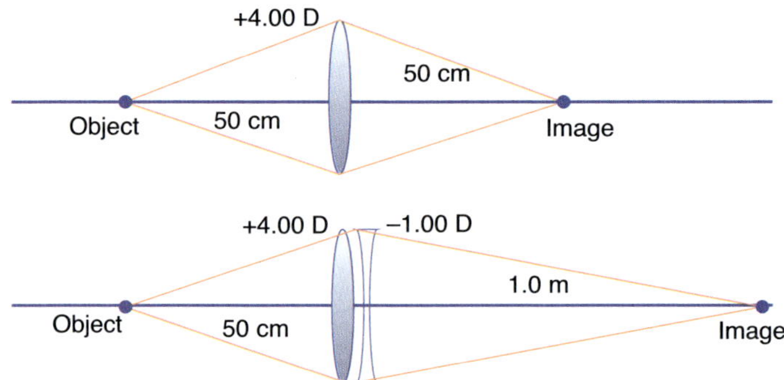

Figure Q-11 Diagram of the vergence of an object at 50 cm and with a +4.00 D lens, compared to a +3.00 D lens combination (+4.00 D and −1.00 D). *(Courtesy of Thomas E. Mauger, MD.)*

Summary Thus Far

Starting with an object a *finite* distance to the left of a convex lens that is strong enough to form an image to the right of the lens (that is, with a focal length *f* shorter than the object distance), there are 2 ways to move the image to the left (closer to the lens): by moving the object to the *left* or by adding an additional convex lens to the lens system. Similarly, there are 2 ways to move the image to the right (farther from the lens): by moving the object to the *right* (as long as it remains farther from the lens than the focal length) or by adding a concave lens to the system.

Images in Denser Media

If the light leaving a lens travels in a medium in which the speed of light is less than its speed in air, such as a watery tissue like the aqueous or vitreous humor of the eye, we must modify the image vergence term in the vergence equation. Here

$$V = n/v$$

where n is the *refractive index* of the denser medium: the ratio of the speed of light in a vacuum (or in air, which is nearly the same) to the speed of light in the denser medium. The refractive index is always a number greater than 1.00, as light travels more slowly in dense media than in air. For the watery tissues in the eye, the value $n = 1.33$ is a useful approximation. (This casual use of the term *denser* has nothing to do with the specific gravity of the medium.)

> **EXAMPLE Q-6**
>
> A nominal value for the power of the human cornea is $P = 43.00$ D. We can calculate the location of the image of a distant star formed by such a cornea in an aphakic eye (an eye with no lens): $U + P = V$, so $0 + 43.00 \text{ D} = 1.33/v$, or $v = 1.33/43 \text{ m} = 0.0309 \text{ m} = 30.9 \text{ mm}$. Because the typical human eye has an axial length of about 23.0 mm (see Chapter 3, Table 3-1), the need for additional refracting power after removal of the crystalline lens is evident.

A Very Much Simplified Model Eye

We now have the background to understand the correction of simple axial refractive errors, which arise from a mismatch between the optical power of the anterior segment (cornea and crystalline lens) and the axial length of the eye.

Emmetropia

Suppose that all the refracting power of the eye is concentrated at a single plane, at the apex of the cornea, and assume the typical axial length of 23.0 mm. If this ultrasimplified model eye is to focus light from distant objects on the retina (Fig Q-12A),the power at the corneal apex must be given by the vergence equation: $0 + P = 1.33/0.023 \text{ m} = 57.82 \text{ D}$.

Myopia

Now suppose that our eye has the standard anterior segment with optical power of 57.82 D but is 1.0 mm longer than normal, so the axial length is 24.0 mm. In such an eye, which is said to be *myopic,* light from a distant point source comes to a focus in front of the retina (Fig Q-12B); the rays then cross and continue for another millimeter before they form a blur circle on the retina. To correct the refractive error, we must shift the image location 1.0 mm toward the back of the eye. One way to do this is with a concave (diverging, or *minus,* power) contact lens of power P placed adjacent to the corneal apex according to the vergence equation: $0 + (P + 57.82 \text{ D}) = 1.33/0.024 \text{ D} = +55.41 \text{ D}$. Thus, the power of the required contact lens is $P = 55.41 \text{ D} - 57.82 \text{ D} = -2.40 \text{ D}$. (In a more precise calculation, the correction would be about –3.00 D for each millimeter of excess axial length.)

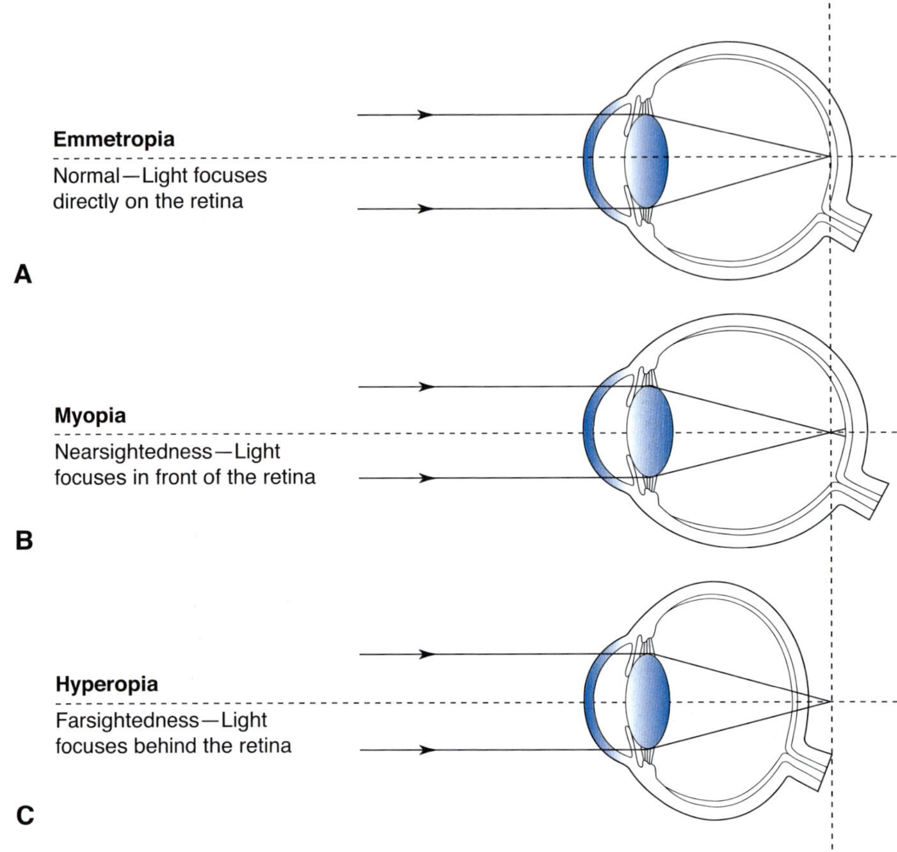

Figure Q-12 The position of light rays focusing. **A,** A normal eye. **B,** A myopic eye. **C,** A hyperopic eye. *(Illustration developed by Scott E. Brodie, MD, PhD.)*

Hyperopia

Similarly, if the axial length of this model eye were reduced by 1.0 mm (to 22.0 mm), distant objects would form an image behind the retina (Fig Q-12C). Such an eye is *hyperopic*. The required contact lens power would be given by the vergence equation: $0 + (P + 57.82 \text{ D}) = 1.33/0.022 \text{ m} = +60.45 \text{ D}$, or $P = +60.45 \text{ D} - 57.82 \text{ D} = +2.63 \text{ D}$, a convex, or *plus*, lens.

> **TAKE NOTE**
>
> *Thus, correction of axial refractive errors requires only the determination of the optimal spherical lens power needed to refocus the light from a distant source on the retina.*

Try It Yourself! Q-1

1. Find a trial lens set with an assortment of plus (+) and minus (–) spherical lenses. (The signs of the lenses will be indicated on the handles or by the color of the lens frames.) Work in groups of 3: the

first person should hold up a small light source (a penlight or the Finoff transilluminator on your instrument stand will work well); the second person should hold the lens or lenses at least 2 or 3 m away; and the third person should hold a small white card, which will serve as a screen to catch the images of the light formed by the lenses (Fig Q-13). Start with, say, a +2.00 D lens, and find the image (a small, round dot of light) about 66 cm farther away from the light source than the lens. (Why is the image not exactly 50 cm from the lens? Because your colleague holding the penlight is not infinitely far away.)

2. Move the light source closer to the lens and find the new image: it will be farther away from the lens.
3. If you have enough room, move the light source farther away from the lens than in step 1, and locate the new image: it will be closer to the lens than when you started.
4. Returning to the setup in step 1, add a second plus spherical lens (say, +1.00 D) and hold the lenses together to act as a single lens system. Locate the image: it will be closer to the lenses than when you started.
5. Remove the added +1.00 D lens and replace it with a –1.00 D lens. Now locate the image: it will be farther away from the lenses than when you started.
6. Compare the location of the image formed by your +2.00 D and +1.00 D lens combination with the location of the image formed by the actual +3.00 D lens from the trial set. They should agree closely.
7. Try comparing the +2.00 D and –1.00 D combination with an actual +1.00 D lens.
8. Verify this "lens arithmetic" with other combinations of plus and minus lenses.

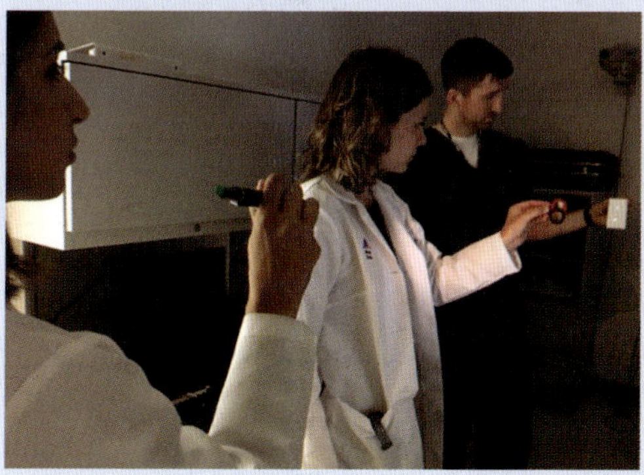

Figure Q-13 Three residents forming a "human optical bench." One holds a penlight, the second compares a +3.00 D sphere with a +4.00 D sphere held together with a –1.00 D sphere, and the third holds a small white card. Notice that the images on the white card are the same. *(Courtesy of Scott E. Brodie, MD, PhD.)*

A net minus lens will not form an image; the white card will show only a dimmer circle of light inside the shadow of the frame than outside it. Why? (Because the minus lens diverges light, reducing the intensity of the illumination/cm^2 of the light that passes through it.)

Astigmatism

In addition to axial refractive errors, we must consider refracting surfaces that lack the circular symmetry that allows spherical lenses to focus all the light emerging from a point source in a single image point. Consider a *toroidal* surface, such as the side of a rugby ball, an American football, or the outer rim of automobile tire inner tube (a *torus*), as in Figure Q-14.

To envision the effect of such a refracting surface, called a *toric lens,* consider the curvature of the intersection of the surface with a plane that rotates about the line perpendicular to the surface at the apex (the *normal line;* Fig Q-15). The orientation of such a plane, or the intersection curve itself, is referred to as a *meridian* of the lens. As this normal plane rotates, the curvature of the intersection varies, from a flattest meridian to a steepest meridian, 90° away (Fig Q-16).

Light rays from a distant point source that land on the steepest meridian are refracted as if they encountered a spherical lens of the same curvature. Light rays that land on the flattest meridian are refracted as if they encountered a spherical lens with less dioptric power. Thus, the focal length varies with the choice of meridian, and the toroidal surface does not image the light from a single point source at a single image point. This situation is referred to as *astigmatism*, derived from the Greek for absence *(a-)* of a (single) point *(stigma),* or focus (Fig Q-17).

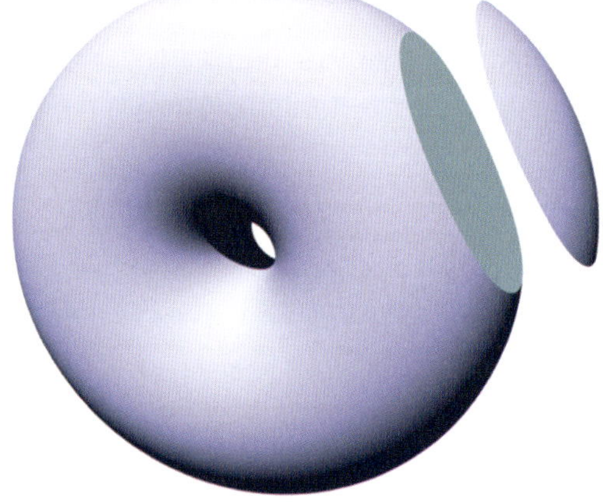

Figure Q-14 The outer rim of a torus forms a toric surface. *(Illustration by Ir. H. Hahn, from Creative Commons.)*

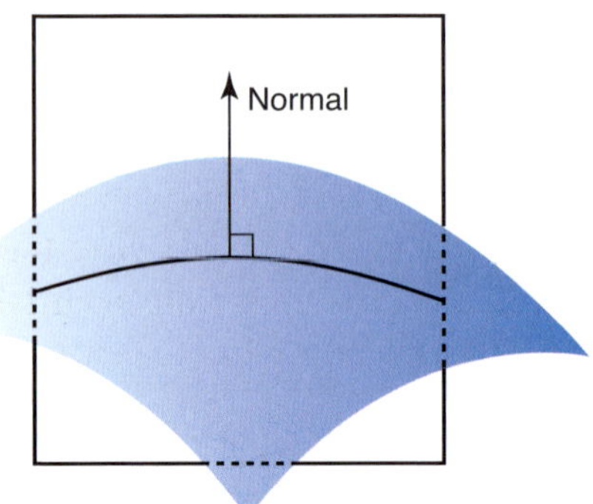

Figure Q-15 A normal plane intersecting a toric surface. The magnitude of the curve where the plane intersects the surface will vary with the orientation of the plane rotated around the apex. Each such curve is a meridian of the surface at that point.

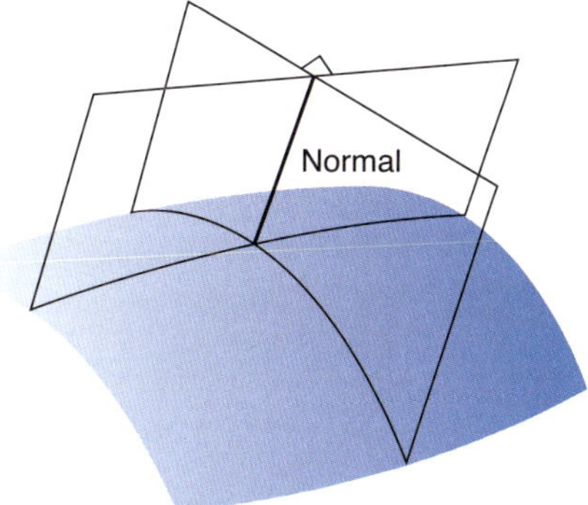

Figure Q-16 Variation of the curvature of a toric surface along 2 different meridians. The meridians for which the curvature is minimal or maximal are 90° apart.

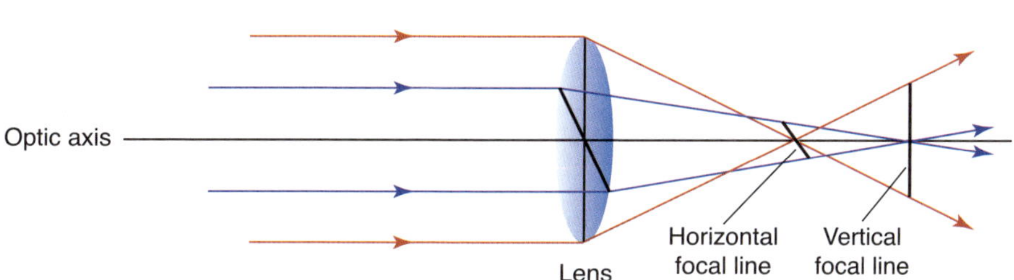

Figure Q-17 Astigmatic image formation by a toric surface. In this example, light rays that land on the horizontal meridian (ie, rays shown in blue) reach a focus farther from the lens than rays that land on the vertical meridian (ie, rays shown in red).

The flattest and steepest meridians lie 90° apart from each other; they are known as *principal meridians*. We can keep track of this situation by drawing a *power cross*, which shows the orientation of the steepest and flattest meridians and indicates their respective refractive powers (Fig Q-18).

In practice, it is often convenient to emphasize the *difference* in the refractive powers between the principal meridians. In this case, we can interpret the refracting surface as the combination of a spherical refracting surface, which refracts equally in all meridians, and a purely cylindrical refracting surface, with maximal power corresponding to one of the meridians indicated in the power cross and no refracting power in the orthogonal direction. Thus, for example, a lens with a power of +1.00 D horizontally and +2.00 D vertically could be described as the combination of a spherical lens with a power of +1.00 D and a cylindrical lens with a power of +1.00 D in the vertical direction. This is notated +1.00 ⊂ +1.00 @ 90°. Alternatively, the same refracting surface could be described as a spherical lens with power +2.00 D combined with a cylindrical lens with power −1.00 D acting in the 180° meridian, notated +2.00 ⊂ −1.00 @ 180°.

Indeed, we can create such lenses in practice by combining spherical lenses with lenses that have cylindrical surfaces, either convex (*plus cylinders*) or concave (*minus cylinders*; Fig Q-19). These cylindrical lenses, which can be found in standard trial lens sets, are marked to indicate the orientation of the original axis of the glass cylinder from which the cylindrical surface was derived. The refracting power of such a cylindrical lens

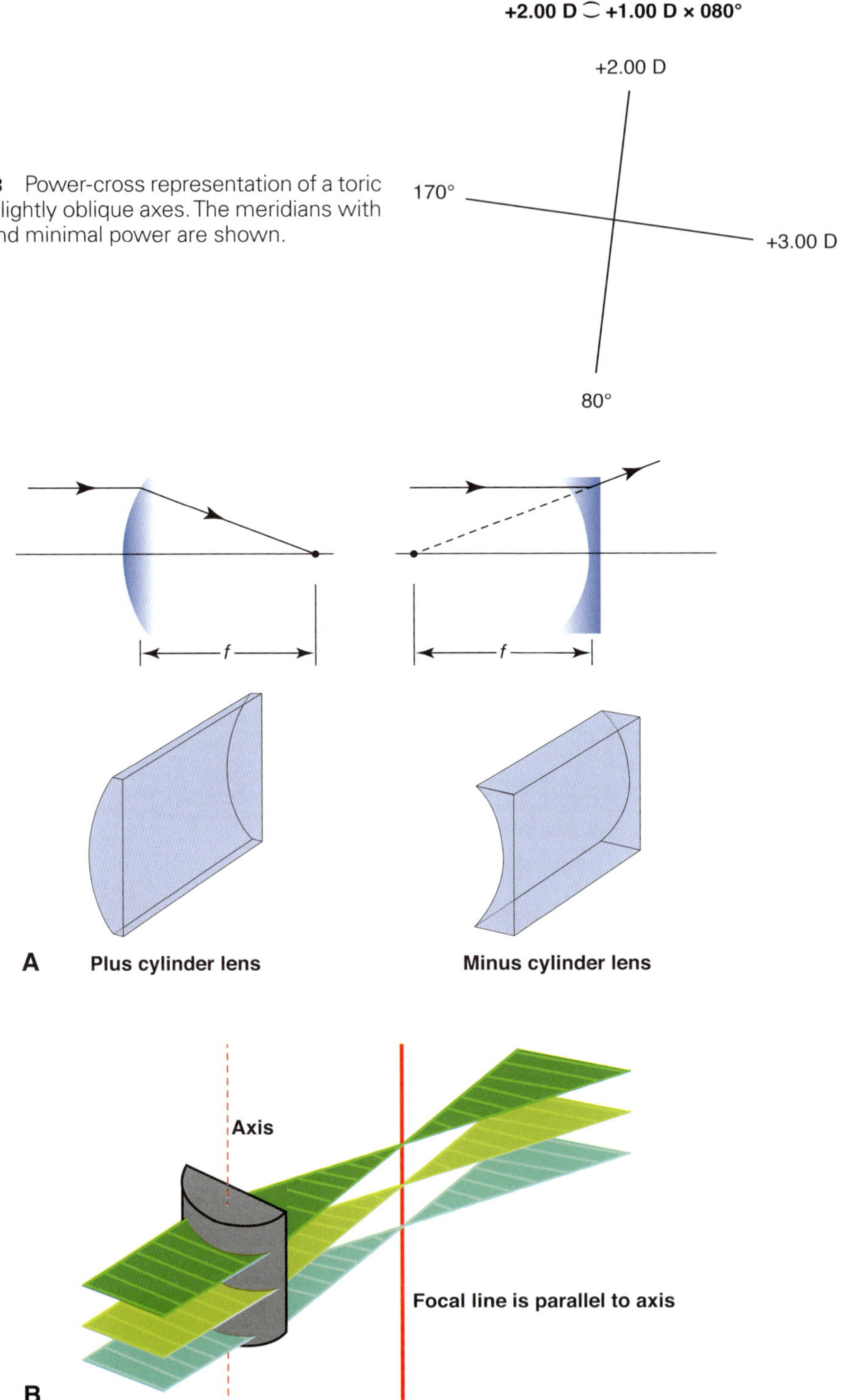

Figure Q-18 Power-cross representation of a toric lens with slightly oblique axes. The meridians with maximal and minimal power are shown.

Figure Q-19 Cylindrical lenses, with curvature in only 1 direction. **A,** Convex (plus cylinder) and concave (minus cylinder) glass lenses. **B,** Refraction through a convex cylinder. *(Courtesy of Kamran Riaz, MD.)*

acts in the direction *perpendicular* to the orientation of the cylinder axis. For example, we obtain a plus cylinder lens with power +1.00 D along the *horizontal* meridian by slicing the surface from a glass cylinder with axis *vertical.* Such a glass cylinder lens is denoted +1.00 × 90°. The notation for combinations of spherical and cylindrical lenses uses the × symbol (× for "axis"). Thus, the lens described in the preceding paragraph can be realized with either a plus cylinder or minus cylinder combination: +2.00 ⊂ −1.00 × 90° or +1.00 ⊂ +1.00 × 180°.

Notice that we use the notation @ (read "at") to denote the meridian (direction) in which a cylindrical lens exerts refractive power. That contrasts with the × notation (read "axis"), which indicates the orientation axis of the cylindrical lens, which will exert its refractive power 90° away from the orientation of the axis.

There are 2 ways to describe the same toric refractive surface: (1) start with the more *plus* sphere power and describe the minus cylinder that provides the difference between the powers of the more plus and more minus meridians, or (2) start with the more *minus* sphere power and describe the plus cylinder that provides the difference between the more minus and more plus meridians. To convert from one description to the other, simply add the sphere and cylinder (keeping track of plus and minus signs) to determine the new sphere power, change the sign of the cylinder, and add or subtract 90° to the axis (to keep the final axis between 0° and 180°). The process of converting between the plus cylinder and minus cylinder descriptions of a toric lens is referred to as *transposition.* This duality occurs in every context in which we consider toric lenses.

Try It Yourself! Q-2

Set up a "human optical bench" as before.

1. Start with a +3.00 D spherical lens and locate the image, perhaps about 40 cm from the lens.
2. Add to this a +1.00 D cylindrical lens, with the axis marks placed horizontally. Observe that this added lens distorts the focal point located in the previous step into a vertical focal line.
3. Gradually move the card closer to the lenses. Observe that the focal line continuously deforms into an ellipse, further rounds up into a circle (the *circle of least confusion*), and then gradually deforms into an ellipse (with horizontal major axis) and, ultimately, into a horizontal focal line.
4. Compare the location of this horizontal focal line to the location of the point image formed by a +4.00 D spherical lens. (They should agree.)
5. Starting again with the +3.00 D spherical lens of step 1, now add a −1.00 D cylinder, again with axis horizontal. The original focal point will again be distorted into a vertical focal line, but now the circle of least confusion will lie farther from the lenses, and the horizontal focal line will be found even farther still.

6. Verify that this horizontal focal line coincides with the location of the point image formed by a +2.00 D spherical lens.
7. Compare the focal lines formed by a +4.00 D sphere together with a −1.00 D cylinder, axis horizontal, to those formed by a +3.00 D sphere together with a +1.00 D cylinder, axis vertical. (They should agree: these 2 spherocylinder combinations are transpositions of each other.)
8. Compare the image formed by combining 2 +3.00 D cylinders, one with axis horizontal and the other with axis vertical, to the image formed by a +3.00 D sphere. (Be careful—you may have to hold the handles of the trial lenses slightly apart to get the axes precisely perpendicular.)

Astigmatic refractive errors

Astigmatic refractive errors of the human eye are not uncommon. Corneal astigmatism is the most common type, but lenticular astigmatism also occurs. In each case, we can consider the net refractive surface as equivalent to a spherical component with a concurrent plus cylinder astigmatic component (corresponding to the forward bulging of the cornea into the surrounding air). For example, the most common pattern of corneal astigmatism seen in younger patients, known as *with-the-rule astigmatism*, suggests a compression of the cornea by the pressure of the eyelids. This compression deforms the cornea, steepening the vertical meridian and flattening the horizontal meridian. This acts as a plus cylinder lens with axis horizontal (Fig Q-20).

The net astigmatic error is corrected by placing a cylinder of equal power and opposite sign over the eye, with the same axis as the intrinsic cylindrical error. For example,

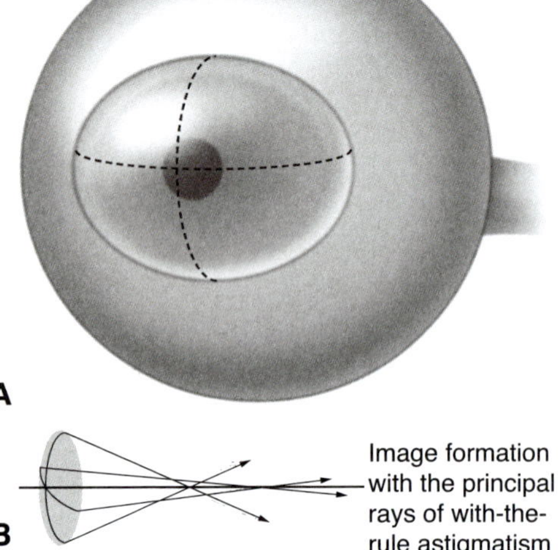

Figure Q-20 Corneal astigmatism. **A,** Schematic drawing of an eye that has with-the-rule astigmatism, with horizontal flattest corneal meridian. **B,** Ray tracing of with-the-rule astigmatism. *(Part A Illustration developed by Scott E. Brodie, MD, PhD; original illustration by Mark Miller. Part B reproduced from the* British Journal of Ophthalmology, *"Astigmatism and the analysis of its surgical correction," Morlet N, Minassian D, Dart J, 2001;185:127–1138, with permission from BMJ Publishing.)*

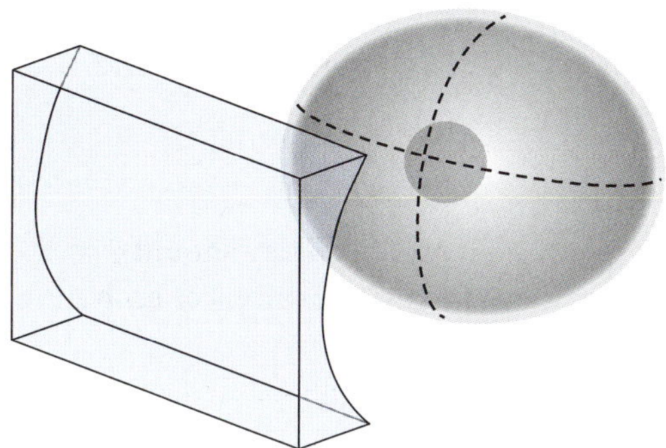

Figure Q-21 Schematic illustration of correction of with-the-rule astigmatism. A minus cylinder is placed with its axis horizontal to compensate for the shape of the cornea, whose vertical axis is steeper than its horizontal axis. *(Illustration developed by Scott E. Brodie, MD, PhD.)*

with-the-rule astigmatism can be corrected with a minus cylinder correcting lens placed with the axis horizontal (Fig Q-21). An equivalent correction can be obtained by placing a plus cylinder lens with the axis vertical and then compensating with a corresponding reduction in the power of the spherical component.

Thus, correction of an eye with an astigmatic refractive error requires the determination of 3 quantities: the power of the correcting cylinder, the axis of the correcting cylinder, and the power of the remaining spherical component. In practice, this task is accomplished as follows:

- Attempt to correct the eye with spherical lenses only or, at least, determine the optimal purely spherical correction.
- Determine whether there is an astigmatic component to the refractive error.
- If astigmatism is present, determine the correcting cylinder axis. This can be done even when the optimal cylindrical correcting power is not yet known.
- Determine the optimal cylindrical correcting power.
- Determine the optimal power to correct any residual spherical error.

Step-by-step instructions for this process are provided in Part 2 of the Quick-Start Guide.

Part 2: Refraction

Highlights

- Many people function with significant visual disability or are effectively blind for lack of a proper refraction.
- Determining best-corrected vision by performing a refraction is an essential step in an ophthalmic examination to differentiate reduced vision caused by refractive error from problems such as cataract or retinal disease.
- The complete process of refracting a patient, including the use of tools such as the phoropter and Jackson cross cylinder, is described in a step-by-step format, complemented by hands-on exercises. After studying this section, the reader should be able to refract a patient.

Glossary

Accommodation The ability of the eye to increase the optical power of the crystalline lens, allowing adjustment of focus for near objects and self-correction of hyperopic refractive errors.

Accommodative control Refraction techniques that suppress accommodation and allow the examiner to determine the refractive state with accommodation relaxed.

Asthenopic complaints Symptoms due to persistent or excessive accommodative effort.

Binary comparison A 2-alternative forced-choice comparison of the clarity of vision between 2 different lenses as, for example, when the examiner asks the patient, "Which is better, 1 or 2?"

Binocular balance Verification that a clinical refraction equally relaxes the accommodation of the 2 eyes.

Clinical refraction The process of measuring the refractive status of a patient's eyes.

Fogging The use of plus lens power to blur the vision in 1 or both eyes, encouraging relaxation of accommodation—a method of accommodative control.

Jackson cross cylinder A lens with cylinders of equal and opposite power, with axes perpendicular to each other, useful for determination of optimal correcting cylinder axis and power.

Manifest refraction The measurement of refractive errors through patients' subjective descriptions of how well they can see.

Monovision A method of correcting presbyopia in which 1 eye is corrected for near vision and the fellow eye for distance vision. It is generally done with contact lenses, refractive surgery, or intraocular lenses in cataract surgery.

Phoropter A refracting instrument (originally a trademarked name, Phoroptor) containing geared spherical and cylindrical lenses for each eye to facilitate subjective refraction.

Pinhole (or pinhole occluder) A device with a small aperture, or an array of small apertures, which reduces the effective aperture of a patient's eye. If pinhole viewing clarifies a patient's vision, this suggests the presence of an uncorrected refractive error.

Overview of Clinical Refraction

Clinical refraction is the process of measuring the refractive status of the eyes of a patient. It is an essential tool in a great many eye examinations: refractive errors are present in nearly half of all adults and children. In most settings, *best-corrected visual acuity* is the gold standard for measuring visual performance. In this section of the Quick-Start Guide, we outline the basic technique of *manifest refraction*—the measurement of refractive errors through patients' subjective descriptions of how well they can see.

Do not confuse performing a manifest refraction with prescribing eyeglasses. The latter is a clinical art, for which refraction is only the first (but critical) step. Guidelines for prescribing glasses are presented in Chapter 4.

Manifest refraction is a subjective process. Success is based on the examiner's ability to elicit the patient's cooperation as much as on their knowledge and skill.

The steps in the process of manifest refraction follow this sequence:

1. Perform the preliminaries (check visual acuity, obtain a visual history).
   a. Indications for refraction: which patients should be refracted?
2. Occlude 1 eye.
3. Make an initial estimate of the refractive error.
   a. Determine the best initial estimate of the refraction, if available, from prior records, old glasses, retinoscopy, or the autorefractor, and place it in the phoropter or trial frame. If there is any known cylindrical correction, go to step 4; if not, go to step 5.

      or
   b. If there is no prior refraction information, retinoscopy, or autorefractor data, begin by refracting only with spherical lenses to obtain the best possible refraction using only spheres. Go to step 3c.
   c. Check for astigmatism by inserting a cylindrical lens, adjusting the sphere to preserve the spherical equivalent, and rotating the cylinder. If this affects image clarity, you have detected some astigmatism. Leave the cylinder in the optimal position (this becomes the starting point for cross-cylinder refinement; go to step 4); if rotating the cylinder has no effect on image clarity, assume there is no astigmatism. Remove the cylinder, restore the original sphere, and go directly to step 5.
4. Refine the cylinder using the Jackson cross cylinder, first in the *axis position* to identify the correct cylinder axis and then in the *power position* to determine the optimal cylinder power. Preserve the spherical equivalent when adjusting cylinder power by adjusting sphere power 1 click (0.25 D) in the opposite direction for every 2-click (0.50 D) change in cylinder power. Go to step 5.
5. Refine the sphere power, first using a 0.50 D difference between the alternatives, bracketing the previous selection, and then using a 0.25 D difference between the alternatives.
6. Reverse the occlusion and repeat for the fellow eye.
7. Check for binocular balance.
8. Refract for near vision.

Additional comments, set off in boxes, are interspersed among the step-by-step instructions. Most of the step-by-step instructions discussed below describe refraction performed with minus cylinder equipment. Equivalent instructions for plus cylinder equipment are so labeled and marked with a tinted background. Recommended language to use with patients is printed in ***boldface italics***.

Step 1. Perform the Preliminaries

Check visual acuity

We use eye charts consisting of *optotypes* (letters or pictures) to test visual acuity. If a patient's visual acuity is known from a prior examination, start at that line of the eye chart. Otherwise, first cover the left eye, and ask the patient to read the 20/40 line on the eye chart with the right eye (Fig Q-22). Go up or down the eye chart to find the line your patient can just barely read. Then cover the right eye and repeat the process to measure the acuity of the left eye.

TAKE NOTE

- *Many patients will balk when instructed to* ***"Read the smallest line you can."*** *You may get the response "But, Doctor, I can't read the smallest line." Expect patients to slow down as they reach the line(s) they can just barely see. Checking visual acuity well takes more time than you would imagine. Think of it as an opportunity to observe your patient's vision, much as a neurologist carefully watches a patient walk into the exam room. Encourage patients to guess at letters they can barely see.*
- *It is customary to perform ophthalmic examinations first for the right eye, then for the left eye. Get into this habit to minimize confusion about which findings go with which eye. Notice systematic errors at the beginning or end of the lines of the eye chart, which might suggest a visual field defect. Craning of the neck may indicate an attempt to cheat in cases of amblyopia. "Searching" may suggest a central scotoma (blind spot). Discourage squinting!*
- *When refracting children, it is preferable to use modern picture optotypes, such as the HOTV character set or the LEA symbols (circle, square, apple, and house) (see Chapter 3, Figs 3-6D and 3-6E, respectively) rather than traditional picture optotypes (Allen symbols: telephone, hand, bird, car, birthday cake, and horse and rider); the latter remain distinguishable even with a great deal of blur and may be confusing. Few children recognize a dial telephone these days!*

If visual acuity is subnormal, try a *pinhole occluder*, which reduces the eye's effective aperture (Fig Q-23). Note: Best-refracted vision may be better than, worse than, or the same as pinhole-corrected vision. Failure to improve with a pinhole does *not* exclude refractive error and does *not* justify omitting the refraction.

For example, pinhole vision is typically worse than best-corrected vision in cases of dense cataracts and in many cases of macular degeneration. Conversely, when looking through a pinhole occluder, patients with early, inhomogeneous cataracts may improve dramatically but may fail to achieve this acuity with spectacles. Using the single pinhole that is provided in the phoropter accessory wheel, a patient may have difficulty finding the eye chart.

If the patient has distance glasses, there is rarely any reason to check the visual acuity without them, unless the patient requests it or acuity with the existing glasses is very poor. In some cases, a patient may inadvertently use reading glasses while attempting to see at distance.

Check visual acuity at near (ie, *reading vision*) routinely only in the following cases: patients who may demonstrate presbyopia (age-related loss of near vision), patients with

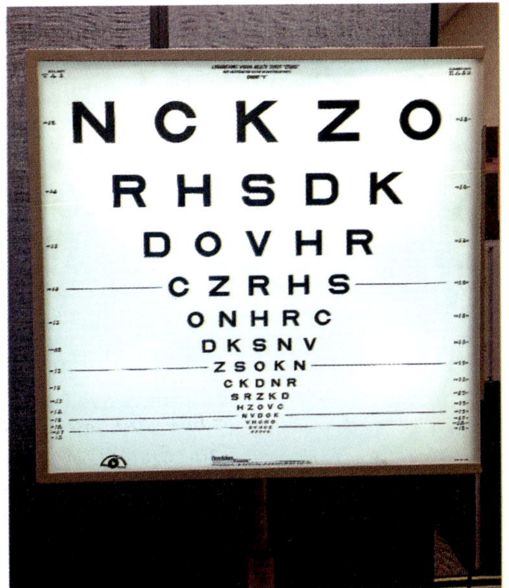

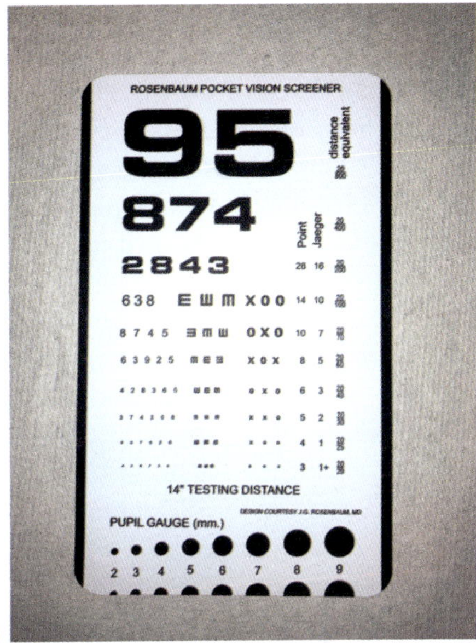

Figure Q-22 Distance and near visual acuity charts. **A,** ETDRS-type chart with Sloan letters. **B,** Near-card with numerals. *(Courtesy of Thomas F. Mauger, MD.)*

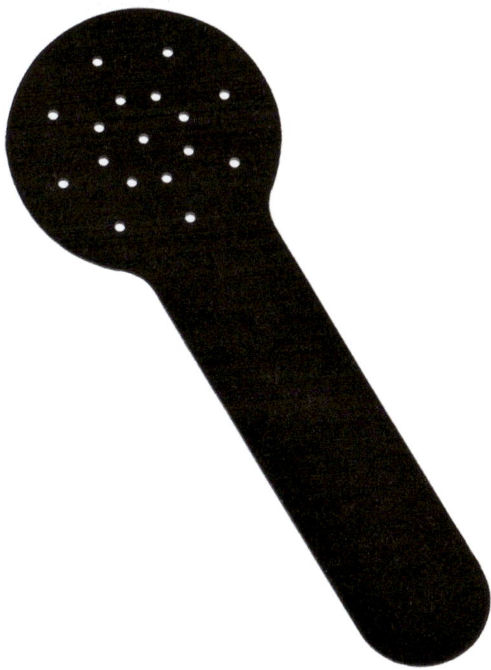

Figure Q-23 Pinhole occluder.

suspected latent hyperopia, patients (especially children) with suspected amblyopia, and those with a near vision or an asthenopic complaint. In amblyopia, near vision may be better than distance vision. However, many patients, especially children, seem to see better at near only because they are permitted to hold the near-vision testing card closer than the calibrated distance (typically 14 inches, or 40 cm). Such compensations are impossible at distance. Asthenopic symptoms include fatigue, headache, "eyestrain," double vision, fluctuating visual acuity, and lengthening of the clearest reading distance. They suggest hyperopic refractive errors, presbyopia, accommodative spasm, or the possibility that the patient's existing glasses contain a stronger myopic correction (or a weaker hyperopic correction) than necessary. These topics are discussed in greater detail in Chapter 4.

Patients older than 40 or so should routinely be checked for presbyopia. It is better to allow such patients to hold the near card at their own preferred reading distance (with or without reading glasses, according to their typical reading habits) and to record the smallest legible line and the distance at which they hold the near card rather than enforcing the standard reading distance. Use Jaeger notation, optotype size in points, or both to record the near vision (eg, "J3 @ 40 cm" or "8-point type @ 15 inches").

Obtain a visual history

As in any patient care encounter, obtaining an accurate history is a vital initial step in clinical refraction. Understanding the patient's visual concerns, if any, is often critical to providing a satisfactory refractive solution. For example, the patient may benefit from glasses suitable for specific activities, such as using a computer, playing a musical instrument, or going shopping; and you may be called on to design spectacles for an occupational or recreational application. Prescribing glasses for a patient without visual concerns or symptoms is rarely helpful.

Seek the following information. If it is not volunteered, ask the patient directly:

- Have you noticed a decrease in visual acuity at distance? At near? Both?
- Do you experience eyestrain or headaches?
- Do you have any difficulty reading at a comfortable distance?
- What is your age?
- What is your occupation? Does it involve a lot of computer work?
- What are your hobbies (eg, music, sewing)?
- Do you use monovision?
- Do you have any current or past eye problems (eg, amblyopia, trauma, glaucoma, prior eye surgery)?

TAKE NOTE

- *Refractive errors are only rarely the cause of headaches. Headaches that wake a patient from sleep or occur early in the morning are almost never due to refractive error.*
- *Be alert for ophthalmic disorders that might limit best-corrected visual acuity.*

Review indications for refraction

Which patients need to be refracted?

- those with subnormal visual acuity (ie, 20/25 or worse, unless a credible refraction documenting a stable best-corrected visual acuity of 20/25 or worse is already in the medical record; those with 20/30 or worse should routinely be refracted)
- those with asthenopic symptoms
- those whose visual acuity has decreased since their previous visit
- postoperative patients (especially after cataract surgery)

> **TAKE NOTE**
>
> *Some cataract surgeons postpone postoperative refractions until there has been sufficient healing to ensure a good visual result. This delay may prevent the detection of an early, vision-threatening complication.*

Step 2. Occlude 1 Eye

Occlude the left eye, refract the right eye first

- Barring exceptional circumstances, begin by occluding the *left* eye, and perform the initial refraction in the *right* eye.
- When using a phoropter, you may dial an opaque occluder (marked "OC") into place using the accessory wheel (Fig Q-24A).
- If the patient is cooperative and does not find it too distracting, it is often preferable to occlude the nonrefracting eye with a plus lens, such as the +1.50 D retinoscopy lens (marked "R") in the accessory wheel of the phoropter (Figs Q-24B, C). This practice is often better at relaxing accommodation in the eye you *are* refracting than using an opaque occluder on the fellow eye. However, this method will not work well on patients with latent hyperopia: first verify that the +1.50 D lens actually reduces the visual acuity. Dial in extra plus lens power if needed. This process is known as *fogging*. If you suspect hyperopia, attempt to relax accommodation by gradually dialing in plus sphere power, 1 click (0.25 D) every 15–20 seconds while talking amiably with the patient, until the visual acuity is substantially reduced.

> **TAKE NOTE**
>
> *Some patients develop nystagmus (rapid involuntary eye movements) when 1 eye is completely occluded. You can sometimes avoid that by using an adequate plus lens, rather than an opaque occluder, to occlude the fellow eye.*

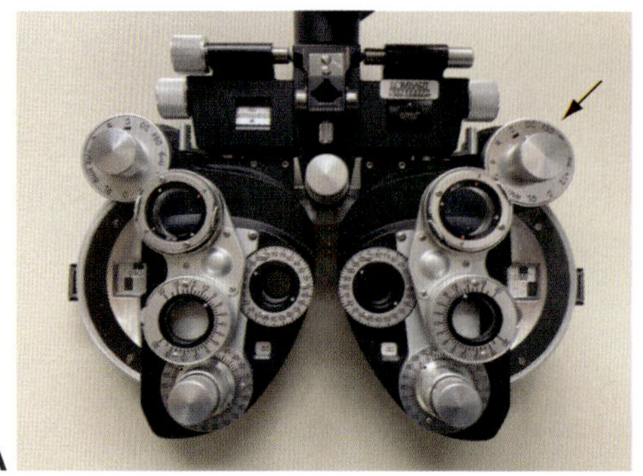

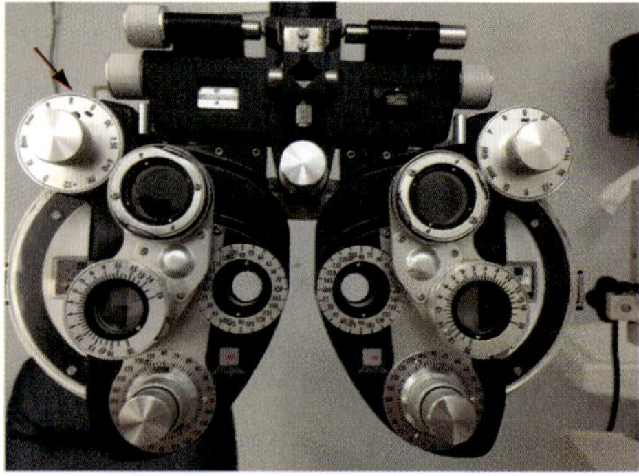

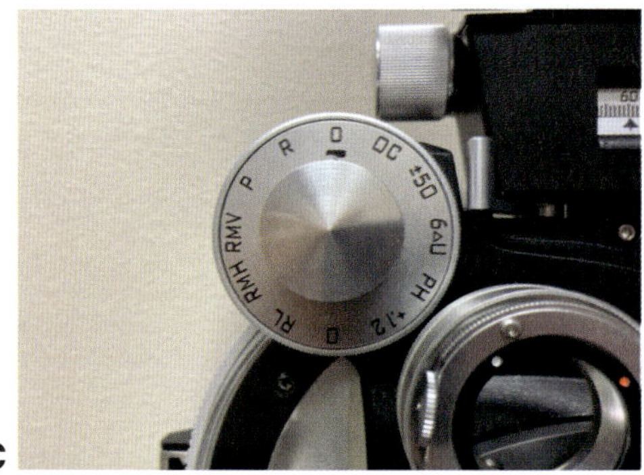

Figure Q-24 Occluding the left side of the phoropter: **A,** Opaque occluder *(arrow).* **B,** +1.50 D "R" accessory lens *(arrow).* Notice the settings of the accessory wheel for the right eye, at the top left of the photos. **C,** Accessory wheel.

Step 3. Obtain Initial Estimate of the Refractive Error

Having established that a patient needs to be refracted, obtain the best-available initial estimate of the refractive correction (if any) and dial it into the phoropter or place it in a trial frame.

TAKE NOTE

Phoropter (Refractor)

The phoropter, also called a refractor, is a device that holds trial lenses on geared wheels to facilitate exchanging lenses in front of the patient's eyes during a manifest refraction (Fig Q-25A). Each side of the device holds lenses for a large range of plus sphere and minus sphere power. The cylinder battery, or array of cylindrical lenses, contains cylinders of only 1 sign, either plus or minus, depending on the individual instrument.

Before beginning a refraction, you must determine whether the phoropter you are using is a plus cylinder or minus cylinder instrument. Note: On many phoropters, minus cylinders are indicated with red numbers (Fig Q-25B), and plus cylinders are indicated with black numbers.

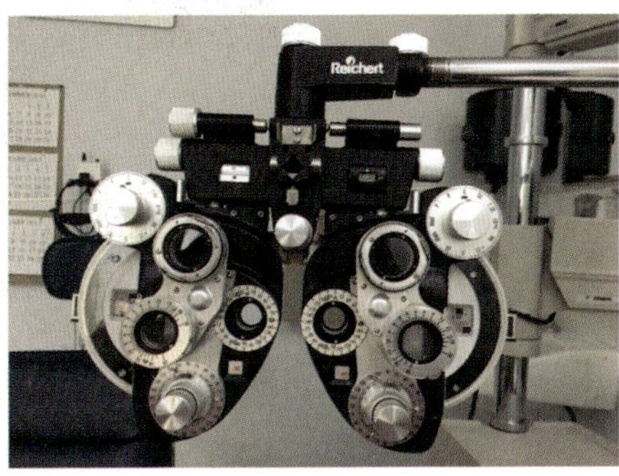

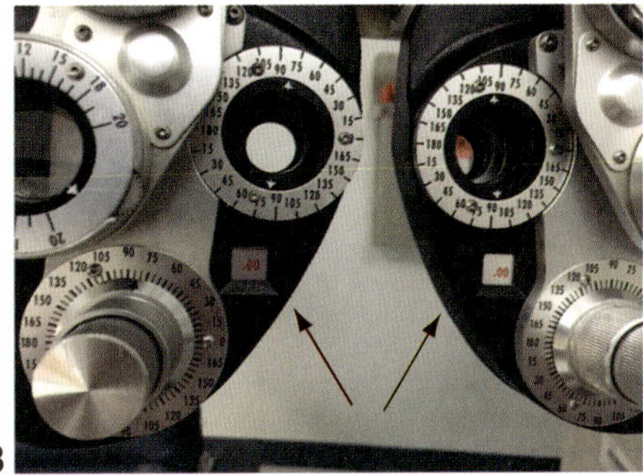

A B

Figure Q-25 Phoropter. **A,** A minus cylinder phoropter. **B,** Close-up view of a minus cylinder phoropter. The red numbers *(arrows)* indicate the cylinder power. Black numbers are used in plus cylinder phoropters.

Perform* either *step 3a or steps 3b and 3c

Step 3a. Use prior information to obtain initial estimate of refractive error

- Measure the patient's current eyeglasses, if available, and dial these values into the phoropter. (Use of the lensometer to measure, or *neutralize*, glasses is described in Chapter 9.) In the absence of glasses, use the results of a previous refraction, such as an earlier prescription for glasses as provided by the patient or as recorded in the patient's medical record.
- Perform retinoscopy (see Part 3 of the Quick-Start Guide, page 40).
  - If lenses in the phoropter are clean, retinoscopy may be performed through the phoropter so that the results of the retinoscopy will be immediately available as the initial phoropter settings for subjective refraction. It is a good habit to write down the retinoscopic findings for comparison with the final refraction.
- Use an autorefractor or a photorefractor. While autorefractors are commonly used, they are not a replacement for retinoscopy, which often allows the examiner to make determinations despite patient movement, small pupils, and media opacity.
- If there is no known astigmatic correction, proceed directly to step 5; if there is an astigmatic correction, go to step 4.

Step 3b. Make direct initial measurement of spherical refractive error

- If no preliminary estimate is available from old glasses, the medical record, retinoscopy, or autorefraction, determine the best spherical correction by offering the patient successive choices of spherical corrections. Starting with the sphere power at 0.00, use the low-power sphere lens wheel on the phoropter (or handheld lenses if using a trial frame) to present the patient with a choice between a spherical lens power of +0.25 D or −0.25 D. This gives the patient a choice between spherical lenses that differ by 0.50 D. (If the patient's visual acuity is very poor, offer a greater difference, such as 1.00 D, between the 2 choices.) Use the language ***"Which is better, 1 or 2?"*** This "forced choice" is referred to as a binary comparison.
  - Make certain the patient is responding to your choice between lens 1 or lens 2, not line 1 or line 2 of the eye chart. If necessary, mask off all but 1 line of the chart.

- Advance the sphere setting 0.25 D toward the preferred alternative, and then offer the next binary comparison to bracket the patient's most recent choice of sphere power setting, again with a 0.50 D difference. (For example, if the patient's initial preference is for the −0.25 D lens, the next choice offered should be between 0.00 and −0.50 D lenses.)
- Repeat this process until the patient suggests that the 2 choices are about the same.
- Recheck this endpoint, using choices that differ by only 0.25 D.
- Generally, try to move most of the time from *more plus* to *less plus* (or from *less minus* to *more minus*). By offering the *more plus* or *less minus* choice first, you will stimulate accommodation only minimally.
  - Try to be sensitive to the patient's responses. As you near the endpoint, responses are typically slower. The patient may simply stop responding rather than volunteering that the choices are about the same. This is still useful information.
- Do not worry about making a mistake by going too far—the method is self-correcting.
- Once the best possible spherical correction has been determined, go to step 3c to determine if there is any astigmatic refractive error.

Step 3c. Detect astigmatism

Now that you have found the optimal spherical correction, determine whether there is any astigmatism, as follows.

Directions for use of a *minus cylinder* phoropter

- Dial in −0.50 D of cylinder.
- Increase the *sphere* power by +0.25 D.
- Rotate the cylinder axis knob slowly once or twice around and ask the patient to tell you to stop when they perceive the clearest vision. (Alternatively, you may ask the patient to turn the knob and leave it where their vision is best.)
- If the patient reports that rotating the dial makes no difference to the visual clarity—even if the vision is rather poor—then you may assume that the patient has *no significant astigmatism* and proceed to step 5. If the patient *can* select a preferred axis, you have detected an astigmatic refractive error. Leave the cylinder dial *at the preferred axis orientation* and proceed to step 4.

Directions for use of a *plus cylinder* phoropter

- Dial in +0.50 D of cylinder.
- Decrease the *sphere* power by −0.25 D.
- Rotate the cylinder axis knob slowly once or twice around and ask the patient to tell you to stop when they perceive the clearest vision. (Alternatively, you may ask the patient to turn the knob and leave it where their vision is best.)
- If the patient reports that rotating the dial makes no difference to the visual clarity—even if the vision is rather poor—then you may assume that the patient has *no significant astigmatism* and proceed to step 5. If the patient *can* select a preferred axis, you have detected an astigmatic refractive error. Leave the cylinder dial *at the preferred axis orientation* and proceed to step 4.

TAKE NOTE

If the visual acuity is very poor, especially if there is a very large astigmatic refractive error, the patient may be unable to detect a difference in visual clarity when the rotating cylinder process is used as described above. If possible, check for astigmatism by retinoscopy, by keratometry, or by use of the stenopeic slit (see Chapter 4).

Step 4. Refine Cylinder Axis and Power

Once you have confirmed that an astigmatic refractive error is present, refine the cylinder *axis* as follows.

Directions for use of a *minus cylinder* phoropter

With the initial estimate of the cylindrical correction dialed into the phoropter, place the *Jackson cross cylinder* in the *axis* position, that is, with an imaginary line connecting the 2 small thumbwheels aligned parallel to the axis of the cylinder battery (Fig Q-26). That alignment is indicated by the arrows on the axis knob and by indicator lines or arrowheads near the aperture of the phoropter. The cross cylinder should click into place.

Present a binary comparison between the 2 positions of the cross cylinder by rotating 1 of the thumbwheels. Notice how this interchanges the indicator dots (red and white) on the cross-cylinder lens. Continue the binary comparisons, and after each, turn the (minus) cylinder axis toward the orientation of the *red* dots on the cross-cylinder lens in the position where the patient reports clearer vision.

The endpoint is often vague ("about the same," "equally bad," and so on). Watch for increased hesitation by the patient or a reversal of the progression of the axis as you make successive binary comparisons. The process is self-correcting—if you go too far in 1 direction, the patient's responses will indicate that the cylinder axis should be brought back to a previous position.

Video Q-1 demonstrates refraction using the Jackson cross cylinder.

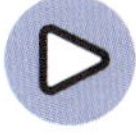

VIDEO Q-1 How to refract tutorial: Jackson cross cylinder technique.
Courtesy of David Guyton, MD.

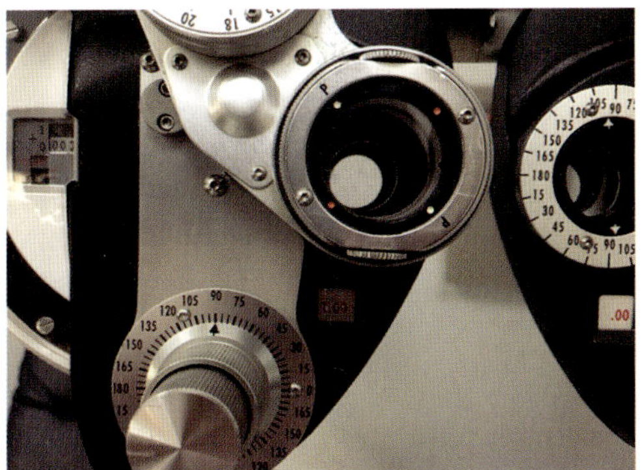

Figure Q-26 Phoropter with Jackson cross cylinder in "axis" position. The cylinder battery has been set with the cylinder axis vertical.

Directions for use of a *plus cylinder* phoropter

Place the Jackson cross cylinder in the *axis* position, that is, with an imaginary line connecting the 2 small thumbwheels aligned parallel to the axis of the cylinder battery (see Fig Q-26). That alignment is indicated by the arrows on the axis knob and by indicator lines or arrowheads near the aperture of the phoropter. The cross cylinder should click into place.

Present a binary comparison between the 2 positions of the cross cylinder by rotating 1 of the thumbwheels. Notice how this interchanges the indicator dots (red and white) on the cross-cylinder lens. Continue the binary comparisons, and after each, turn the plus cylinder axis toward the orientation of the *white* dots on the cross-cylinder lens in the position where the patient reports clearer vision.

The endpoint is often vague ("about the same," "equally bad," and so on). Watch for increased hesitation by the patient or a reversal of the progression of the axis as you make successive binary comparisons. The process is self-correcting—if you go too far in 1 direction, the patient's responses will indicate that the cylinder axis should be brought back to a previous direction.

Next, refine the cylinder *power.*

Directions for use of a *minus cylinder* phoropter

Turn the cross-cylinder turret 45° to the *power* position, as indicated by an imaginary line connecting the "P" marks on the cross-cylinder lens rim running parallel to the cylinder axis you have just determined (Fig Q-27). Flip the cross cylinder to provide a binary comparison. Notice how either the red dots or the white dots on the cross cylinder will line up along the cylinder axis. If the patient's preferred position of the cross cylinder places the *red* dots along the cylinder axis, *increase* the minus cylinder power. If the preferred position of the cross cylinder places the line through the *red* dots *perpendicular* to the cylinder axis, so the line connecting the white dots lies parallel to the cylinder axis, *reduce* the minus cylinder power.

Repeat until you reach an endpoint where the views through the alternate positions of the cross cylinder are "about the same." (Note that at this stage, the view may still not be very good.) When in doubt, go with the numerically weaker choice of minus cylinder power.

KEY STEP For each 0.50 D (2-click) *increase* in *minus cylinder* power as determined by these cross-cylinder flips, *add* +0.25 D (1 click) of plus *spherical* power. After you have

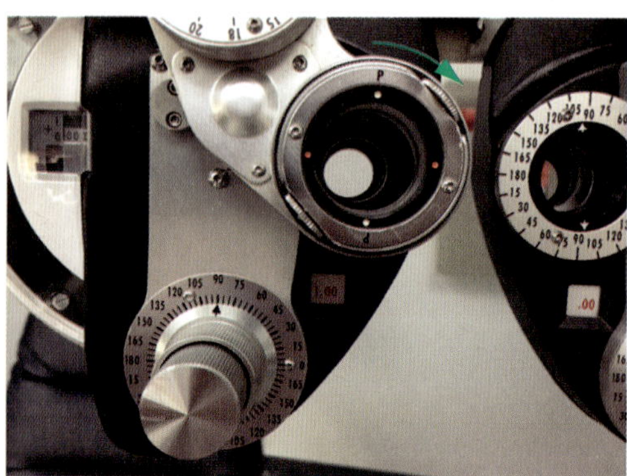

Figure Q-27 Phoropter with Jackson cross cylinder in "power" position. The cylinder battery remains set with the cylinder axis vertical. The green arrow demonstrates rotation of the Jackson cross cylinder from the "axis" position to the "power" position. *(Courtesy of Scott E. Brodie, MD, PhD.)*

located the endpoint, remove the cross cylinder from the optical pathway. If all is well, the patient should experience a considerable improvement in visual acuity.

Once the optimal cylinder axis and power have been determined, proceed to step 5.

Directions for use of a *plus cylinder* phoropter

Turn the cross cylinder turret 45° to the *power* position, as indicated by an imaginary line connecting the "P" marks on the lens rim running parallel to the cylinder axis you have just determined.

Flip the cross cylinder to provide a binary comparison. Notice how either the red dots or the white dots on the cross cylinder will line up along the cylinder axis. If the patient's preferred position of the cross cylinder places the *white* dots along the cylinder axis, *increase* the plus cylinder power. If the preferred position of the cross cylinder places the line through the *white* dots *perpendicular* to the cylinder axis, so the line connecting the red dots lies parallel to the cylinder axis, *reduce* the plus cylinder power.

Repeat until you reach an endpoint where the views through the alternate positions of the cross cylinder are "about the same." (Note that at this stage, the view may still not be very good.) When in doubt, go with the numerically weaker choice of plus cylinder power.

KEY STEP For each 0.50 D (2-click) *increase* in *plus cylinder* power as determined by these cross cylinder flips, *add* +0.25 D (1 click) of minus power to the sphere (or subtract +0.25 D of plus power, as the case may be). After you have located the endpoint, remove the cross cylinder from the optical pathway. If all is well, the patient should experience a considerable improvement in visual acuity.

Once the optimal cylinder axis and power have been determined, proceed to step 5.

TAKE NOTE

If you are using loose trial lenses in a trial frame instead of a phoropter, you will have to align the handheld Jackson cross cylinder (Fig Q-28) with the tentative axis of the correcting cylinder in the trial frame by yourself. To refine the cylinder axis, hold the cross cylinder with the handle parallel to the correcting cylinder axis. After each binary comparison, rotate the cylinder axis toward the preferred position of the red or white dots on the cross cylinder, depending on whether you are working with minus cylinder or plus cylinder trial lenses, respectively.

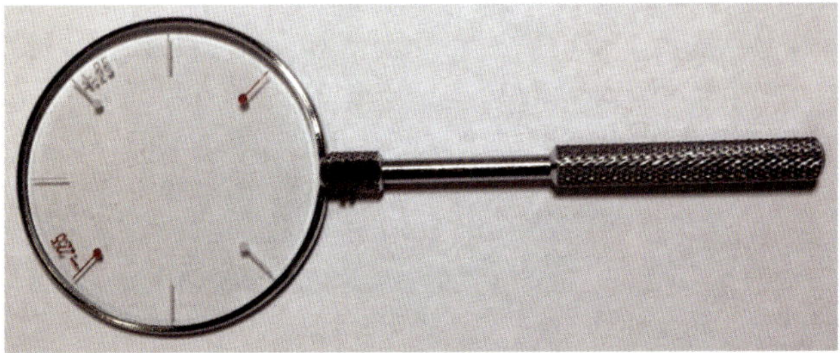

Figure Q-28 Handheld Jackson cross cylinder. Notice the red and white dots that straddle the axis of the handle. *(Courtesy of Scott E. Brodie, MD, PhD.)*

For the next binary comparison, you will have to adjust the orientation of the cross-cylinder handle to align with the new position of the trial cylinder axis. (This realignment of the cross cylinder takes place automatically on most phoropters.) To refine the cylinder power, hold the handle of the cross cylinder 45° away from the axis of the trial cylinder. This will align the lines between the red and white dots on the cross cylinder either parallel or perpendicular to the axis of the trial cylinder. Then proceed as above.

After optimizing the cylinder power, you may find it useful to recheck the cylinder axis. If the cylinder axis is substantially changed, recheck the cylinder power as well.

Step 5. Refine Sphere Power

Once you have achieved the optimal cylinder axis and power, recheck the sphere power, as in step 3b.

Step 6. Occlude the Right Eye, Refract the Left Eye

You have completed refraction of the right eye. To refract the patient's other eye, repeat the process of steps 3 through 5 for the fellow eye.

Try It Yourself! Q-3

- **Refract the wall.** A good way to see how the logic of cross-cylinder refraction works is to try this simple exercise. Position the phoropter parallel to a wall about 20 cm away (Fig Q-29A). Occlude 1 side of the phoropter. Tape a random cylinder trial lens to the back of the other side; the metal clip will help hold it in place. (About 1.50 D works well. Start with a cylinder of the sign opposite to the sign of the cylinders in your phoropter.) Ask a friend to hold a penlight or Finoff transilluminator several feet away, pointing it toward the open aperture of the phoropter. You should see a small elliptical spot projected on the wall behind the phoropter (Fig Q-29B).
- **Refract with spheres.** Using binary comparisons, find the optimal spherical "correction" for the wall. This will be a *circular* image (the circle of least confusion).
- **Is astigmatism present?** Set the cylinder battery to 0.50 D of cylinder power and adjust the sphere power 0.25 D in the opposite direction. Then slowly rotate the cylinder axis knob and observe the changes in the diameter of the blur circle on the wall. You should be able to set the axis to the optimal position (with the smallest, brightest image) within a few degrees or so. For practice, set it about 10° away from the optimal setting.
- **Refine the cylinder axis.** Swing the cross cylinder in place, in the axis position. Use binary comparisons to optimize the cylinder axis. You should be able to find the optimal axis within a degree or so.

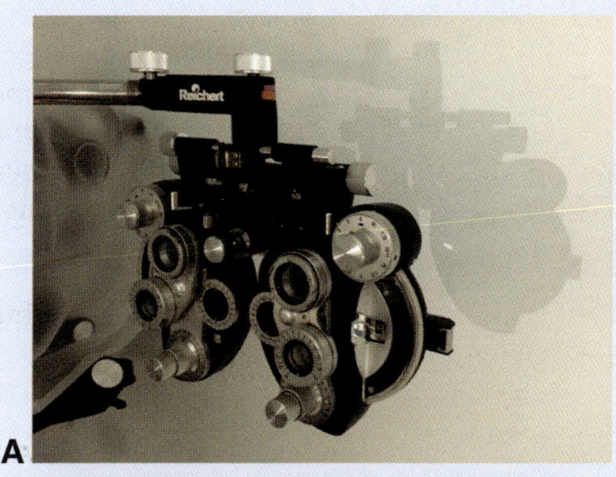

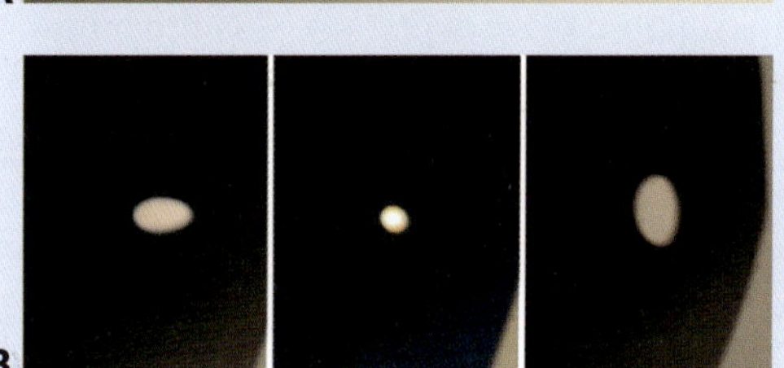

Figure Q-29 Refracting the wall. **A,** Notice the elliptical image of a distant penlight on the wall behind the phoropter. **B,** The conoid of Sturm demonstrated by the images of a penlight showing on the wall through the aperture of the phoropter. *(Courtesy of Scott E. Brodie, MD, PhD.)*

- **Refine the cylinder power.** Rotate the cross-cylinder turret 45° to the power position. Use binary comparisons to refine the cylinder power. Notice how the process of adjusting the sphere power 0.25 D for each 0.50 D change in cylinder power (as described in the Key Step) is necessary to keep the image optimal. When you reach the endpoint, you may see the image flip between small elliptical spots—you are seeing the residual astigmatism that the cross cylinder itself introduces into the optical pathway.
- **Remove the cross cylinder and refine the sphere power to obtain the smallest, brightest image.**
- **Check your work.** The final cylinder correction should closely approximate the power of the "error cylinder" you introduced at the start, with the same axis. (Be careful as you compare axes from the 2 sides of the phoropter!) The final sphere power should be slightly greater than the dioptric equivalent of the distance between the phoropter and the wall, because your light source is not infinitely far away.
- **Try this exercise with another error cylinder of the same sign as your phoropter cylinders.** The final correcting cylinder will be of nearly the same power, perpendicular to the error cylinder.

Step 7. Accommodative Control and Binocular Balance

Accommodation is the ability of the eye to increase the focusing power of the crystalline lens, mainly to allow clear vision for near objects. In general, the primary goal of clinical refraction is to determine the refractive error, if any, with the accommodation fully relaxed. That means the eyes are focused for distant targets; the patient has the full use of the accommodative amplitude to focus over as large a range of nearer objects as possible. In addition, accommodation should be equally relaxed for the 2 eyes—a state referred to as *binocular balance*.

However, in practice, the patient might not spontaneously attain this fully relaxed state of accommodation, which complicates the task of the refractionist. Many factors, such as hyperopic refractive errors (which can often be corrected by a patient's own accommodative effort), awareness of near objects (including the refracting instruments and lenses), and accommodative spasm, can induce an increase in accommodative tone, steering the refractive process toward undercorrection of a hyperopic error or overcorrection of a myopic error. In some cases, patients seem to prefer the high-contrast, minified image seen by accommodating to compensate for a myopic overcorrection. It is thus important to make every effort to use *accommodative control* techniques that relax the accommodation during the refraction process and guard against inadvertent stimulation of accommodation and overminusing the patient as a result. Using a plus lens occluder instead of an opaque occluder and biasing the binary comparisons to offer the more plus choice first will help prevent spurious accommodation.

TAKE NOTE

It is good practice to double-check the accommodative control as the final step in a routine refraction to guard against these errors, at least in patients younger than 50 or 60 years. (Accommodation is discussed more fully in Chapter 3.)

The "Rule-1" test is a quick and easy way to check accommodative control. You can perform this test for each eye separately or binocularly if the vision is comparable in the 2 eyes.

- Dial in +1.00 D sphere power above the final refractive correction. Visual acuity should fall at least 2 lines on the eye chart. (For example, if the final refraction brings the acuity to 20/20, adding +1.00 D sphere to both eyes should reduce the acuity to 20/30 or worse.)
- If the acuity does not drop 2 lines as expected, continue to increase the plus sphere power until the acuity is reduced by 2 lines.
- Next, remove the excess added plus sphere power 1 click (0.25 D) at a time until the acuity returns to the optimal level. (Ask, ***"Is this step definitely better, or are the letters just smaller and blacker?"***) The final endpoint should be the last step that permits the patient to read *additional* letters. Disregard the patient's enthusiasm for any additional minus sphere (or reduced plus sphere) power that does not allow more letters to be read.

If you perform this procedure for each eye separately, it also serves as a check of binocular balance—that is, confirming that the 2 eyes are accommodating to the same degree. The Lancaster red–green (duochrome) test (not to be confused with the Lancaster red–green test for strabismus, described in BCSC Section 6, *Pediatric Ophthalmology and*

Strabismus) is recommended for patients with 20/40 or better best-corrected acuity. It can be performed monocularly or binocularly. When each eye is evaluated separately, this test functions as an effective check of binocular balance.

- Bring up the duochrome slide or filter on your chart projector. This will display one side of the chart against a bright red background and the other side against a bright green background.
- Ask, ***"Which side of the chart has the clearer, crisper, blacker letters: the red side or the green side?"*** (If the patient is confused by the intense colors, add ***"Concentrate on the letters, not on the backgrounds. Look at the smallest letters you can read."***
- If the patient reports that the letters seen against the *red* background are clearer, more *minus* sphere power is needed; if the *green* side is preferred, more *plus* sphere power is indicated.
- The goal is to leave both sides of the chart equally clear. When in doubt, leave the patient with the more plus (or less minus) sphere choice (ie, with a slight preference for seeing against the red background), which will better relax the accommodation.

The duochrome test is based on the chromatic aberration of the human eye. This test works just as well in color-blind patients as in patients with normal color vision, as long as you describe the alternatives as left versus right instead of red versus green.

Try It Yourself! Q-4

Refract a friend or colleague to become familiar with the process (and let him or her refract you in turn).

- If he or she has little or no refractive error, introduce an error cylinder by taping a cylindrical trial lens to the back of the phoropter. Pay attention to how the ability to provide evaluations of the binary comparisons slows as you approach the endpoints and the differences in appearance of the targets become subtler. This is an important clue for you as the refractionist.
- Try deliberately overminusing your subject. Notice how far beyond the real refractive endpoint you can go without blurring the vision. Ask your subject to say whether the optotypes start becoming "smaller and blacker."
- With your subject clearly overminused, slowly dial back the refraction toward the correct endpoint. Notice that the accommodative tone is "sticky"—you will likely return to optimal acuity before returning to the original endpoint. Beware: this can happen with your patients, too!
- Refract yourself. Sit behind the phoropter and reach around to operate the knobs in the front. Notice how easy or difficult are the various comparisons you will be asking your patients to make.

Step 8. Refract for Near Vision

Refracting at near (ie, determining the optimal correction, if any, needed for near vision) is not routinely done on patients younger than 40 years unless they have a specific near-vision concern.

- Begin with the current distance correction in place in the phoropter or trial frame. If you do not know the distance refraction with confidence, perform a careful distance refraction even if the patient volunteered *no* complaints at distance. This step is critical to detect latent hyperopia.

  Converge the phoropter such that the optics point toward the near eye chart—use the 2 small levers just below the top of the instrument (Fig Q-30). Install the near eye chart on the stick and holder provided for near work at a working distance of 40 cm (Fig Q-31). (The multipaneled Rotochart provided with the phoropter is excellent for near-vision testing. The Rosenbaum card also works well.) If neither is available, the patient can hold a near-vision testing card at the appropriate distance. Be sure to provide suitable illumination.
- Add plus sphere power over the distance correction until near acuity is optimized, with the zone of clear vision centered at 40 cm or at the patient's preferred reading

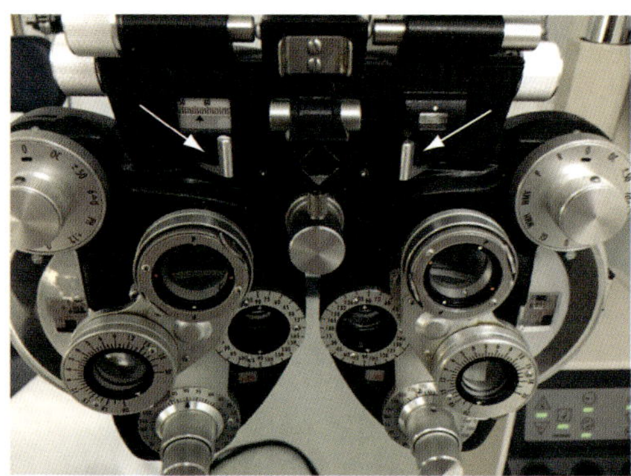

Figure Q-30 Converging the phoropter. Notice the position of the small vertical levers *(arrows)* near the top; compare with Figure Q-24. *(Courtesy of Scott E. Brodie, MD, PhD.)*

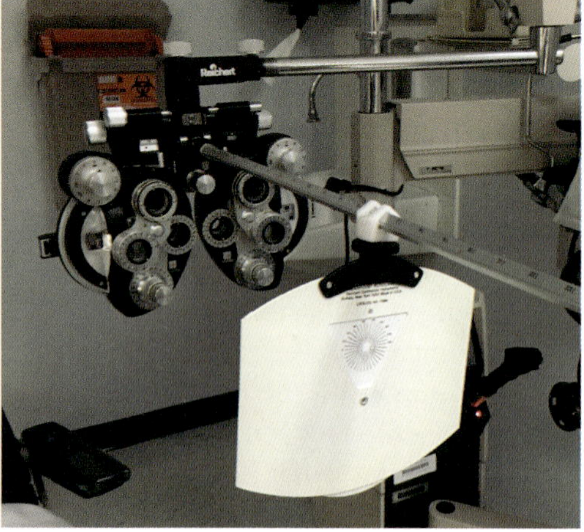

Figure Q-31 Phoropter with near-point chart in place, 40 cm away. *(Courtesy of Scott E. Brodie, MD, PhD.)*

distance. (Check this by sliding or moving the near card toward and away from the patient.) Rough near-point add guidelines according to age are as follows: 40 years, +1.00 D to +2.00 D; 50 years, +1.50 D to +2.50 D; 60 years and older, +2.00 D to +2.75 D.

Patients frequently prefer higher adds. Try to resist this bias—the higher adds not only require that text be held unnaturally close to the eyes but also decrease the range over which the material can be seen clearly (decreasing intermediate vision). This decreased range of comfortable reading positions hastens fatigue during reading. When in doubt, choose the lesser add. It should rarely be necessary to use an add greater than +2.75 D, except as a low vision aid.

> **TAKE NOTE**
>
> *Corrected acuity at near should roughly correspond to the same Snellen fraction as the distance acuity. A significant discrepancy in either direction suggests the presence of ocular pathology.*

Final Remarks

At the core of ophthalmic practice is the ability to assess a patient's visual function. Thus, your capacity to perform an efficient, accurate refraction is critical. Subjective refraction is a clinical art—it takes time to develop facility. Learn to refract well.

- There are many excuses to avoid refracting almost any patient you see. Refract every patient who needs it. Just because a refraction is not easy does not mean that it is not important to the patient or that successful refraction would not greatly benefit the patient. Difficult refractions are an inevitable part of ophthalmology. If necessary, reschedule the patient to allow the additional time.
- Carefully adjust the pace of the refraction to the ability of the patient to respond. The patient should not feel rushed, but you should offer the binary comparisons crisply to encourage the patient to respond based on his or her initial visual impression. The amount of time between choices will vary among patients. It may be as brief as 1 or 2 seconds for some patients but longer for others. The pace should discourage the patient from attempting to accommodate before deciding on the better lens choice.
- Cycloplegia (paralysis of accommodation with anticholinergic eyedrops) is indicated whenever there is uncertainty about the accommodative status. This technique should be routine for children younger than 10 years. (See Chapter 4.)
- Many healthy young adults can see 20/15 if given the chance. Don't settle for 20/20, let alone 20/25. Children younger than 6 or even 7 years are frequently uninterested in reading past the 20/30 line, even though more sophisticated testing methods have shown that they may possess 20/20 acuity. (That is why many "picture" eye charts stop at the 20/30 line.)

- For children under the age of 6 or 7 years, use a chart with "tumbling" E, Landolt C, or picture targets. Do not rely on a parent's assurance that their child knows the letters of the alphabet.
- There are few opportunities in clinical ophthalmology to improve your patient's visual function as convincingly as the chance to prescribe a good pair of glasses. Competent refraction is a key tool for developing a patient's confidence in you.

Part 3: Retinoscopy

Highlights

- Retinoscopy provides useful estimates of refractive error for all patients.
- Retinoscopy is particularly valuable in infants and small children, and in patients who cannot cooperate with manifest refraction.
- Retinoscopy provides important clues to the presence of ocular disease, including cataract, keratoconus, and retinoblastoma.

Glossary

Blur Unequal clarity of the streak images viewed parallel to the principal axes of the eye—a sign of uncorrected astigmatism.

Break Apparent discontinuity of the streak image as it crosses the pupillary margin—a sign of uncorrected astigmatism.

Gross retinoscopy The total power of the lenses that generate a neutral retinoscopic reflex, regardless of the working distance.

Neutral reflex The appearance of the retinoscopic reflex after all refractive errors have been corrected; the pupil appears to fill uniformly with light, and no motion is seen as the streak is moved.

Net retinoscopy The difference between the gross retinoscopy and the power of the working lens. This is the retinoscopic estimate of the lens combination that corrects the eye's refractive error.

Peephole A small aperture in the retinoscope through which the user views the retinoscopic reflexes.

Pseudoneutral reflex A dull, motionless reflex seen in highly myopic eyes.

Reflex The image of the retinoscope filament as projected onto the retina and viewed by the examiner through the peephole of the retinoscope.

Retinoscope A handheld instrument for measuring refractive errors.

Skew Apparent disparity between the direction of motion of the streak image as seen within the pupil and as projected onto the surface of the eye; a sign of uncorrected astigmatism.

Sleeve A movable part on the retinoscope that controls the orientation and vergence (focus) of the projected slit beam.

Streak retinoscope A type of retinoscope in common use that projects a streak of light into the eye, facilitating measurement of astigmatism as well as axial refractive errors.

Working distance The distance from the retinoscope to the patient's eye, as chosen by the examiner—often 0.66 m (66 cm).

Working lens A spherical plus lens with dioptric power equal to the reciprocal of the working distance in meters that may be placed in front of the patient's eye during retinoscopy, for example, +1.50 D lens for a working distance of 66 cm.

The Role of Retinoscopy

The retinoscope is a simple, handheld optical instrument that allows for objective measurement of refractive errors. Although it has been supplanted in many clinics by computerized automated refracting instruments, it remains an essential tool in many situations.

Perhaps its most important use is in pediatric ophthalmology, when refractive errors must be measured even in patients who will not still in front of automated instruments or fixate on projected targets on request. It is also essential for refraction of patients under general anesthesia. Retinoscopy is valuable in adult practice as well: the ophthalmologist can use it to quickly determine a starting point for subjective refraction, detect vision-limiting opacities in the optical pathway, and refract patients who are nonverbal or do not speak the same language as the examiner.

In addition, the retinoscope has a unique ability to detect the optical effects of irregularities of the cornea and lens that are not otherwise evident. It can also be used to quickly check existing glasses or to identify a change in the refraction after cycloplegia in patients suspected of latent hyperopia.

Types of Retinoscopes

Retinoscopes are frequently found in well-equipped examination lanes, often placed in charging wells along with a direct ophthalmoscope and a transilluminator (it is a good habit to keep your retinoscope in its charging well between uses). Most clinics have instruments similar to those pioneered by Welch-Allyn, featuring a small, fixed pointlike light source, with a rotating slit aperture and a movable lens controlled by a sleeve. With these instruments, most retinoscopy is done with the sleeve in the fully *lowered* position. There is usually enough friction in the mechanism to prevent the sleeve from automatically dropping to the lowered position—you must purposely ensure that it is fully lowered.

You might occasionally encounter an alternative design pioneered by Jack Copeland, the inventor of the modern streak retinoscope, although these are no longer being manufactured. With Copeland scopes, most retinoscopy is done with the sleeve in the fully *elevated* position. In many cases, there is a weak spring and a slight click to encourage keeping the sleeve maximally elevated, but it is always a good idea to check before starting to examine a patient.

Fundamental Concepts

In the simplest terms, retinoscopy is a process that allows an examiner to assess the refractive state of an eye by determining the sphere power (and cylinder, as appropriate) of the lens (or lenses) needed to correct any refractive error present. This is accomplished by watching the motion of an image of the retinoscope light source as lenses are changed in front of the eye. The process is continued, with addition and subtraction of lens power, until the image is stationary, indicating that the refractive error has been *neutralized.*

The basic idea behind the retinoscope can be demonstrated—even without the retinoscope—by using loose lenses from a trial set *(hand neutralization).* Explore this concept in Try It Yourself! Q-5.

Try It Yourself! Q-5

Hand Neutralization of Spherical and Cylindrical Lenses

Take a +1.00 D and a −1.00 D spherical lens from a trial set. Hold the +1.00 lens in front of your eye, and sight through it to view a distant object. Move the lens slowly up and down in front of your eye and note that the image of the distant object appears to move in the *opposite* direction from the motion of the lens: when the lens moves upward, the image appears to move downward, and vice versa.

Next, sight the same object through the −1.00 D lens, move the lens up and down, and note that the image appears to move in the *same* direction that you move the lens. It is thus possible to determine the sign of an unknown lens. Now view the distant object through the combination of the +1.00 and −1.00 lenses held adjacent to each other; as you move the combined lenses, the image of the distant object will remain stationary.

In a similar fashion, one can determine the power of any unknown spherical lens—it is simply equal in power and opposite in sign to whichever lens from your trial set cancels the motion of a distant object as seen through the two lenses held together and moved up and down.

One can hand-neutralize cylindrical lenses as well. Rotate a 2.00 D cylindrical lens in front of your eye, and observe a distant vertical object, such as a doorframe or bookcase. The vertical feature will rotate clockwise and counterclockwise compared with true vertical. Observe that when the axis of your trial lens is itself accurately vertical, the distant vertical feature also appears straight up-and-down. Now place a trial cylindrical lens of equal and *opposite* power adjacent to the first lens, with axes accurately aligned. Rotating this combination of lenses together will show no skewing of the distant target, confirming neutralization of the original cylinder. Note that one can also neutralize the rotation by placing a cylindrical lens of the *same* sign and power as the original, but oriented with axis *90° away*.

In the case of retinoscopy, we project a moving luminous object (the *streak*) onto the retina and interpret the apparent motion of this object as it is projected back out through the optics of the eye, as viewed through a small aperture (the peephole of the retinoscope). If the emerging light rays converge on the peephole, there is no apparent motion of the streak image (a *neutral* retinoscopic reflex); the pupil appears to fill uniformly with light, which flashes on or off as the streak moves across the pupil.

If the eye has a net hyperopic refractive error (relative to the location of the peephole), the emerging rays will cross *behind* the retinoscope (that is, farther from the eye), and the observer will see the streak image within the pupil move in the *same* direction as the motion of the source (*with* motion). Conversely, if the eye has a net myopic refractive error (relative to the location of the peephole), the emerging rays will cross *between* the eye and the retinoscope, and the observer will see the streak image within the pupil move in the direction *opposite* to the motion of the source (*against* motion). See Chapter 4 for further details.

Preliminaries for Retinoscopy

Retinoscopy is most easily performed when the patient's pupils are mid-dilated. A dim room is preferred, with a distant fixation target. In infants and the elderly, pupils are physiologically constricted, but they are usually adequate for retinoscopy in patients between the ages of 10 and 60 years or so. Retinoscopy in infants should routinely be performed under cycloplegia; in older adults, cycloplegia is optional. Cycloplegia may also be helpful when fixation is unsteady, leading to variable retinoscopy findings, and in cases of potential latent hyperopia, such as young patients with asthenopic complaints, premature presbyopia, or possible accommodative spasm.

The examiner should sit facing the patient, at eye level. As with direct ophthalmoscopy, the examiner's right eye should be used to examine the patient's right eye, with the instrument held in the right hand, and vice versa ("right-right-right; left-left-left"). This will allow the patient to sight the distant target with the fellow eye, allowing better control of accommodation, without the examiner's head getting in the way.

If the patient's eye is emmetropic, it will project an image of the fovea to optical infinity; thus, for practical purposes, it is necessary to correct for a finite working distance between the examiner and the patient. A working distance of 0.66 m (66 cm) is often convenient. In this case, a working lens of +1.50 D is placed in front of the patient's eye, in addition to any correcting lenses, to bring the fovea conjugate to the peephole of the retinoscope. Those with shorter arms may wish to work closer to the patient. In any case, the working lens (in diopters) should be the reciprocal of the working distance in meters (eg, +2.00 D for a working distance of 50 cm).

If a specific working lens is used, it can simply be removed from the stack of correcting lenses that neutralize the retinoscopic reflex, with the remaining lenses representing the estimated refractive correction. This is particularly convenient with the phoropter, which contains a +1.50 D lens in the accessory lens wheel (labeled "R") for this purpose. (Just remember to revert to the open position on the accessory dial ["0"] upon completion of the retinoscopy.) Alternatively, you can ignore the correction for the working distance during the retinoscopy and then algebraically subtract the dioptric equivalent of the working distance (eg, +1.50 for a working distance of 66 cm) from the apparent result (the *gross retinoscopy*) to obtain the *net retinoscopy,* which will represent the estimated correction.

Video Q-2 demonstrates the retinoscopy technique.

VIDEO Q-2 Retinoscopy: basics.
Courtesy of Thomas F. Mauger, MD.

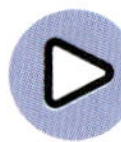

Basic Retinoscope Operation

Set the retinoscope sleeve as appropriate for your instrument (sleeve down for Welch-Allyn type scopes, sleeve up for Copeland scopes). If desired, place the appropriate working lens in front of the patient's eye to correct for the working distance. As usual, start with the right eye. Place the instrument in front of your right eye—you may rest it lightly against your brow or your eyeglasses. Aim the streak at the patient's eye and align it carefully so as to illuminate the pupil. (This is trickier at first than it sounds.)

Whatever orientation you find the streak, *always* move it back and forth across the pupil in a direction *perpendicular* to the orientation of the streak. (If the streak is horizontal, move it up and down across the pupil; if vertical, move side to side.) Compare the direction of motion of the streak as seen within the pupil with the direction of motion of the streak as projected onto the eye.

With *motion: hyperopic refractive errors*

If the streak image within the pupil tracks in the same direction as the motion of the streak projected onto the eye, this is referred to as *with* motion—the streak image moves with the projected streak. This indicates a hyperopic refractive state. Neutralize this refractive error by inserting additional plus lens power in front of the patient's eye. Eventually, the streak image in the pupil will become wider and wider until it entirely fills the pupil, and no motion is seen. This is called the *neutral reflex,* which indicates that the lenses now in front of the eye correct the refractive error.

Against *motion: myopic refractive errors*

If the streak image within the pupil moves in the opposite direction from the motion of the streak projected onto the eye, this is referred to as *against* motion—the streak image moves against the projected streak. This indicates a myopic refractive state. Neutralize this refractive error by inserting additional minus lens power in front of the patient's eye. As in the hyperopic eye, the streak image will eventually stop moving and fill the entire pupil; the neutral reflex shows that the myopia has been corrected.

Note that the *against* reflex is not precisely comparable to the *with* reflex. The *with* reflex is seen as a stripe or bar within the pupil, moving in parallel with the streak projected on the eye (Fig Q-32A). The *against* reflex begins as a pupil completely filled with light, which "empties" in the direction *opposite* to the direction of the motion of the projected streak. Thus, if the streak projected onto the eye is vertical and is moved from the left of the eye toward the right, the pupil will initially appear filled with light, and then a dark band will appear beginning at the *right* of the pupil, and gradually enlarge toward the left, until the pupil is completely dark (Fig Q-32B). Gain experience observing these reflexes using a commercial retinoscopy "practice eye" (Fig Q-33), or make one using the instructions in Try It Yourself! Q-6.

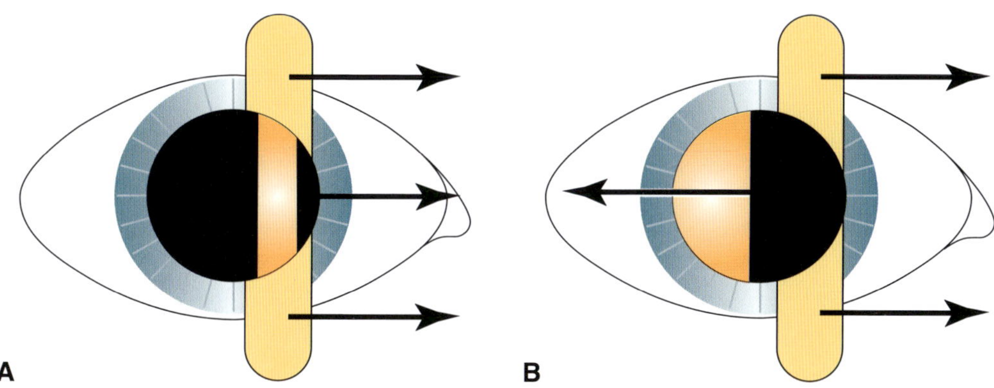

Figure Q-32 Retinoscopy streak and retinal reflex. **A,** *With* motion. **B,** *Against* motion. *(Illustration by C. H. Wooley.)*

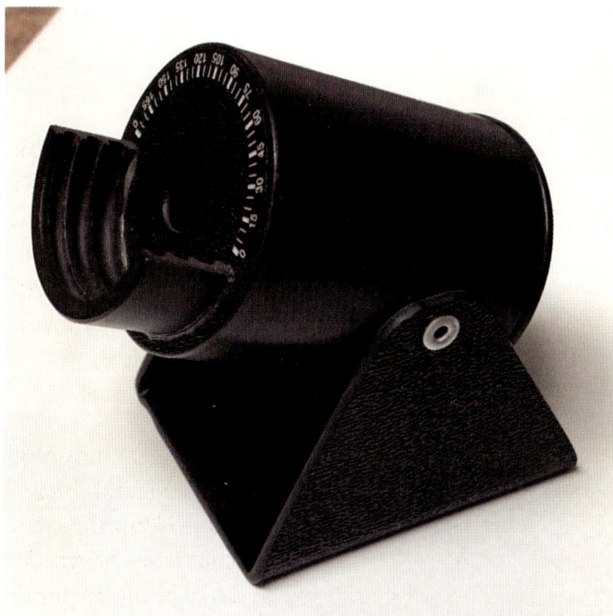

Figure Q-33 Commercial model eye for retinoscopy practice. *(Courtesy of Thomas F. Mauger, MD.)*

Try It Yourself! Q-6

Making a Practice Eye

Start with an empty 35-mm film canister (about 5.5 cm in length) or a small plastic cylindrical medication vial (about 7 cm in length). Tape a yellow or orange circle of paper to cover the bottom of the inside of the container and occlude the top of the container with an opaque cover with a central circular perforation 5–6 mm in diameter. Place a plus spherical trial lens of power equal to the reciprocal of the length of your cylinder (about +18.00 D for a film canister, about +14.00 D for a medication vial) in the small clip behind the aperture of one side of a phoropter, and tape the cylinder behind the trial lens, with the central perforation centered in the aperture of the phoropter (Fig Q-34).

Sit opposite the phoropter as you would in front of a patient and view the retinoscope streak image within the artificial pupil you have set up behind the phoropter. Adjust the spherical lens settings in the phoropter to view the with, against, and neutral reflexes in your simple model eye. Confirm that you can convert the neutral reflex to a readily appreciable *with* reflex by moving several inches closer to the phoropter than your usual working distance.

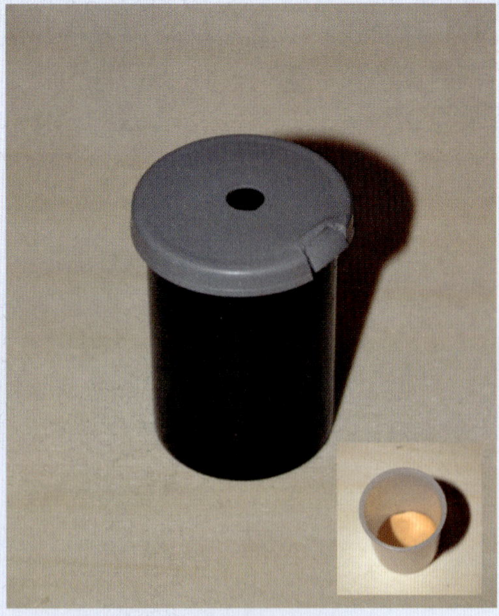

Figure Q-34 Film cannister modified for use as a model eye for retinoscopy practice. The hole punched in the lid should be about 5–6 mm in diameter; it is helpful to tape an orange disk of paper at the bottom of the canister *(inset)* to create more realistic reflexes. *(Courtesy of Scott E. Brodie, MD, PhD.)*

Pseudoneutral reflex in high myopia

In patients with very high myopia, the retinoscopic reflex will initially appear very dull and motionless. This *pseudoneutral reflex* should not be confused with the neutral reflex seen in emmetropia—it does not convert to *with* upon moving a few inches closer to the patient.

If a pseudoneutral reflex is observed, move the sleeve of the retinoscope to the opposite of the usual position (fully elevated with Welch-Allyn type scopes, fully lowered with Copeland scopes). This will reverse all the retinoscopic reflexes—in particular, the unrecognizable *against* of highly myopic patients will be converted to a readily appreciable *with* reflex. In this case, add sufficient *minus sphere* lens power to convert the reflex, with the sleeve reversed, to a readily apparent *with* reflex. Return the sleeve to its usual position and note that the reflex will likewise revert to a clear *against* reflex. Continue to add minus sphere power until the reflex is converted to *with*, and then back off from this overcorrection to finally approach neutrality from the *with* direction, as with typical myopic refractive errors. This situation is discussed in more detail in Chapter 4, and in Video Q-3.

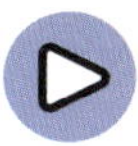

VIDEO Q-3 Retinoscopy: pseudoneutralization.
Courtesy of Thomas F. Mauger, MD.

Detection of astigmatism

If the patient's eye has only spherical refractive errors, the retinoscopic reflexes will be comparable in appearance and in apparent motion regardless of the orientation of the retinoscope streak projected onto the eye. However, if astigmatism is present, this symmetry is broken, allowing the detection of the astigmatic refractive error. Following are 3 indicators of the presence of astigmatism:

- *Blur.* This is a variation in the sharpness of the streak image within the pupil with a change in the orientation of the streak. The difference is most pronounced between the 2 (perpendicular) principal meridians of the eye (Fig Q-35).

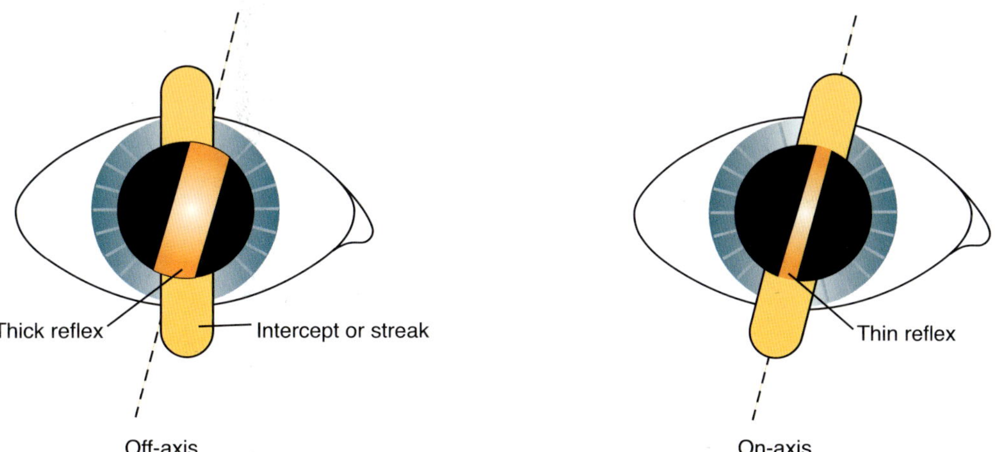

Figure Q-35 "Blur." The retinal reflex is thick and blurred when off-axis *(left)* compared with when on-axis *(right)* to the retinoscopy streak. *(Illustration by C. H. Wooley.)*

- *Break.* This is a visible discontinuity of the streak as it crosses the pupillary border. This discontinuity is apparent only when the streak is *not* aligned with one of the principal meridians (Fig Q-36).
- *Skew.* This is a dynamic version of the misalignment between the streak image within the pupil and the projected streak on the eye, appreciated as a disparity in the *direction of motion* between the streak image and the projected streak. As with break, skew is apparent only when the streak is *not* aligned with a principal meridian of the eye. The skew phenomenon may be more readily apparent than break in eyes with a modest degree of astigmatism (Fig Q-37).

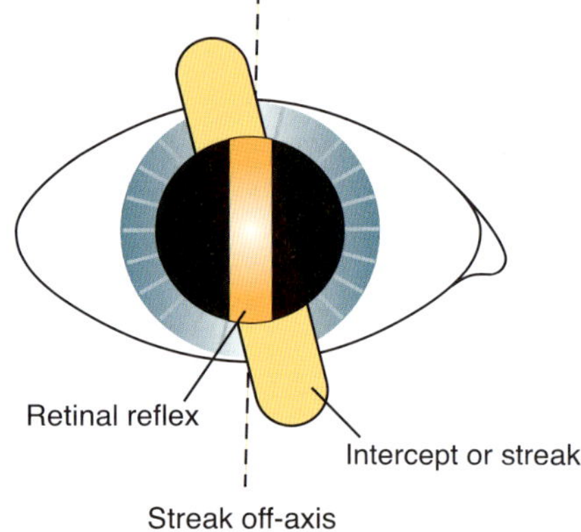

Figure Q-36 "Break." The retinal reflex is not aligned with the retinoscopy streak when the streak is not aligned with 1 of the 2 major axes. *(Illustration by C. H. Wooley.)*

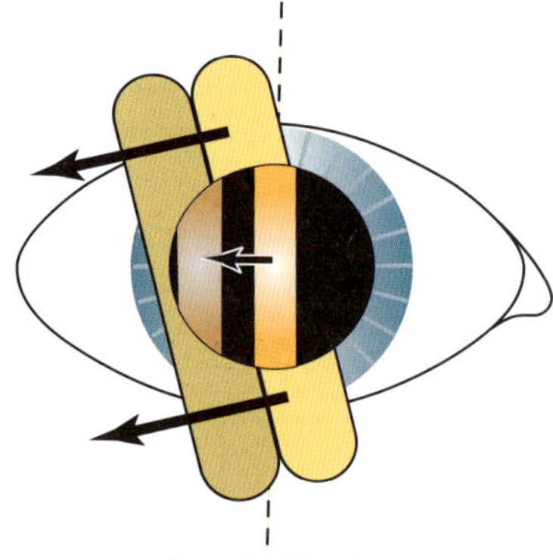

Figure Q-37 "Skew." Disparity in the direction of movement between the streak and the reflex when the streak is not aligned with a major axis. *(Illustration by C. H. Wooley.)*

Try It Yourself! Q-7

Detection of Astigmatism

- Set up a practice model eye as in Try It Yourself! Q-6. Adjust the sphere power to obtain a neutral reflex, and then dial in an additional –1.50 D of sphere power to make your model eye mildly hyperopic. Observe the resulting *with* reflex in all meridians by rotating the sleeve of the retinoscope as you move the streak, always perpendicular to its current orientation. The reflexes should appear the same in all meridians.

- Use the cylinder adjustment of the phoropter to dial in +1.00 or −1.00 D of cylinder power, whichever kind of cylinders are provided in your phoropter, with cylinder axis horizontal. Examine the various meridians by rotating the streak as above. Note that the clearest, brightest streak image is seen in either the horizontal or the vertical meridian, with the broadest, least clear streak image 90° away from the clearest meridian. These are the principal meridians of the astigmatic error you have just introduced. This disparity in streak image quality is the blur phenomenon, indicating the presence of the astigmatism.
- Next, turn the streak about 20° away from the meridian with the clearest, brightest streak. Note the break and skew phenomena as you move the streak, perpendicular to its own length, in this orientation.
- When you can readily perceive the blur, break, and skew induced by the 1.00 D cylinder, reduce the cylinder strength to 0.50 D. Examine the reflexes in all meridians as above. With care, you should be able to appreciate the subtler indications of blur, break, and skew for this degree of astigmatism as well.
- Try it again with a 0.25 D cylinder. Don't be discouraged if you are unable to detect this very minor degree of astigmatism. (A disparity of 0.25 D in a cylindrical correction is rarely of clinical significance.)

Activity Q-1 makes use of an online retinoscopy simulator.

ACTIVITY Q-1 Retinoscopy simulator.
Courtesy of Faruk H. Örge, MD, and K. David Epley, MD.

Putting It All Together

1. Dim the lights in the refracting lane, and direct the patient's attention to a distant fixation target.
2. If desired, place a working lens in front of the right eye. If convenient, use the +1.50 D "R" lens in the phoropter accessory wheel. You may wish to fog the fellow eye with the +1.50 D "R" lens as well.
3. If using handheld trial lenses (as with infants and small children), it may be preferable to omit the working lens and correct for the working distance algebraically. This reduces the number of lenses that must be held simultaneously in front of the patient's eye, as well as the number of distracting reflections.
4. With the retinoscope sleeve down (for Welch-Allyn type scopes) or up (for Copeland scopes), examine the retinoscopic reflexes in all meridians by rotating the sleeve.

5. If reflexes are the same in all meridians, with no apparent blur, break, or skew, assume that there is no astigmatism.
   a. If all reflexes are *with*, slowly add plus sphere or reduce the minus sphere to approach the neutral reflex from the *with* direction.
   b. If all reflexes are *against*, add sufficient minus sphere to convert the *against* reflexes to *with* reflexes, and then proceed as in step 5a, above.
   c. Confirm neutrality by moving several inches closer to the patient, converting the neutral reflex back to *with*.
   d. Skip ahead to step 7.
6. If the reflexes are dissimilar, perhaps *with* in some meridians and neutral or *against* in others—or if you see blur, break, or skew—assume that astigmatism is present.
   a. If necessary, add sufficient minus sphere to convert all reflexes to a readily recognizable *with*.
   b. Identify the meridian where the reflex is clearest, narrowest, and brightest. We will refer to this as the *strong* meridian. The break and skew phenomena will not be visible along the strong meridian.
   c. Rotate the streak 90° away from the strong meridian, revealing a dimmer, broader *with* reflex along the *weak* meridian.
   d. Neutralize the weak meridian with *plus sphere* lens power.
   e. Rotate the streak 90° to coincide once again with the strong meridian. The *with* reflex will be less clear and bright than that originally apparent in step 6b above, as it has been partially neutralized by the plus sphere applied in step 6d.
   f. If *plus cylinder* lenses are available, align the axis of the cylinder battery with the strong meridian (currently indicated by the orientation of the retinoscope streak), and neutralize the remaining *with* reflex by gradually increasing the *plus cylinder lens power*.

      If only *minus cylinder* lenses are available (for example, if you are working with a minus cylinder phoropter), align the cylinder battery *perpendicular* to the strong meridian. Neutralize the remaining *with* reflex by gradually increasing *plus sphere lens power*—and compensating by adding 0.25 D of *minus cylinder power* for each 0.25 D increase in *plus sphere power*. This sequence allows you to approach neutrality from the *with* direction when only minus cylinders are available.
   g. Verify the neutral reflex in all meridians.
7. Correct for the working distance by removing the working lens or by algebraically subtracting the reciprocal of the working distance in meters from the total of the lenses selected in steps 5 or 6, above. What remains is the retinoscopic estimate of the refractive error for the right eye.
8. Repeat steps 2 through 7 for the left eye.

A complete retinoscopy using plus cylinder is demonstrated in Video Q-4.

VIDEO Q-4 Retinoscopy plus cylinder technique: full tutorial with phoropter.
Courtesy of David Guyton, MD.

It is frequently asked whether one can simply neutralize the strong and weak meridian separately using only spherical lenses. While this is possible, the technique outlined above is preferred for 2 reasons: (1) Neutralizing both meridians with spheres requires a subsequent additional calculation step to convert the power-cross information into spherocylindrical notation to proceed with subjective refinement or to write the spectacle prescription. It is easy to mix up the axis that goes with the cylinder. (2) Working with cylindrical lenses allows use of the technique of *straddling* to refine the estimate of the cylinder axis (see Chapter 4 for details). Straddling is not possible with spherical lenses alone.

The retinoscopic refractive results can be used directly for prescribing glasses if no other refractive information is available or as a starting point for subjective cross-cylinder refinement as described in Part 2 of the Quick-Start Guide. If you are working with a phoropter, the retinoscopy results will be in place automatically at the completion of the retinoscopy, once the "R" working lens is removed, and you will be ready to begin cross-cylinder refinement.

Subjective Retinoscopy Findings

In addition to its use in objective measurement of refractive errors, the retinoscope is a valuable tool in assessing the optical quality of the eye. It will instantly identify patients with media opacities (including cataract and vitreous hemorrhage), thereby averting a fruitless attempt at subjective refraction. In patients with dilated pupils, the retinoscope can dramatically illustrate the optical degradation caused by cortical, nuclear, or posterior subcapsular lens opacities, which are seen clearly in silhouette against the red reflex of the fundus—more clearly than with other optical instruments. (In particular, the indirect ophthalmoscope is particularly unsuitable for this evaluation, as it creates a virtual pinhole effect that minimizes the impact of the optical imperfections.)

The retinoscope is also an excellent way to appreciate the optical effects of subtler irregularities in the optics of the eye, such as irregular astigmatism, keratoconus, and central lens densities (such as "oil-droplet" cataracts) and anterior or posterior lenticonus, which may not otherwise be visualized at all. (See Chapter 4 for details.)

Final Remarks

Retinoscopy is a novel skill for beginning ophthalmologists. As with the stethoscope, developing your facility with the instrument and your ability to interpret the findings comes only with practice. The time you spend at the beginning of training acquiring the skill of retinoscopy will be paid back many times over during the rest of your training and throughout your entire career.

- Many residents put off learning retinoscopy until they begin their rotations in pediatric ophthalmology, where retinoscopy is an essential skill and can no longer be avoided. This is an unfortunate strategy—it is far better to arrive for your pediatric rotation as a skilled retinoscopist, ready to proceed efficiently and with confidence.
- After experiencing the various reflexes with a model eye, as described in the Try it Yourself! exercises above, it is helpful to begin practicing on your fellow residents

before you start working with actual patients. You can slip trial lenses into the clip behind the phoropter to simulate refractive errors.

- Try to take at least a quick look at the retinoscopic reflexes of every patient you examine. Even just noting media opacities and irregular optics will steer the remainder of the clinical encounter more productively than simply forging ahead with subjective refraction or other examinations.
- Purchasing your own retinoscope is a sound investment in your future. It may become an essential tool, for example, if you find yourself practicing in an outlying location such as a nursing home or satellite clinic, or if you undertake an eye care mission far from your training program. Used retinoscopes are frequently available on the Internet at a very modest cost.

CHAPTER 1

Geometric Optics

This chapter includes related videos. Go to www.aao.org/bcscvideo_section03 or scan the QR code in the text to access this content.

Highlights

- According to the *theory of geometric optics,* light rays traveling in a straight line can undergo refraction, reflection, or both when they encounter an object, such as a lens or mirror.
- Snell's law of refraction relates to the angle of incidence, the angle of refraction, and the refractive indices of the media through which the light rays travel.
- Light rays passing through a prism undergo refraction toward the *base* of the prism; for an observer, the image will appear to be shifted toward the *apex* of the prism.
- For any given source object, the *vergence equation* can be used to determine the location, orientation, size, and type (real or virtual) of the corresponding image. The *lensmaker's equation* can be used to determine the power of a lens and how the lens power is affected by a change in media (ie, change in index of refraction).
- Ray tracing can be used to visualize light rays as they pass through a lens (or mirror) system.
- According to the *wavefront theory of light,* light travels in waves and undergoes optical aberrations as it passes through a surface such as the cornea or crystalline lens. The most significant wavefront aberrations for clinical or surgical practice are spherical aberration, coma, and trefoil.

Glossary

Aberration Any deviation of an optical system from stigmatic imaging.

Angle of incidence The angle between a ray incident to a mirror and the surface normal at the point of incidence.

Angle of reflection The angle between a ray reflected off a mirror and the surface normal at the point of incidence.

Astigmatism The disparity in focal length for rays from a single object point that are incident at different meridians of the lens.

Axial magnification The ratio of the axial extent (depth) of the image of an extended source object to the depth of the object, as measured along the optic axis.

Chromatic aberration A variation in the power of a lens system with the wavelength of incident light.

Coma A disparity in focal length for rays from a single off-axis object point that are refracted at different distances from the center of the lens.

Conjugate points Points that share an object–image relationship.

Conoid of Sturm A geometric figure traced by the refraction of a single point source object by an astigmatic lens.

Critical angle The angle at which a light ray passing from one medium to another with a lower refractive index undergoes total internal reflection.

Curvature of field A disparity in focal length for objects at different distances from the optic axis.

Defocus An aberration corresponding to an axial refractive error, that is, a disparity between the power and the axial length of the eye.

Depth of field The range of locations of a source object for which an optical system forms acceptably sharp images.

Depth of focus The range of image locations over which an optical system forms acceptably sharp images of a fixed source object.

Distortion A disparity in transverse magnification for objects at different distances from the optic axis.

Effectivity of lenses The adjustment in the power of a lens necessary to compensate for changes in the distance between the lens and the desired image location.

Fermat's principle Among alternative paths between 2 points, light rays will travel along the path with the shortest total travel time.

Galilean telescope A telescope with a convex objective lens and a concave ocular lens.

Gaussian optics An efficient mathematical treatment for the paraxial optical regime by means of linear algebra.

Geometric optics Optical phenomena that are effectively described in terms of light rays that travel along straight lines unless deviated by lenses or mirrors.

Jackson cross cylinder A lens superimposing cylindrical lenses of equal and opposite power, placed with axes perpendicular to each other.

Keplerian (or astronomical) telescope A telescope with convex objective and ocular lenses.

Law of reflection The statement that the angle of incidence equals the angle of reflection.

Lensmaker's equation A mathematical formula for the power of a curved refracting surface.

Nodal points The conjugate points on the optic axis through which incident and exiting light rays form equal angles with the optic axis.

Paraxial (or paraxial ray) The optical regime in which light rays travel close to the optic axis and form only small angles with the optic axis. Rays conforming to this description are termed *paraxial rays.*

Point spread function The distribution of light from a point source in the image plane, which characterizes the aberration of an optical system.

Power cross A graphical depiction of the action of a toric lens, showing the orientation of the principal axes and the power along each axis.

Power-versus-meridian graph A graph showing the power of an astigmatic lens at each meridian.

Prentice position An orientation for an ophthalmic prism such that incoming or exiting light rays strike 1 of the prism surfaces perpendicularly.

Principal plane One of 2 planes at which the refraction of a general lens system appears to take place.

Principal point The intersection of either principal plane with the optic axis.

Prism diopter (Δ) A unit describing the deflection of light by an ophthalmic prism equal to 100 times the tangent of the angle of deflection.

Ray tracing The graphical localization of images by drawing rays of light from the source object through the focal points and nodal points of an optical system.

Real image An image formed by the actual convergence of light rays.

Real object An object that serves as the source of light rays in an optical system.

Reduced optical system A simplified optical system equivalent to a general multielement optical system characterized by the power and the locations of the principal planes and the nodal points.

Reduced vergence The product of object or image vergence and the refractive index of the medium through which the light travels.

Reference sphere The hypothetical spherical wavefront surface that corresponds to a perfect point image.

Refractive index The ratio of the speed of light in a vacuum to the speed of light in a material medium.

Seidel aberrations A series of common aberrations of simple optical systems, such as spherical aberration, coma, astigmatism, curvature of field, and distortion.

Snell's law A mathematical description of the deflection of light as it passes between media with different refractive indices.

Spherical aberration A disparity in focal length for rays from a single axial object point that are refracted at different distances from the center of a lens.

Spherical equivalent The power of a spherical lens equal to the average power of the principal meridians of an astigmatic lens.

Stigmatic imaging Imaging by a lens system that focuses the light from a point source at a single image point.

Surface normal The line perpendicular to a surface through a point of interest.

Thin-lens approximation An approximate treatment appropriate for thin lenses that ignores the spacing between the front and back lens surfaces.

Total internal reflection The reflection of a light beam directed from one medium with a higher refractive index to another with a lower refractive index when the angle of incidence exceeds the critical angle, and no emerging ray can satisfy Snell's law (ie, no refraction occurs).

Transverse magnification The ratio of the height of an image to the height of the source object, as measured perpendicular to the optic axis.

Vergence The reciprocal of the distance between a source object or image and a lens or mirror.

Vergence equation A mathematical relationship between object vergence, the power of a lens or mirror, and the resultant image vergence.

Virtual image An apparent image inferred as the source of a divergent bundle of light rays.

Virtual object An intermediate image formed by an optical system that serves as the apparent source of a bundle of light rays, which in turn is imaged by a subsequent optical element.

Wavefront A surface connecting the points of equal travel time for rays of light emerging from a single point source.

Zernike polynomials A standard mathematical system of polynomial functions used to describe the deviation of a wavefront from the reference sphere as a description of the aberration of an optical system.

Introduction

Geometric optics refers to those optical phenomena that are effectively described in terms of light rays, which travel along straight lines unless deviated by lenses or mirrors. Other phenomena such as diffraction, polarization, and interference, which illustrate the wave properties of light (ie, the wavefront theory of light), and fluorescence, phosphorescence, and amplification by stimulated emission (as in lasers), which illustrate quantum properties of light (quantum electrodynamics), are discussed in Chapter 2.

Geometric optics governs many facets of ophthalmic clinical practice (eg, contact lenses, prismatic correction of strabismus) and surgical practice (eg, intraocular lens [IOL] calculation formulas, ray tracings in dysphotopsias). The mastery of this subject is an important part of modern ophthalmology.

The basic principles of geometric optics can be summarized in 4 simple rules:

1. Light rays travel in straight lines through uniform media.
2. The paths of light rays can be altered only by *reflection* (when they encounter a smooth reflective surface such as a mirror) or by *refraction* (when they travel at different speeds from one medium to another), according to the law of reflection and Snell's law, respectively.
3. When light rays pass through more than 1 refractive surface, the image formed by each surface in turn becomes the source object for the action of the next refracting surface the rays encounter.
4. The paths of light rays are reversible.

The basic ideas of refraction with lenses were introduced in Part 1 of the Quick-Start Guide, in the section Imaging Nearby Objects: Vergence and the Vergence Equation. If you are not familiar with this material, it would be helpful to review that chapter now, before proceeding with the more detailed treatment that follows.

Refractive Index

The speed of light in a vacuum (299,792,458 m/s) is one of the fundamental constants of nature. The speed of light in air is essentially the same. It is convenient to refer to the speed of light in other materials by comparison to the speed of light in a vacuum: the ratio of the speed of light in a vacuum to the speed of light in another medium is referred to as the *refractive index* of the medium. We abbreviate the refractive index *(n)* as

$$n = \frac{\text{Speed of light in a vacuum}}{\text{Speed of light in a medium}}$$

and use subscripts to designate different media as appropriate. Because the speed of light in a vacuum is *always greater* than its speed in any material medium, the refractive index of any material medium is *always greater* than 1.0.

A material's chemical composition and, sometimes, other factors strongly influence its refractive index. For example, by incorporating small amounts of various additives, manufacturers can vary the refractive index of optical glass from less than 1.4 to more than 1.9. The refractive indices of various materials of interest are listed in Table 1-1. The refractive index values of air, water, and the cornea should be committed to memory.

Although it is occasionally critical to determine the refractive index to several decimal places, approximate values are sufficiently accurate for most clinical purposes. For

Table 1-1 Refractive Indices of Some Clinically Important Media[a]

Medium	Refractive Index	Refractive Index (Approximate)
Vacuum	1.00000 (exactly)	
Air at STP	1.000277	1.000
Water at 25°C	1.3325	1.33, or 4⁄3
Aqueous and vitreous humors	1.336	1.33, or 4⁄3
Cornea	1.376	1.37
PMMA	1.49	1.50, or 3⁄2
HEMA (monomer)	1.4505	1.45

Abbreviations: HEMA = hydroxyethyl methacrylate; PMMA = polymethyl methacrylate; STP = standard temperature and pressure.

[a] The approximate values are used in this text. The values may depend on conditions. For instance, the refractive index of water varies with temperature. The refractive index of HEMA polymer depends on its water content and differs somewhat from that of HEMA monomer.

example, the refractive index of the vitreous humor is 1.336, but the approximate value of 4⁄3 is much easier to remember and introduces negligible error.

Recently, the index of refraction of various ocular structures (eg, cornea, aqueous, crystalline lens) has garnered more attention for the purpose of biometry in IOL calculations. Historically, an assumed refractive index, determined by the given manufacturer, was used for measuring the eye's axial length by optical biometry devices. It has been suggested that a "sum of segments" axial length measurement, incorporating the measurement of each intraocular structure according to its specific refractive index, may yield more accurate measurements for the required IOL power.

Flat Refracting Surfaces: Snell's Law

The optics of a flat refracting interface, such as the surface of a still pool of water or a flat slab of glass, is easy to describe. As light passes from a medium with lower refractive index (greater speed of light) to a medium with higher refractive index (lesser speed of light), light rays *bend toward* the line perpendicular to the interface at the point of entry (the *surface normal,* or just the "normal line"), according to *Snell's law of refraction* (Fig 1-1):

$$n_1 \sin \theta_1 = n_2 \sin \theta_2$$

If light travels from a denser medium to a less dense medium, light rays bend *away* from the surface normal. This redirection of light at a flat interface produces an apparent object displacement, such as that seen when you look into a body of water (Fig 1-2) or that provided by an ophthalmic prism.

Prisms

You are probably already familiar with dispersing prisms that produce rainbows or spectra. Refractive index varies with the frequency (or wavelength) of light, a phenomenon known as *dispersion.* Light rays typically contain a mixture of frequencies; when a light ray

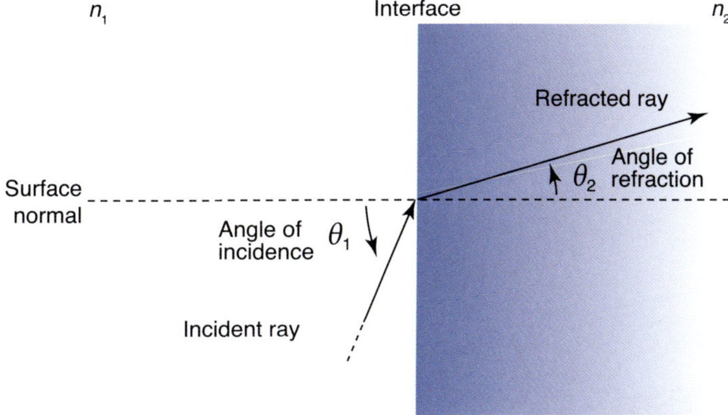

Figure 1-1 Snell's law. The angle of incidence θ_1 is defined by the incident ray and the surface normal *(dashed line).* The angle of refraction θ_2 is defined by the refracted ray and the surface normal. The 4 variables n_1, n_2, θ_1, and θ_2 are related by Snell's law: $n_1 \sin \theta_1 = n_2 \sin \theta_2$. When $n_1 < n_2$ (ie, the speed of light is reduced when rays cross the interface from left to right), the refracted ray bends toward the surface normal; when $n_1 > n_2$, the refracted ray bends away from the normal. *(Illustration developed by Edmond H. Thall, MD.)*

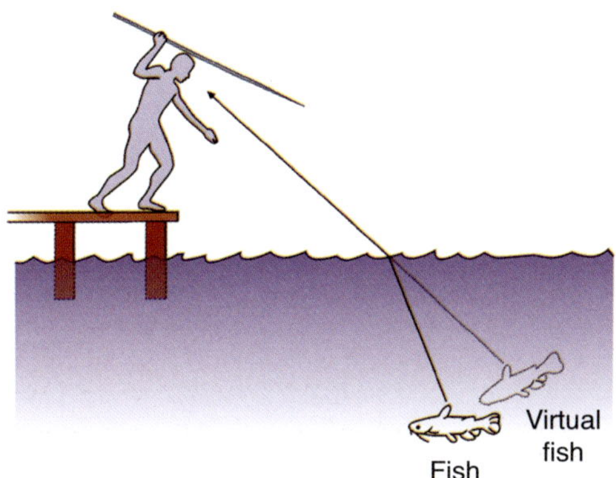

Figure 1-2 Image displacement. Light rays emanating from the fish will be bent *away* from the norm as they undergo refraction at surface normal (between the air and water) and pass from a medium of higher index of refraction (water) into a lower one (air). From the fisherman's point of view, the virtual image of the fish will be *behind* the fish. Thus, the fisherman must throw his spear *in front of* the virtual image that he sees (ie, to the left of the virtual fish in this 2-dimensional diagram). *(Illustration developed by Kevin M. Miller, MD, rendered by Jonathan Clark, and modified by Neal H. Atebara, MD.)*

traverses a dispersing prism, each frequency is deviated by a different amount, producing a spectrum of colors *(chromatic aberration).* Ophthalmic prisms help minimize the separation of colors by using materials that have nearly the same refractive index for all frequencies so that all the light is deviated by essentially the same amount.

When a light ray traverses a prism, the ray is deviated in accordance with Snell's law toward the base of the prism (Fig 1-3). For the observer on the other side of the prism, as we see with the example of the fisherman in Figure 1-2, the light ray will be *perceived* as coming from a point closer to the apex *(virtual image)* because the light ray bends toward the base. Understanding this concept will be useful when we discuss ray tracings with lenses. A convex (plus) lens can be thought of as simply 2 prisms matched base to base, and a concave (minus) lens as 2 prisms matched apex to apex. For both types of lenses, incoming light rays will be refracted toward the "base" of one of these prisms.

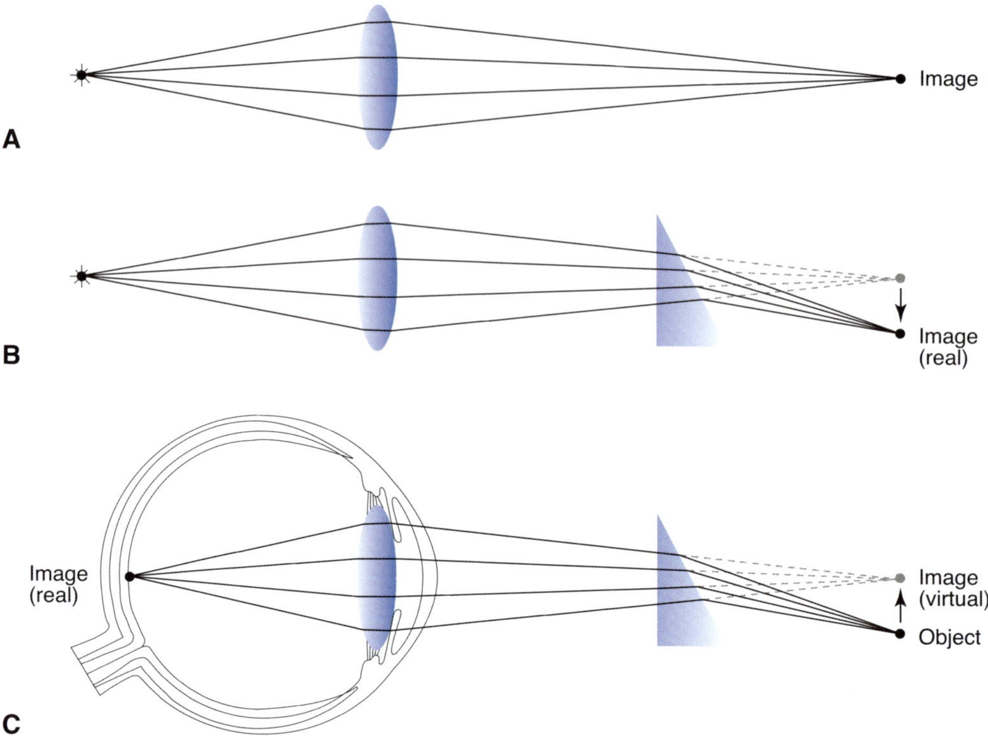

Figure 1-3 Effect of prisms on image position. **A,** Original real image formed by a lens. **B,** Base-down prism added. Because light passing through a prism is always refracted toward the prism's base, the original real image is also displaced toward the base, in this case, downward. **C,** By turning the light around, we see that a virtual image viewed through a prism is always shifted toward the apex of the prism. *(Reproduced from Guyton DL et al.* Ophthalmic Optics and Clinical Refraction. *Prism Press; 1999.)*

Any prism can produce a range of deviations, depending on the angle of the incoming light ray. The angle of deviation is least when light passes through the prism symmetrically (the *minimum deviation position*).

Prism Power

Prisms are labeled with a *prism power*—its strength, or amount of deviation produced as a light ray traverses the prism. That power is correct only if the prism is positioned in front of the patient in a manner consistent with its labeling. Glass prisms should be held in the *Prentice position,* in which light enters or leaves the prism perpendicular to 1 face of the prism (Fig 1-4A), and plastic prisms or plastic prism bars in the *minimum angle of deviation (MAD) position* (Fig 1-4B), as they are calibrated to be used in these positions. You can approximate the MAD position by holding the prism with its back surface perpendicular to the direction of the fixation object, which for distant objects corresponds to the frontal plane position (Fig 1-4C). Plastic prisms are more commonly used in clinical practice. Note that the Prentice position is not to be confused with the Prentice rule; the

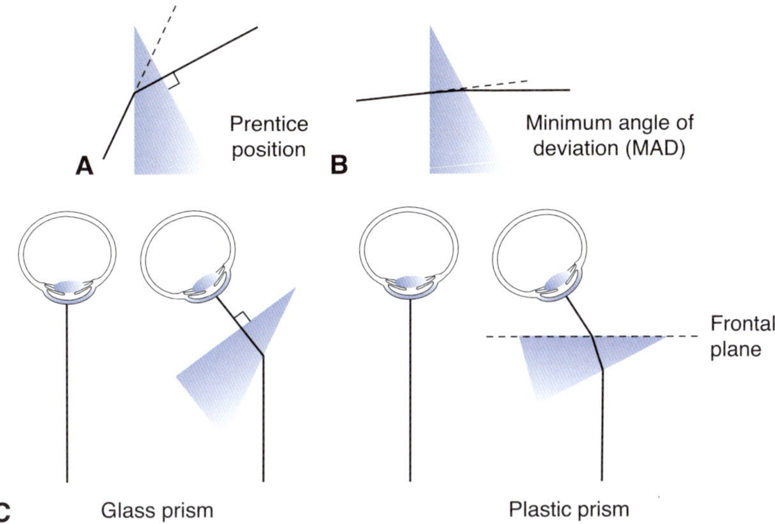

Figure 1-4 Positioning of prisms. **A,** Prentice position. The prism is held with its back surface perpendicular to the line of sight. This position is used for glass prisms. **B,** Minimum deviation position (minimum angle of deviation, MAD). The prism is held such that the line of sight makes an equal angle with 2 faces of the prism. **C,** *Left,* Glass prisms should be used in the Prentice position, perpendicular to the line of sight in the deviating eye. *Right,* Plastic prisms should be held in the frontal plane position. The prism is held with its rear surface in the frontal plane (perpendicular to the direction of the fixation object). This position approximates the minimum deviation position, which is difficult to estimate. *(Parts A and B are courtesy of Edmond H. Thall, MD; part C was developed by Edmond H. Thall, MD, and Kevin M. Miller, MD, and rendered by C. H. Wooley.)*

latter describes the amount of prismatic deviation experienced when looking away from the optical center of a lens (see Chapter 5, Eyeglasses).

The power of prisms combined with surfaces adjacent is *not* additive (Fig 1-5A). To verify this, look at the interface between 2 such combined prisms (Fig 1-5B). Notice, however, that the net effect of 2 prisms placed over the 2 eyes separately *is* additive. Thus, it is preferable to split the prisms between the 2 eyes when you measure large strabismic deviations.

The angular deviation produced by a prism is often measured not in degrees or radians but in prism diopters. A *prism diopter,* indicated by a delta symbol (Δ), is the number of centimeters of deviation undergone by a light ray when measured at 100 cm from the prism (Fig 1-6). This is equal to 100 times the tangent of the angle of deviation. Thus, a prism of strength 15Δ will deviate a light ray by 15 cm when measured at 1 m.

As mentioned previously, a prism deviates light toward its base (Fig 1-6). The orientation of a prism is designated by the position of its base: base up, base down, base in, or base out. A patient may have both a vertical and a horizontal deviation (eg, in cranial nerve [CN] IV palsy), in which case prism power adds as vectors. For instance, a 4Δ base-out prism combined with a 3Δ base-up prism in front of the right eye produces a net 5Δ base at the 143° meridian, base up and out. (Meridians are discussed in the Quick-Start Guide, in the section on Astigmatism.) Clinically, it is rarely necessary to be

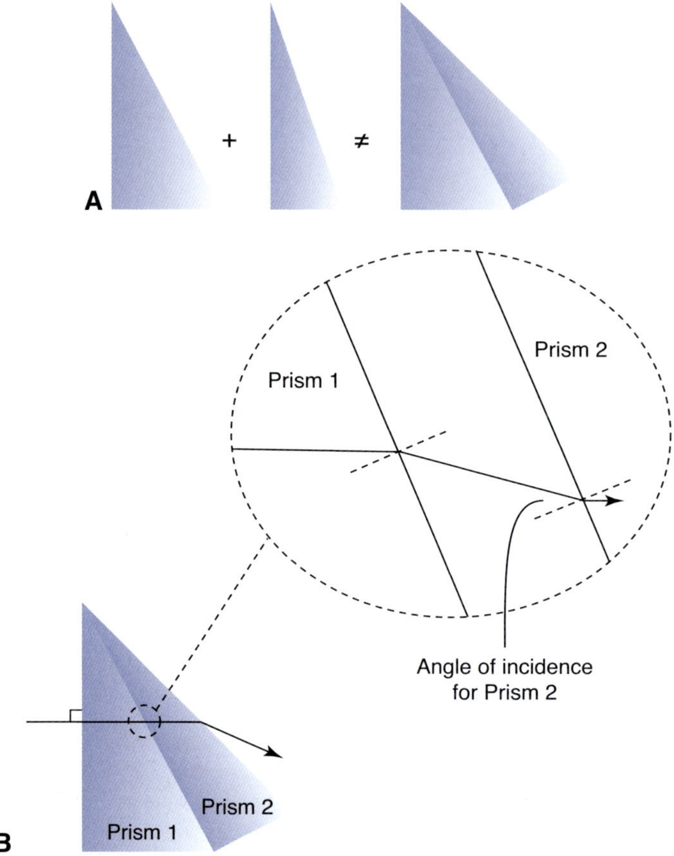

Figure 1-5 Prism power is not additive. **A,** The power of 2 prisms in contact is not equal to the sum of the powers of the individual prisms. The resulting deviation is much larger. Prisms should never be combined in this way. **B,** Look at the interface between 2 stacked glass prisms: with prism 1 in the Prentice position, the light ray is perpendicular to the first surface of prism 1; with prism 2 nowhere near the Prentice position, the light ray enters at an angle far from perpendicular. *(Part A developed by Edmond H. Thall, MD; part B from Irsch K. Optical issues in measuring strabismus.* Middle East African J Ophthalmol. *2015;22:265–270.)*

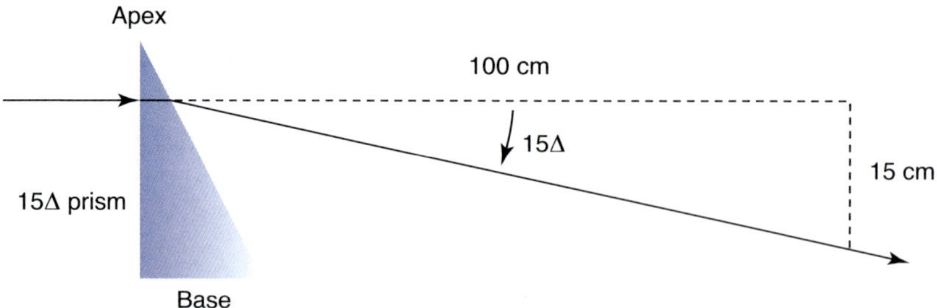

Figure 1-6 Definition of a prism diopter (Δ). One prism diopter is a deviation of 1 cm at a distance of 100 cm from a prism. This prism is a 15Δ prism, so light is deviated 15 cm toward the base, when measured 100 cm (1 m) away from the prism. *(Courtesy of Kristina Irsch, PhD.)*

concerned with this detail. You can prescribe the prism by specifying the individual base-up and base-down powers; the optician will perform the calculation. However, be aware that the lens will be ground with a single prism at an orientation that is neither base up nor base down.

EXAMPLE 1-1

Apply Snell's law to calculate the power of a prism (index of refraction, n = 1.5) in Prentice position (Fig 1-E1).

The prism is oriented such that the incident ray (A) is perpendicular to the first surface of the prism and parallel with the normal (N) of that surface. The ray (B) is not deviated by this surface and is transmitted to the second surface. The exiting ray is not perpendicular to this second surface or parallel with its normal (E). The ray is therefore deviated *away* from the normal because it is traveling from a medium of greater index of refraction ($n_1 = 1.5$) to air ($n_2 = 1.0$). The amount of the deviation is defined by Snell's law, $n_1 \sin \theta_1 = n_2 \sin \theta_2$.

We can use Snell's law to calculate the strength of the prism if we know the incident angle. For example, for a prism vertex angle θ_1 of 30°, Snell's law gives (1.5) (0.5) = (1.0) (sin θ_2), so sin θ_2 = 0.75, or θ_2 = 48.6°. Thus, the angle between the incoming ray and the deviated ray exiting the prism is $\theta_2 - \theta_1$ = 18.6°. Because tan (18.6) = 0.3365, the strength of the prism is 33.65Δ (recall that the strength of a prism is equal to 100 times the tangent of the angle of deviation).

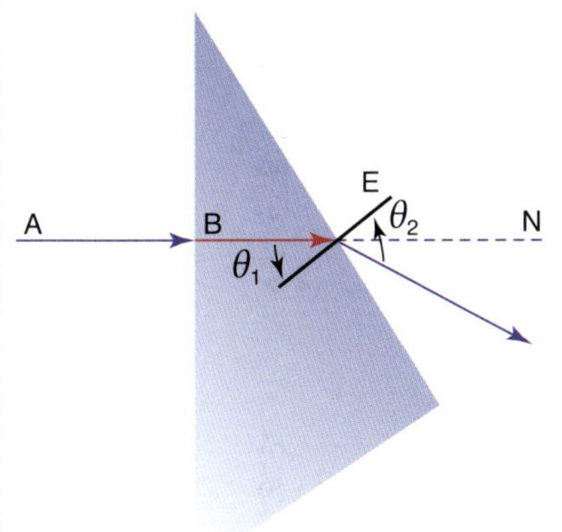

Figure 1-E1 Calculating the power of a prism in Prentice position.

Fresnel Prisms

The power of a prism is related to the angle formed by its sides, not its thickness. Nevertheless, when ground into a spectacle lens, a prism can make 1 edge of the lens quite thick. An alternative is a Fresnel prism (Fig 1-7), in which the angled surface is broken up into a series of much smaller prismatic surfaces at the same angle.

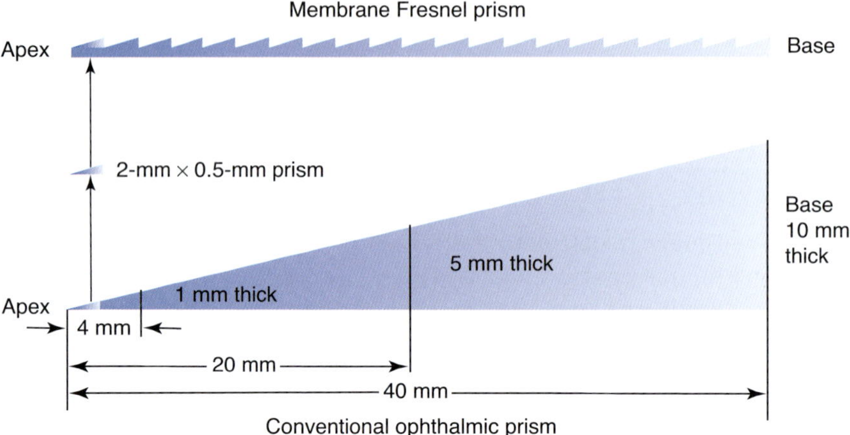

Figure 1-7 Fresnel prism versus conventional prism. A Fresnel prism is a collection of small prisms placed parallel to each other. Both prisms depicted here have the same power, but the Fresnel prism is thinner. *(Redrawn from William Tasman, ed.* Duane's Foundations of Clinical Ophthalmology. *1st edition. Lippincott Williams & Wilkins; 1993.)*

A Fresnel Press-On prism (3M), made of flexible plastic, can be applied to a spectacle lens with the base in any orientation. The optical quality of a press-on prism is not as good as that of a prism ground into a spectacle lens. However, a ground-in prism is expensive and increases the weight and thickness of the spectacle lens. Moreover, in many cases, a prism is required only temporarily, especially in adults (for example, when used on a trial basis in the office for the management of a non–pupil-involving CN III palsy), or its strength may need to be changed frequently. Fresnel Press-On prisms can be quite useful in these situations.

Disadvantages of Fresnel prisms include the potential to become smudged or dislodged from the spectacle lens and possible unsatisfactory cosmetic appearance. In addition, higher prism powers require thicker materials, which may further blur visual acuity, and chromatic aberration may reduce best-corrected visual acuity.

Reflection

Critical Angle and Total Internal Reflection

Most applications of Snell's law involve the refraction of light traveling from a less dense (lower n) medium, such as air, into a more dense (higher n) medium, such as water or glass. In this situation, as we have seen, the light bends *toward* the surface normal. If the direction of light transmission is reversed, the light will bend *away from* the surface normal as it enters the less dense medium (Fig 1-8A).

However, light rays can be reflected at the surface normal based on several factors, such as the incoming angle (angle of incidence). The *critical angle,* which varies depending on the given medium, refers to the angle at which Snell's law of refraction cannot be satisfied; the light remains in the optical interface (Fig 1-8B). If the angle of incidence exceeds the critical angle specified by the formula sin $\theta_{crit} = n_2/n_1$, given that no angle has a sine greater than 1.0, then the light ray will undergo reflection. Specifically, this is termed *total internal reflection (TIR)*—the light is totally reflected at the interface and cannot pass from the denser medium to the less dense medium (Fig 1-8C). For an interface between air and an aqueous tissue, the critical angle is about 48°. This prevents a view of the anterior chamber angle from the exterior of the eye without the use of optical devices, such as a goniolens (Fig 1-9).

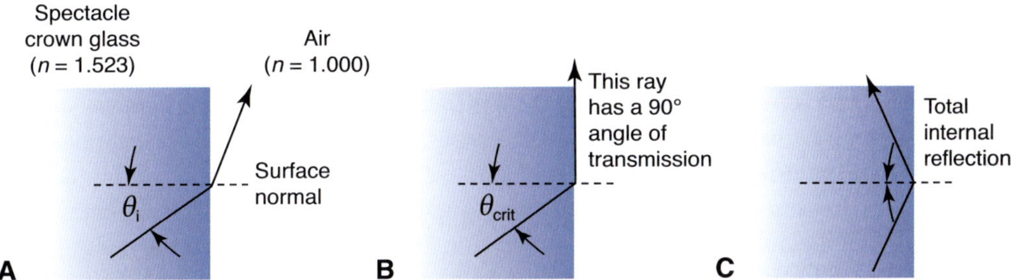

Figure 1-8 Total internal reflection. **A,** When light travels from one medium to a less dense (lower-*n*) medium, the rays bend away from the surface normal (refraction). **B,** At the critical angle, θ_{crit}, the refracted light ray undergoes neither pure refraction nor reflection; instead, it travels in the optical interface. **C,** Beyond the critical angle, all light is reflected by the interface. In A and B, light is also reflected by the interface (not shown). *(Illustration developed by Kevin M. Miller, MD, and rendered by C. H. Wooley.)*

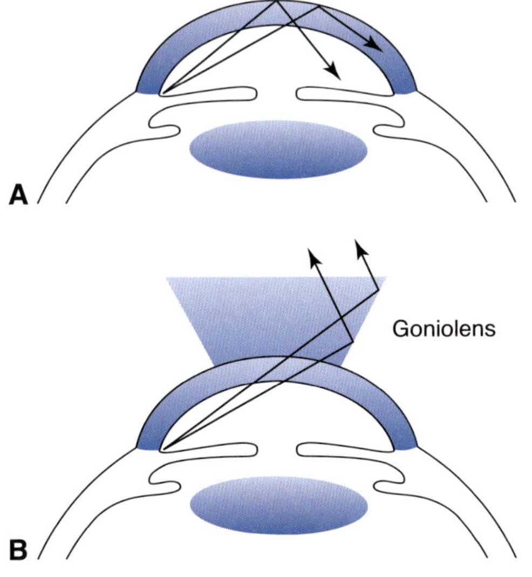

Figure 1-9 Total internal reflection at the cornea–air interface. **A,** Light from the anterior chamber angle undergoes total internal reflection (TIR) at the air–tear film interface. **B,** A goniolens placed in contact with the cornea prevents TIR and allows visualization of the angle structures. *(Illustration developed by Kevin M. Miller, MD, and rendered by C. H. Wooley.)*

Section Exercise 1-1

1.1 Compute the critical angle for the air–tear film interface. The formula for the critical angle is sin $\theta_{crit} = n_2/n_1$. For the air–tear film interface,

$$\sin\theta_{crit} = \frac{n_2}{n_1} = \frac{1.00}{1.33} = 0.75$$

so

$$\theta_{crit} = 48.75°.$$

Refraction by a Single Curved Surface

The next simplest refracting system (Fig 1-10) is that in which an incident light ray undergoes refraction by a single curved surface that separates 2 regions with different refractive indices. We will assume that the curved surface is perfectly symmetric and is oriented perpendicular to the general direction of the incoming light. An incident light ray emanating from a point on the optic axis undergoes refraction and is directed toward the image point, likewise located on the optic axis. For example, as noted in the Quick-Start Guide, for a source object infinitely far away, the image point will be located at the focal point of the lens at a distance equal to the reciprocal of the lens power. This construction of an object–lens system will be helpful for ray tracing and the vergence equation discussions that follow.

If we assume that the rays of light travel in close proximity to the optic axis and make only small angles with the optic axis (the *paraxial regime*), we may deduce the following 2 equations from Snell's Law, simple geometry, and the small-angle trigonometric approximations (for more detail, see Appendix 1-1):

$$\frac{n_1}{u} + P = \frac{n_2}{v} \quad \text{(vergence equation)}$$

$$P = \frac{(n_2 - n_1)}{r} \quad \text{(lensmaker's equation)}$$

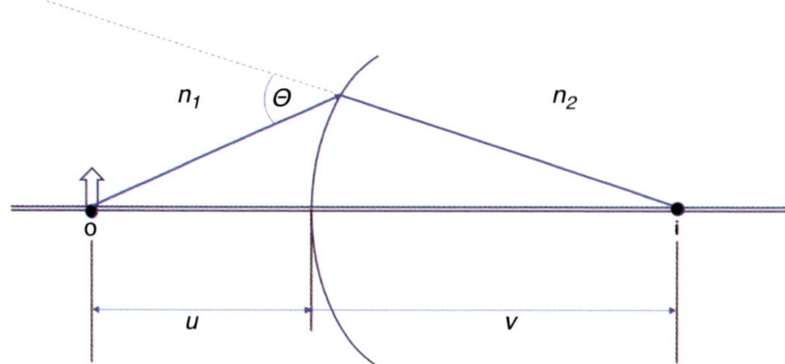

Figure 1-10 Refraction by a single curved surface. The incident ray emanating from an object (o) located at a given distance *(u)* undergoes refraction by a single curved surface (eg, a simple plus lens of negligible thickness). The refracted ray is directed toward an image point (i), which is located at a distance, *v*, along the optic axis. *(Courtesy of Kamran M. Riaz, MD.)*

Here, n_1 and n_2 are the refractive indices of the regions to the left and to the right, respectively, of the refracting interface; u is the (signed) distance from the source object point to the refracting interface; v is the (signed) distance from the refracting interface to the image of the source object point; and r is the (signed) radius of curvature of the refracting interface. The sign convention for u, v, and r is that distances to the left of the interface are taken as negative numbers; distances to the right of the interface are taken as positive numbers. Light is assumed to travel from left to right. The quantity P is referred to as the *power* of the refracting interface. Note that some texts may alternatively refer to P as D.

If either medium is air, the term n_1/u or n_2/v reduces to a simple reciprocal—$1/u$ or $1/v$, respectively—and is referred to as the *object vergence* or *image vergence.* If the refractive index of either medium is greater than 1.0, the quantity n_1/u or n_2/v is referred to as the *reduced vergence* (even though these quantities are larger than the simple reciprocals). In either case, the vergences (or reduced vergences) are frequently abbreviated as $n_1/u = U$ or $n_2/v = V$, and the vergence equation takes the simple form:

$$U + P = V$$

The unit of measure for both the vergences U and V and the refractive power P is reciprocal meters, which in this context is called the *diopter (D)*. In many cases, especially regarding the human eye, measurements must *always* be converted to units of meters for the purpose of the vergence equation, although typical distances are more conveniently measured in centimeters or millimeters. The distance equivalents of some common dioptric values are listed in Table 1-2.

This simple geometry, with a single curved refracting surface separating 2 regions of different refractive index, seldom arises in practice. An important exception involves the aphakic eye. Because such an eye has no lens, as a first approximation, we may ignore

Table 1-2 Some Common Dioptric Values and Their Distance Equivalents

Diopters	Distance	Approximate Distance
0.25	4 m	
0.50	2 m	
1.00	1 m	
1.25	80 cm	
1.50	⅔ m	66–67 cm
2.00	50 cm	
2.50	40 cm	
3.00	⅓ m	33–34 cm
4.00	25 cm	
5.00	20 cm	
6.00	⅙ m	16–17 cm
7.00	⅐ m	14.0–14.5 cm
8.00	12.5 cm	
9.00	⅑ m	11.0–11.5 cm
10.00	10 cm	

the interface between the cornea and the aqueous humor, which decreases the refractive power of the air–cornea interface by about 10%. (See Example Q-6 in the Quick-Start Guide.)

EXAMPLE 1-2

Apply the lensmaker's equation to compare the power of an IOL in air and in an aqueous medium ($n = 1.33$).

$$P = \frac{n_2 - n_1}{r} \qquad \text{(lensmaker's equation)}$$

Consider an IOL that is planoconvex, with the convex side facing the cornea, and has a radius of curvature of the curved surface of 8.0 mm. The index of refraction of the IOL is 1.5 (n_2).

The power of the anterior surface in air (n_1) is

$$P_{air} = \frac{1.5 - 1.0}{0.008\ \text{m}} = +62.50\ \text{D}$$

The power of the posterior surface of the same lens in air is 0, so the net power of the lens is +62.50 D.

If the same lens is placed in aqueous humor, with $n_2 = 1.333$, the power of the anterior surface is

$$P_{aqueous} = \frac{1.5 - 1.333}{0.008\ \text{m}} = +20.90\ \text{D}$$

and the power of the flat posterior surface is again 0. Therefore, an IOL in air has approximately 3 times the nominal labeled power of the IOL (which is labeled with the assumption that the IOL will be placed in the eye and bathed in aqueous).

Section Exercises 1-2 through 1-6

Vergence equation problems. Thin lenses in air: In each case, given the values of u (the distance from source to lens) and P (lens power), find v (the distance from lens to image). (The symbol for infinity [∞] is used here and elsewhere in this chapter's Section Exercises.)

$$\frac{n_1}{u} + P = \frac{n_2}{v} \qquad \text{(vergence equation)}$$

$$U + P = V \qquad \text{(vergence equation, simple form)}$$

1-2 $U = \infty$, P = +4.00 D

In air, $U = 1/u$ *and* $V = 1/v$, so

using the simple vergence equation, $U + P = V$

$(1/\infty) + (+4.00\ \text{D}) = V$

$0 + 4.00\ \text{D} = V;\ v = 1/V$

$v = 1 / 4.00\ \text{D} = +0.25\ \text{m}$

1-3 $u = -4$ m, $P = +2.00$ D
Again, in air, $U = 1/u$ *and* $V = 1/v$, so
$(1/-4 \text{ m}) + (+2.00 \text{ D}) = 1/v$
$+1.75 \text{ D} = 1/v$
$v = 1/1.75 \text{ D} = +0.57 \text{ m}$

1-4 $u = -1$ m, $P = +2.00$ D
$(1/-1 \text{ m}) + (+2.00 \text{ D}) = 1/v$
$+1.00 \text{ D} = 1/v$
$v = +1 \text{ m}$

1-5 $u = -0.5$ m, $P = +2.00$ D
$(1/-0.5 \text{ m}) + (+2.00 \text{ D}) = 1/v$
$-2.00 \text{ D} + (+2.00 \text{ D}) = 0 = 1/v$
$v = \infty$, meaning that no image is formed.

1-6 $u = -0.4$ m, $P = +2.00$ D
$(1/-0.4 \text{ m}) + (+2.00 \text{ D}) = 1/v$
$(-2.50 \text{ D}) + (+2.00 \text{ D}) = -0.50 \text{ D} = 1/v$
$v = 1/-0.50 \text{ D} = -2 \text{ m}$

Section Exercises 1-7 through 1-10

Vergence equation problems. Thin lenses in water: Rework Section Exercises 1-3 through 1-6 but with the image space filled with an aqueous medium ($n_2 = 1.33$).

1-7 $u = -4$ m, $P = +2.00$ D
Because the image space is filled with an aqueous medium, we have to use the full vergence equation.
Therefore, $V = 1.33/v$, so
$(1/-4 \text{ m}) + (+2.00 \text{ D}) = 1.33/v$
$-0.25 \text{ D} + (+2.00 \text{ D}) = +1.75 \text{ D} = 1.33/v$
$v = 1.33/+1.75 \text{ D} = 0.76 \text{ m}$

1-8 $u = -1$ m, $P = +2.00$ D
$(1/-1 \text{ m}) + (+2.00 \text{ D}) = 1.33/v$
$-1.00 \text{ D} + (+2.00 \text{ D}) = +1.00 \text{ D} = 1.33/v$
$v = 1.33/1.00 \text{ D} = 1.33 \text{ m}$

1-9 $u = -0.5$ m, $P = +2.00$ D
$(1/-0.5 \text{ m}) + (+2.00 \text{ D}) = 1.33/v$
$(-2.00 \text{ D}) + (+2.00 \text{ D}) = 0 = 1.33/v$
$v = 1.33/0 = \infty$

1-10 $u = -0.4$ m, $P = +2.00$ D
$(1/-0.4 \text{ m}) + (+2.00 \text{ D}) = 1/v$
$(-2.50 \text{ D}) + (+2.00 \text{ D}) = -0.50 \text{ D} = 1.33/v$
$v = 1.33/-0.50 \text{ D} = -2.66 \text{ m}$

Two-Sided Lenses

More typical than the 1-sided lenses we have discussed earlier are 2-sided lenses, with front and back refractive surfaces (eg, the cornea). These surfaces separate the denser medium of the lens from the surrounding medium, usually air or a watery substance such as aqueous or vitreous humor. In many cases, if the distance between the front and back surfaces is small, we may treat the lens as a single refracting object with power $P = P_1 + P_2$, where P_1 and P_2 are the powers of the front and back lens surfaces (make sure to include the signs). This is referred to as the *thin-lens approximation*. Note: For a typical biconvex lens in air, both the front surface and the back surface have positive power, while both the numerator and the denominator in the lensmaker's equation for the back surface are negative numbers.

In some cases, such as the crystalline lens of the normal human eye or an IOL, we cannot ignore the separation between the front and back surfaces of a lens. The power of such a "thick lens" for paraxial rays is given, to a first approximation, by the formula

$$P = P_1 + P_2 - \left(\frac{t}{n}\right) P_1 P_2$$

where P_1 and P_2 are the powers of the front and back surfaces of the lens, respectively, t is the distance between them (ie, the thickness of the lens) in meters, and n is the refractive index of the lens material. This formula reduces to the thin-lens approximation as the lens thickness approaches 0.

EXAMPLE 1-3

Derive the thick-lens formula for a 2-sided lens in air:

$$P = P_1 + P_2 - \left(\frac{t}{n}\right) P_1 P_2$$

Suppose that the front surface has power P_1, the lens has refractive index n and thickness t, and the back surface has power P_2 (Fig 1-E3). At the front surface, a paraxial ray with zero vergence is refracted and intersects the optic axis at v, where $0 + P_1 = n/v$, or $v = n/P_1$. The reduced vergence of the refracted ray as it reaches the back surface is $n/(v - t) = n/[(n/P_1) - t]$. After the ray is refracted at the back surface, it meets the optic axis at distance v_2 from the back surface of the lens, and the exiting vergence is

$$\frac{1}{v_2} = \frac{n}{\left(\frac{n}{P_1}\right) - t} + P_2 = \frac{nP_1}{n - tP_1} + P_2$$

$$= \frac{P_1}{\left[1 - \left(\frac{t}{n}\right) P_1\right]} + P_2$$

$$= \frac{1}{\left(1 - \left(\frac{t}{n}\right) P_1\right)} \left\{ P_1 + P_2 \left[1 - \left(\frac{t}{n}\right) P_1\right] \right\}$$

$$= \frac{1}{\left[1 - \left(\frac{t}{n}\right) P_1\right]} \left[P_1 + P_2 \left(\frac{t}{n}\right) P_1 P_2 \right]$$

For small values of t, this approaches $P = P_1 + P_2 - (t/n)P_1P_2$.

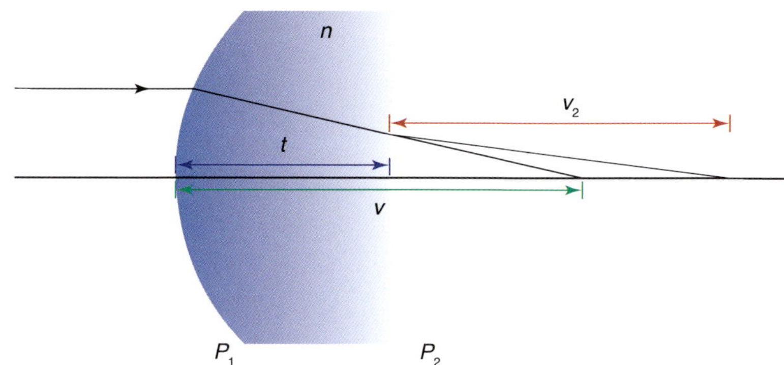

Figure 1-E3 Calculating the power of a thick lens. Here, v is the distance from the front lens surface to the point where the ray refracted by the front lens surface intersects the optic axis. The powers of the front and back surfaces are P_1 and P_2, respectively. *(Courtesy of Scott E. Brodie, MD, PhD.)*

Principal Planes and Ray Tracing

The thin-lens approximation treats the front and back lens surfaces as if they coincide, and we use their common location as the position of the lens to calculate the object and image vergences (U and V, respectively), as we did in the Quick-Start Guide. However, if we are not dealing with a thin lens, we do not immediately know how to measure the distance from a source object to a thick lens (or from the lens to the image location) in order to apply the vergence equation. It is helpful to use a diagram, together with the principles of ray tracing, to help visualize the refraction undergone by light rays as they pass through a lens (Fig 1-11). Recall from the Quick-Start Guide that the focal point F_2 of a lens is the location of the image of light from a very distant object (at a distance $f = 1/P$).

In this case, parallel rays from a distant object at left are brought to a focal point F_2 on the right side of the lens. But careful inspection shows that the refraction takes place in 2 steps: (1) as the rays cross the front surface of the lens and (2) as they cross the back surface. If we extend the incident rays and the exiting rays (shown by the dashed lines in Figure 1-11), they cross at an apparent single refracting surface—the second, or "back," *principal plane*—located within the lens substance. That plane, indicated by the vertical line, passes through the optic axis at H_2. Similarly, rays that originate from the front focal point, F_1, and emerge from the lens as parallel rays appear to have been refracted at a different internal plane—the first, or "front," principal plane)—which passes through the optic axis at H_1 (Fig 1-12).

These apparent refracting planes provide the appropriate locations for the calculation of object and image vergence, respectively. The intersections H_1 and H_2 of the principal planes with the optic axis are known as the first and second (or front and back) *principal points.*

The location of the principal planes depends on the lens design and on the refractive indices of the material in the object space, lens, and image space. For meniscus lenses, such as those used for spectacles, with 1 convex surface and 1 concave surface, the principal planes may lie outside the lens itself (Fig 1-13).

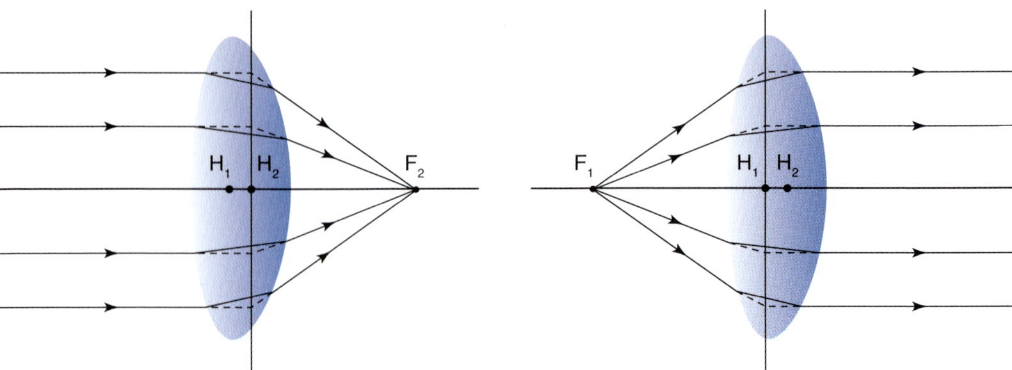

Figure 1-11 Ray tracing for parallel incident light rays striking a thick convex lens. Notice that the rays appear to bend at an internal plane at H_2. *(Redrawn from Creative Commons illustration by Bob Mellish.)*

Figure 1-12 Ray tracing for rays emerging from the first focal point, F_1, striking a thick convex lens. Notice that the rays appear to be refracted at a different plane than the incident parallel rays shown in Figure 1-11. *(Redrawn from Creative Commons illustration by Bob Mellish.)*

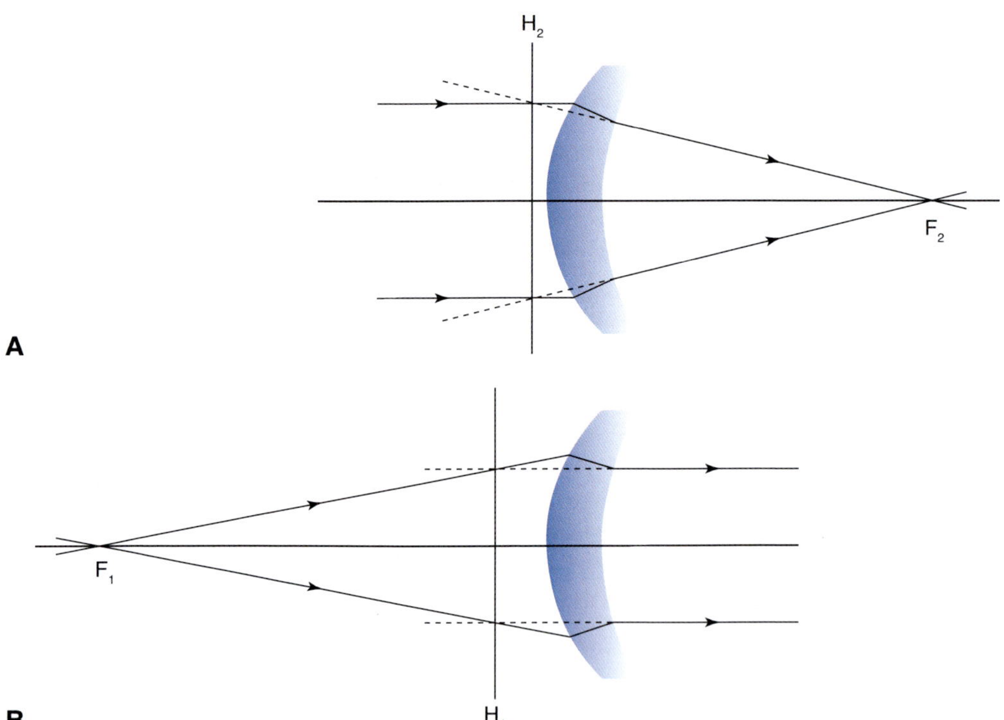

Figure 1-13 Ray tracing for a meniscus lens in air. Notice that the principal planes H_1 and H_2 lie outside the lens. **A,** Parallel rays from a distant object at left focus at a focal point (F_2) located on the right side of the lens. **B,** Rays from the first focal point (F_1) undergo refraction and emerge from the lens as parallel rays to the right.

Calculations of the location of the principal planes are beyond the scope of this book. Fortunately, for most purposes involving ophthalmic lenses in air, such as spectacle corrections and contact lenses, the thin-lens approximation is adequate. However, most calculations of refraction within the eye, where the thickness of the lens is a large fraction of the axial length, may require more detailed treatment. Hence, some newer IOL calculation formulas (eg, Olsen, Barrett Universal 2, etc) incorporate lens thickness into calculations to improve accuracy of the calculated IOL power.

In addition, ray tracing can provide a helpful check on computations based on the vergence equation. For a thin convex lens in air, it is convenient to depict the source object as a vertical arrow, with its tail on the optic axis and its head at a distance—say, *h*—from the optic axis (Fig 1-14A). We can take a central vertical line to be the common location of the front and back principal planes. The ray from the tip of the arrow passes through the center of the lens on the optic axis without deviation. To locate the image of the arrow, we can trace 2 rays that originate at the tip of the arrow. The ray that propagates parallel to the optic axis is bent at the common principal plane and passes through the back focal point, F_2. The ray emerging from the tip of the arrow and passing through the front focal point, F_1, is bent at the common principal plane and redirected to continue parallel to the optic axis, where it eventually crosses the (refracted) path of the previous ray, locating the image of the tip of the arrow. In general, we can also use a third ray, from the tip of the arrow through the (common) principal point on the optic axis (the center of the lens) to confirm the construction. By symmetry, this ray will emerge from the lens as if undeviated (though in fact it makes a slight zigzag as it enters and exits the lens) and should also intersect the point of intersection of the previous 2 rays.

The various cases of interest with the source object arrow located at 4 different distances from a thin convex lens (very far left of F_1, slightly to the left of F_1, at F_1, and between F_1 and the lens) are illustrated in Figure 1-14, parts A–D, respectively. The ray tracing for a thin concave lens in air is given in Figure 1-15 for the 2 cases in which the source object is located to the left of F_2 or between F_2 and the lens. See Appendix 1-4.

Section Exercises 1-11 through 1-14

Draw the ray-tracing diagrams for Exercises 1-2 through 1-5.

1-11 See Figure 1-14A.
1-12 See Figure 1-14B.
1-13 See Figure 1-14C.
1-14 See Figure 1-14D.

Depth of Focus and Depth of Field

The preceding discussion has tacitly implied that there is 1 exact image location. Anyone who has focused an optical instrument has noticed that the best focus is a small region, rather than a point, where the image neither improves nor blurs. This typically

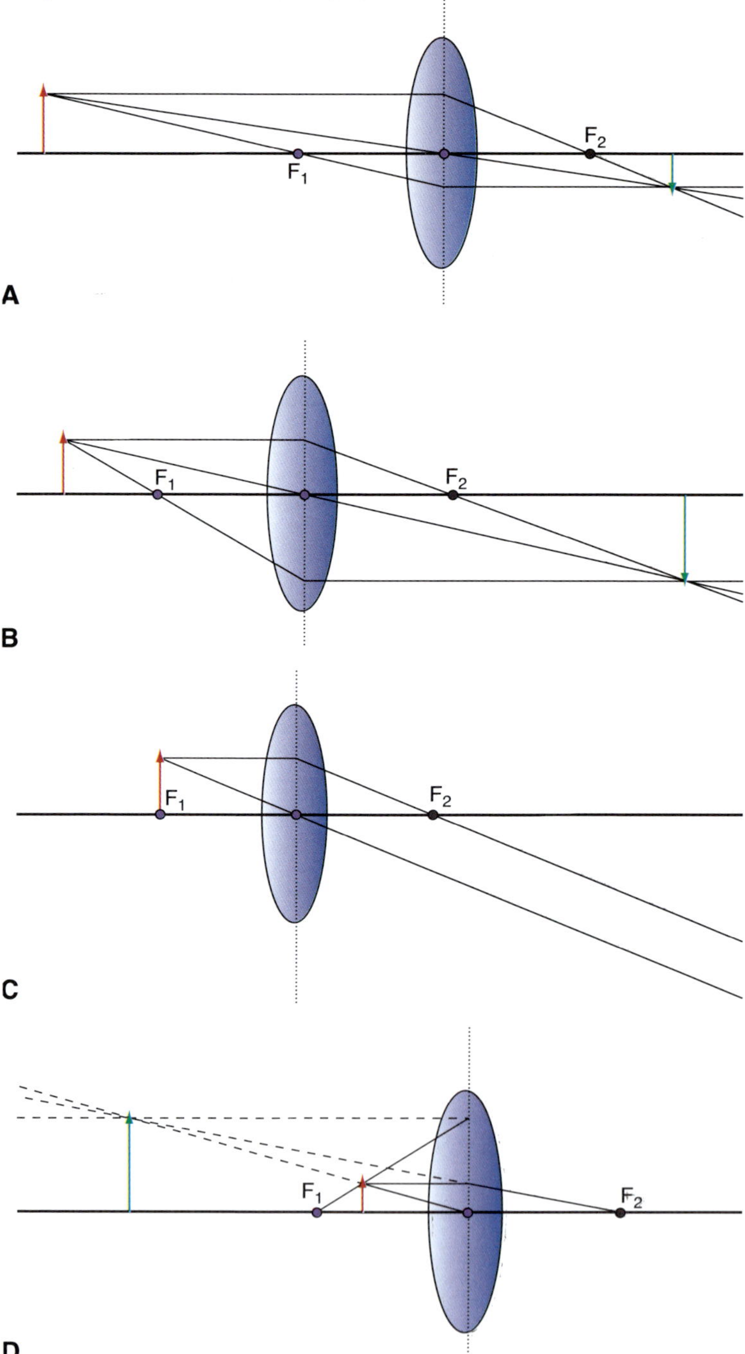

Figure 1-14 Ray tracings for a simple convex lens in air. The red arrow represents the source object; the green arrow shows the corresponding image location and size. Points F_1 and F_2 are the front and back focal points of the lens, respectively. The optic axis is represented by the heavy line and the principal plane by the dotted line. The principal point (optical center of the lens) is shown at the intersection of the optic axis and the principal plane. The first and second focal points are shown on the optic axis. Solid lines show paths of actual light rays, and dashed lines show paths of virtual light rays. **A,** Source object far to left; real image (inverted and minified) is on opposite side of lens. **B,** Source object at left, near first focal point; real image (inverted and magnified) is on opposite side of lens. **C,** Source object coincides with first focal point; "image" is at infinity. **D,** Source object between first focal point and lens; virtual image (upright and magnified) is seen to left of source object. *(Illustration developed by Scott E. Brodie, MD, PhD.)*

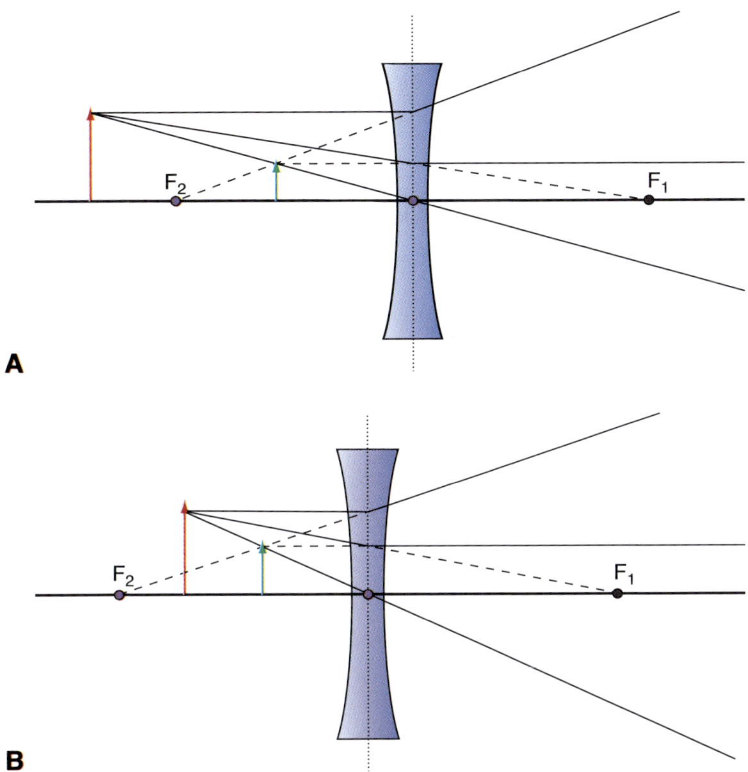

Figure 1-15 Ray tracing for a concave lens in air. The red arrow represents the source object; the green arrow shows the corresponding image location and size. The optic axis is represented by the heavy line and the principal plane by the dotted line. The principal point (optical center of the lens) is shown at the intersection of the optic axis and the principal plane. The first and second focal points, F_1 and F_2, are shown on the optic axis. Solid lines show paths of actual light rays, and dashed lines show paths of virtual light rays. **A,** When the source object is located to the left of the focal point, a virtual, upright, and minified image is formed between focal point and the lens. **B,** Moving the object between focal point and lens produces a similar virtual and upright image, though with less image minification. *(Illustration developed by Scott E. Brodie, MD, PhD.)*

small but definite region is the *depth of focus* (Fig 1-16). We can conveniently describe it in terms of the range of effective correcting lens powers (in diopters) that permit adequate image clarity.

Depth of focus is a *property of the imaging system,* not of the image, and it varies from lens to lens. As discussed in the Quick-Start Guide (see "The Camera Obscura: Pinhole Imaging"), a pinhole has an infinite depth of focus; lenses have a far more restricted depth of focus.

Whereas depth of focus is the range of *image* locations over which an object remains sharply focused, *depth of field* is the range of *object* locations that will be sharply focused at a single image location (Fig 1-17). Clinically, depth of field is important for prescribing

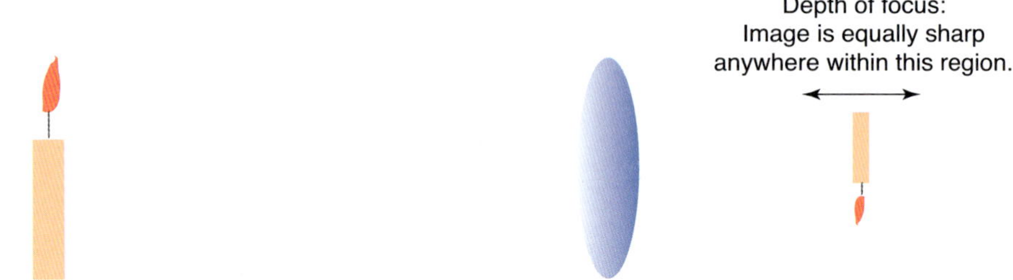

Figure 1-16 Depth of focus. An image is equally sharp anywhere within the indicated region. *(Courtesy of Edmond H. Thall, MD.)*

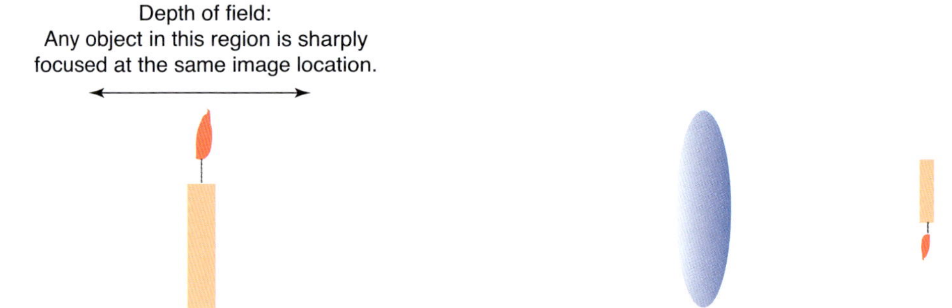

Figure 1-17 Depth of field. Any object within the depth of field will appear sharply focused in the image. *(Courtesy of Edmond H. Thall, MD.)*

bifocals and trifocals for presbyopia. Even when the depth of focus is small, the depth of field can be large, depending on various factors.

General Refracting Systems

Refracting systems can be built up from multiple combinations of lenses of arbitrary thickness and various compositions of optical media, such as types of glass with different refractive indices. Regardless of the complexity, for paraxial rays, such systems can be characterized by a single pair of principal planes and a single refractive power, *P*.

This is a remarkable simplification. We can ignore everything that takes place at the numerous optical interfaces within such an optical system and proceed by simply determining the object vergence *(U)* at the first principal plane, adding the power *P*, and then locating the image by referencing the exiting vergence *(V)* to the second principal plane (Fig 1-18). In this figure, notice that the entire 3-lens system can be simplified to a single pair of principal planes (H_1 and H_2). In addition, Gaussian optics allows for an elegant reduction of the individual events within the lens system (see box on page 79).

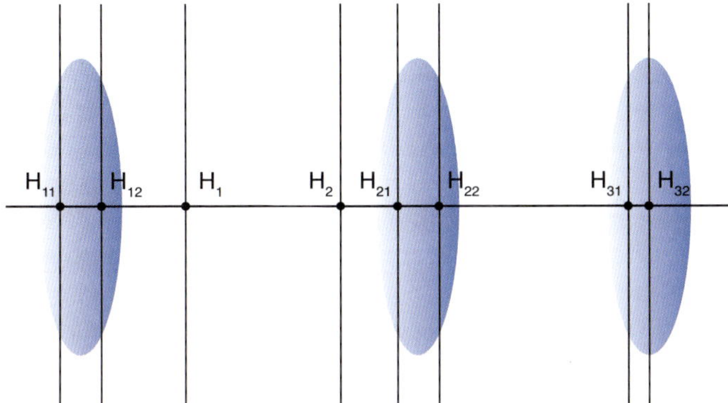

Figure 1-18 References for a compound optical system. Each lens has its own power and pair of principal planes, as indicated by subscripts 11 and 12, 21 and 22, and 31 and 32. The combined system has an equivalent, or net, power and a single pair of principal planes representing the entire system, indicated by H_1 and H_2. *(Courtesy of Edmond H. Thall, MD.)*

EXAMPLE 1-4

Principal planes. Redo Section Exercises 1-3 through 1-6 for a complex lens system with principal planes separated by 1.0 cm = 0.01 m and net power $P = +2.00$ D.

Assume that the object distances are referenced to the front principal plane. Then the image distances are the same as before, when referenced to the second principal plane, and are thus 1.0 cm greater than the answers to Section Exercises 1-3 through 1-6: +0.58 m, +1.1 m, infinity, and −1.9 m, respectively.

Section Exercises 1-15 through 1-18

Redo Section Exercises 1-3 through 1-6 for a lens system with net power $P = +10.00$ D.

1-15 $u = -4.0$ m, $P = +10.00$ D
$v = 1/9.75$ D = 0.10256 m from the second principal plane

1-16 $u = -1.0$ m, $P = +10.00$ D
$v = 1/9.00$ D = 0.111 m from the second principal plane

1-17 $u = -0.5$ m, $P = +10.00$ D
$v = 1/8.00$ D = 0.125 m from the second principal plane

1-18 $u = -0.4$ m, $P = +10.00$ D
$v = 1/7.50$ D = 0.1333 m from the second principal plane

EXAMPLE 1-5

Principal planes and distant objects. The Gullstrand mathematical model closely approximates the human eye. (The Gullstrand model eye is discussed in Chapter 3.) The net power of the entire refracting system of the model eye is $P = +58.64$ D; the refractive index of the vitreous humor is 1.336, and the second (back) principal plane is located 1.602 mm behind the anterior corneal surface. Locate an image of a distant object as formed by the Gullstrand model eye with relaxed accommodation.

The image is located according to the vergence equation: $U + P = V$. Since the object is located extremely far away, $U = 0$. Therefore, $0 + 58.64$ D $= 1.336/v$, so $v = 0.02278$ m, or $1.602 + 22.78 = 24.382$ mm from the anterior corneal surface. While the axial length varies among patients, this calculated number indicates that the focal point of the image will fall nearly exactly on the retina in many eyes.

EXAMPLE 1-6

Effectivity of lenses. Suppose that a lens of power P in air places the image of a distant object at a distance v to the right of the lens. To move the lens t meters to the right while preserving the image location, how must you adjust the power of the lens?

In its new position, the lens will form the image at a distance $v_2 = v - t$ to the right of the lens (as $u = 0$). Thus, the power P_2 of the moved lens should be $P_2 = 1/(v - t) = 1/(1/P - t) = P/(1 - tP)$. Indeed, the same formula applies to divergent lenses, with the initial image location to the left of the lens, as long as the proper sign conventions are observed. This adjustment is referred to as the correction for the *effectivity of lenses.*

The effectivity of lenses comes into play, for example, when we convert a spectacle correction to the corresponding contact lens correction. For example, a hyperopic correction will place the image of a distant object at the far point of the eye (the location conjugate to the fovea with relaxed accommodation; see the Quick-Start Guide). In this case, the far point is behind the retina, and the effectivity calculation requires that the power of the correcting contact lens be greater than the power of the equivalent spectacles. For example, for a spectacle correction of +4.00 D worn at the standard vertex distance of 13.75 mm from the corneal apex, the power of the equivalent contact lens is +4.00 D/[1 − (0.01375 m)(4.00 D)] = +4.232 D, which suggests that the contact lens power should be increased by 0.25 D. This correction is negligible for lenses weaker than about 3.00 D.

Gaussian Optics

To calculate the location of the principal planes, we must know the details of the refractive events within the lens system. In practice, this is usually done by means of an elegant formalism known as *Gaussian optics* (or *Gaussian reduction*). The details are beyond the scope of this book, but the basic idea is as follows: the paraxial approximation is effectively a linearization of Snell's law. We can therefore express the approximation in terms of 2 types of linear operators. (1) The *translation operator* describes the propagation of a light ray through a medium of refractive index n over a distance t. This is, in essence, equivalent to the step of recalculating the vergence of light from a source object (or image created by a previous refracting surface) as referenced to the next refracting surface in an optical system. (2) The *refraction operator* describes the change in vergence at a curved optical interface of radius r between media of refractive indices n_1 and n_2. It is the equivalent of adding P to find the vergence of light exiting from a refractive interface. We can represent each of these operators in an appropriate coordinate system by a suitable 2×2 matrix. We can then use matrix multiplication to calculate the net action of a sequence of refractive events at the various refractive surfaces in a complex optical system.

Characteristics of Objects and Images: Real and Virtual

In analyzing the action of a (perhaps complex) sequence of refracting surfaces, we have seen that we can treat each surface in turn by considering the image formed by each surface in the sequence as the source object for the next. From the point of view of the next refracting surface in the sequence, it makes no difference whether the source is an actual source of emitted (or reflected) light or the image of such a source formed by the previous refracting surfaces in the system. We cannot tell by looking at such a beam of light whether it comes from a physical object or the image formed by the previous optics. Nevertheless, it is often helpful to keep track of whether the rays that form an image actually converge at the image location *(real images),* such as the image of a distant object formed by a converging lens, or only appear to diverge from the image location *(virtual images),* such as the image of a distant object formed by a diverging lens (see the Quick-Start Guide sections Convex Lenses and Concave Lenses).

We can make a similar distinction between the apparent objects that are imaged by successive refractive surfaces. A *real object* is one from which light emanates (diverging light, indicating that U is negative) as it approaches a lens (or mirror) surface; an apparent object toward which light appears to converge (as with imaginary or extended rays on ray tracing) as it approaches a refracting surface is a *virtual object* for that surface (Fig 1-19). Evidently, the distinction between "real" and "virtual" objects depends on the context—that is, the location of the lens surface that will form the next image of the object in turn.

We can also make a distinction between images formed by successive refractive surfaces. An image is *real* if it is located on the same side of the lens as the image rays (that is, with the light traveling from left to right, to the right of the lens that forms it; mathematically, V is positive), and *virtual* if it is located on the other side of the lens where the image rays do not exist (mathematically, V is negative).

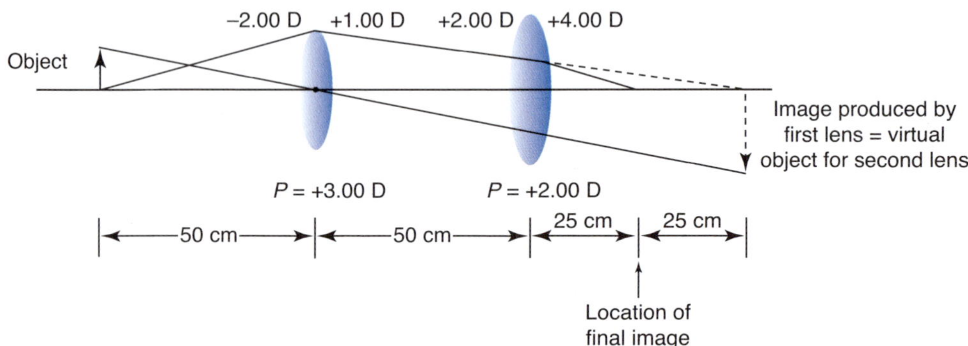

Figure 1-19 Ray tracing for a system of 2 convex lenses in air. The real image formed far to the right by the first lens becomes a virtual object for the second lens. *(Courtesy of Edmond H. Thall, MD.)*

Consider the 2-lens system in Figure 1-20, which shows an object located 50 cm to the left of a +3.00 D lens. Using the vergence equation, $U + P = V$, $-2 + 3 = +1$. The first image (real image) is located 1 m to the right of the first lens, which also happens to be 50 cm to the right of the second lens. For the second lens, this real image becomes a virtual object: hence, U will be *positive.* We can again use the vergence equation to obtain $+2 + 2 = +4$. The second image will form 25 cm to the right of the second lens. Because V is positive, this second image is a *real image.*

Mathematically, the elegance of the vergence equation allows us to determine real and virtual objects by looking at the signed values of U and V. A negative U indicates a real object; a positive U indicates a virtual object. Conversely, a positive V indicates a real image; a negative V indicates a virtual image. In addition, we can use ray tracing to visually confirm the presence of real versus virtual objects and images in a given lens system.

EXAMPLE 1-7

For Section Exercises 1-3 through 1-6, determine which images are real and which are virtual. Images in 1-3 and 1-4 are real, and image 1-6 is virtual. The "imaging" in 1-5 is afocal—that is, the optical system does not form an image at a finite location.

Transverse Magnification

Optical systems are frequently employed to obtain images of a more convenient size or location for study than the original objects. Magnifiers and microscopes provide enlarged images of inconveniently small objects; telescopes and binoculars provide smaller, more conveniently located images of immense objects that are very far away. The relocation of images is described by the vergence equation. Magnification is also readily determined in this context. For objects of finite size and distance, *transverse magnification*—the ratio of the height (or distance from the optic axis) of an image to the height of the original source object—is the most appropriate description. Transverse magnification (sometimes

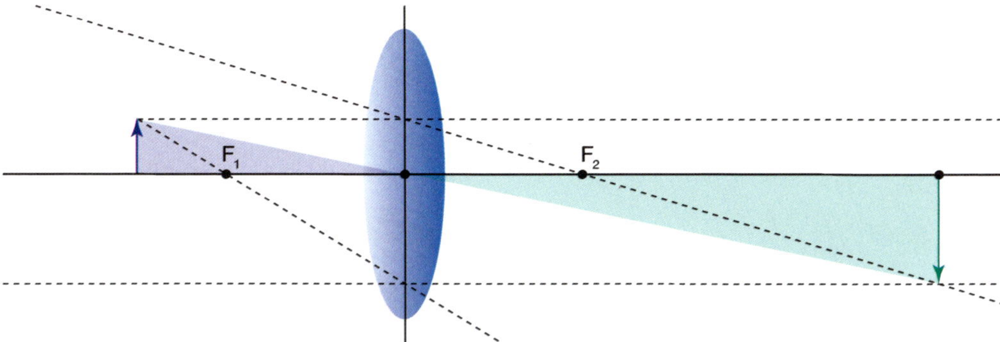

Figure 1-20 Ray tracing for a convex lens used in air. Notice how the principal ray through the central point of the lens creates similar triangles, indicating that the transverse magnification is proportional to the ratio of image distance to object distance. *(Illustration developed by Scott E. Brodie, MD, PhD.)*

referred to as *lateral magnification* or *linear magnification*) is denoted by M_T. For lenses in air, a simple calculation with similar triangles (Fig 1-20) gives $M_T = h_2/h_1 = v/u$. Here, u and v carry the same sign conventions as used in the vergence equation. This can also be calculated using the vergence equation values of $M_T = U/V$ (notice the capitalization).

If the lens separates media of refractive indices n_1 and n_2, the corresponding formula is $M_T = n_1 v / n_2 u$. The refractive index for the object medium multiplies the image distance and vice versa. Negative values of M_T indicate images that are upside down (inverted), not images that are reduced in size ("minified"); magnification is indicated by an M_T less than 1 in absolute value.

Section Exercises 1-19 through 1-22

Compute the transverse magnification for the following object–lens systems in air:

1-19 Object located 0.5 m to the left of a +5.00 D lens
$U + P = V$
$-2 + 5 = 3$; $v = 1/V = 0.33$ m (real image)
$M_T = v/u = 0.33/-0.5 = -0.66$. Note that using U/V will also yield the same result ($-2/3 = -0.66$)
The image is inverted and 66% of the size of the object.

1-20 Object located 1 m to the left of a +2.00 D lens
$u = -1$ m, $P = +2.00$ D, $v = 1$ m
$M_T = v/u = 1\text{ m}/-1\text{ m} = -1$
The image is inverted and the same size as the object.

1-21 Object located 0.5 m to the left of a +2.00 D lens
$u = -0.5$ m, $P = +2.00$ D
$-2 + 2 = 0$; $v = 1/V = 1/0 = \infty$

$M_T = v/u = \infty/-0.5 \text{ m} = \text{null}$
The image is "infinitely" magnified mathematically, but in practical terms, magnification is null.

1-22 Object is located 0.4 m from a +2.00 D lens
$u = -0.4 \text{ m}, P = +2.00 \text{ D},$
$-2.5 + 2 = -0.5; v = 1/V = 1/-0.5 = -2 \text{ m}$
$M_T = v/u = -2 \text{ m}/-0.4 \text{ m} = +5$
The image is upright and 5 times the size of the object.

Axial (Longitudinal) Magnification

As we have seen, a thin lens in air produces a transverse magnification described by the simple equation $M_T = v/u$. If the source "object" is in fact an assemblage of objects, or an extended object with an axial dimension (measured along the optic axis), the image will also exhibit an axial extent, or apparent thickness. We can show (for example, by differentiating the vergence equation) that the apparent thickness of the image—the *axial,* or longitudinal, *magnification* for a refracting system in air—is given by

$$M_L = (M_T)^2$$

Axial magnification is illustrated in Figure 1-21.

This effect leads to a substantial distortion of the images seen by direct or indirect ophthalmoscopy. Although it is difficult to appreciate image depth with the monocular view through the direct ophthalmoscope, the aerial image seen with the indirect ophthalmoscope is generally seen stereoscopically. Depending on the power of the condensing lens used, the distortion factor may vary as much as fourfold in changing from a 14.00 D lens to a 30.00 D lens. The overall stereoscopic effect is reduced by the small interpupillary

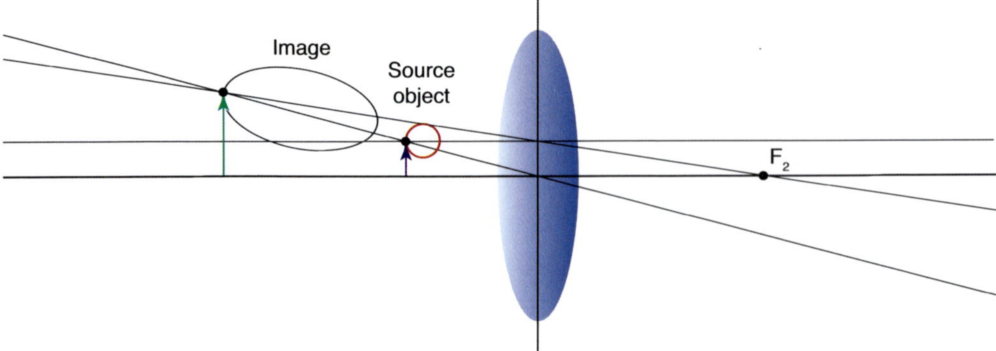

Figure 1-21 Ray tracing for a convex lens in air demonstrating comparison of transverse magnification and axial (longitudinal) magnification. Note that because of the proximity of the object to the lens, imaginary extensions of the refracted rays and central ray can be extended backward to determine the location of the virtual image. The source object is the red circle; its image is the blue ellipse. Notice the considerable distortion caused by the disparity between transverse and axial magnifications. *(Illustration developed by Scott E. Brodie, MD, PhD.)*

distance of the periscopic viewing system; but, nevertheless, the perceived shape of fundus features, such as tumors or optic disc excavation, is typically somewhat exaggerated.

EXAMPLE 1-8

Compute the relative apparent thickness of the retinal features as seen by indirect ophthalmoscopy with a 15.00 D, 20.00 D, 30.00 D, and 90.00 D condensing lens. (Assume a total power for the eye of 60.00 D.)

The transverse magnification of an indirect ophthalmoscope is equal to the ratio of the power of the eye (about 60.00 D) to the power of the condensing lens (similar to the formula for the power of a Keplerian telescope). The axial magnification is given by $M_L = (M_T)^2$. Although the apparent thickness (or depth) of retinal features is reduced by the periscopes built into the indirect ophthalmoscope (which reduce the effective interocular distance of the examiner) compared with normal viewing, the *relative* depth of fundus features is unaffected. The ratio of the transverse magnification provided by each lens can be determined by dividing the power of the eye by the power of the lens. Thus, transverse magnification with the 15.00 D, 20.00 D, and 30.00 D condensing lenses is then 4×, 3×, and 2×, respectively, so the relative axial magnifications are in the ratios of 16:9:4, respectively. Thus, the apparent retinal thickness as seen with a 15.00 D condensing lens is nearly double that seen with the 20.00 D lens, and 4 times that seen with the 30.00 D lens. Note that while clinically difficult to use in this setting, the 90.00 D lens will form an image approximately 44.4% of the thickness of a retinal source object.

Conjugate Points

Points that form an object–image pair are said to be *conjugate* to one another, or to form a conjugate pair. Because the paths of light rays are reversible, each point in a conjugate pair is the image of the other. In the case of a source object infinitely far to the left of an optical system, this "point at infinity" is considered conjugate to the back (second) focal point, F_2, to the right of the lens. Similarly, the front (first) focal point, F_1, is conjugate to the point infinitely far to the right of the lens. Notice that the front and back focal points are *not* conjugate to each other. In air, the front and back focal points are located at a distance $f = 1/P$ from the front and back principal planes, respectively.

Nodal Points

Consider a thick lens (Fig 1-22). It can be shown (for example, by means of Gaussian reduction) that there is a pair of conjugate points on the optic axis for which an object ray directed at one of these points, N_1, making an arbitrary small angle, θ, with the optic axis will, on exiting the lens, appear to emerge from the other point, N_2, at the same angle θ with the optic axis.

The points N_1 and N_2 are referred to as the front (or first) and back (or second) *nodal points*, respectively. They serve, for ray tracing with thick lenses in a general optical system, as an analogue for the central point in a thin lens and have a role similar to that of

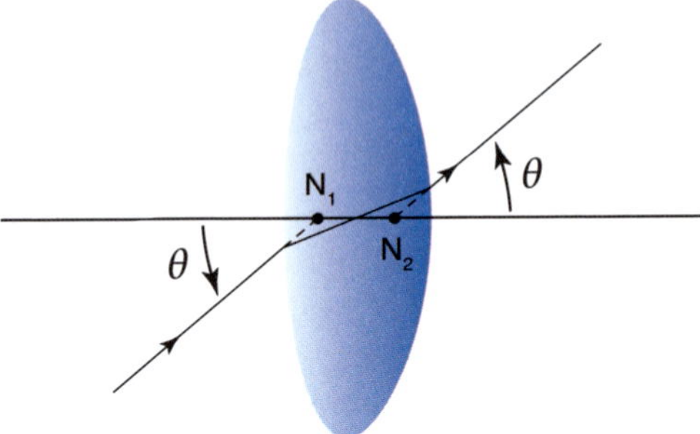

Figure 1-22 Nodal points of a thick convex lens in air. The inclination of an incident ray through the first nodal point (N_1) equals the inclination of the exiting ray as it apparently emerges from the second nodal point (N_2). *(Redrawn from Creative Commons illustration by Bob Mellish.)*

the front and back principal planes for determining object and image vergence. When the refractive indices n_1 and n_2 are equal, the nodal points coincide with the principal points. Nodal points are particularly useful for determining image size (Example 1-9).

It is tempting to draw an analogy between the role of the nodal points in ray tracing and the fulcrumlike action of a pinhole aperture, as described in Part 1 of the Quick-Start Guide (see the section The Camera Obscura: Pinhole Imaging). In both cases, the angles between the incident and emergent rays and the optic axis for rays passing through the pinhole or nodal points are equal. But this analogy is potentially misleading for optical systems with finite apertures. For these systems (unlike simple pinholes), it is *not* true that all the light passes through the nodal points, only that the unique rays that *do* pass through the nodal points preserve the same simple geometry as the rays passing through a pinhole aperture. In particular, a small posterior subcapsular lens opacity does not cause a disproportionate reduction in visual acuity by virtue of its proximity to the posterior nodal point of the eye. (Such an opacity may, however, be an effective scatterer of light, greatly reducing a patient's contrast sensitivity.)

EXAMPLE 1-9

In the reduced model eye, the eye's refracting surfaces are replaced by idealized air–water interfaces. Suppose that the nodal point of the reduced model eye is 17 mm in front of the retina and 7 mm behind the cornea. Using this nodal point, calculate the retinal image size of a target of light 1.0 cm in diameter on a bowl-shaped background (as in the Goldmann perimeter) viewed at 33 cm. (The reduced schematic eye is discussed in Chapter 3.)

We can use similar triangles to solve for the retinal image size. It Is important to make sure that we *compare similar parts* of the triangles, as well as to ensure that the *units of measurement are the same.* We can replace the 1.0 cm with 10 mm to ensure uniformity among the units of measurement. By similar triangles, image height/10 mm = 17 mm/337 mm = 0.50 mm.

The Reduced, or Equivalent, Optical System

A complex multiple lens system can always be analyzed sequentially, but the process is tedious and must be repeated from the beginning for each source object location.

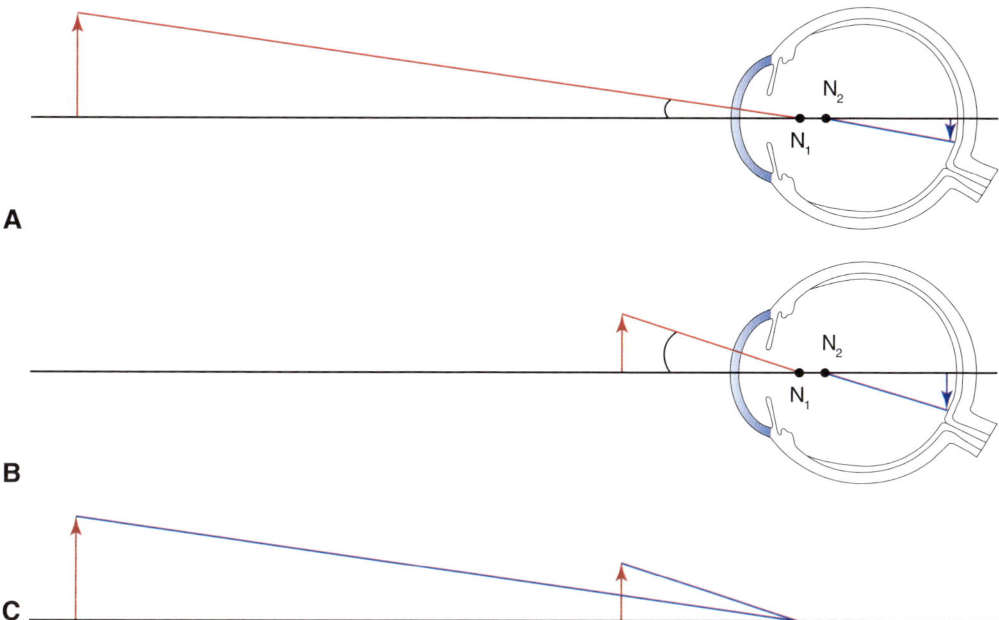

Figure 1-23 Reduced optical system for the human eye. The retinal image size (apparent size) of an object depends in part on the angle subtended at the object nodal point N_1. A small object close to the eye can subtend a larger angle than a large but distant object. This is the basis of the magnification produced by a telescope. The object in part **A** is twice the size of the object in part **B.** However, the object in part B is 4 times closer to N_1 than the object in part A. Therefore, the angle that the object in part B subtends is twice as large as the angle that the object in part A subtends. **C,** The 2 angles are directly compared. *(Courtesy of Edmond H. Thall, MD.)*

However, we can calculate an equivalent optical system consisting of just 1 pair of principal planes, 1 pair of focal points, 1 pair of nodal points, and 1 power. The paraxial properties of this equivalent system, called the *reduced optical system,* are identical in every respect to the original system consisting of multiple lenses. Thus, once the equivalent system is determined, we need only a single vergence equation calculation to locate the image of any object. A simplified reduced model for the human eye (Fig 1-23) is discussed in Chapter 3.

EXAMPLE 1-10

Draw the ray tracing for the general case of a thick lens with positive power and distinct principal planes and nodal points.

Suppose that the source object is more distant from the front of the lens than the anterior focal point and that the lens sits with air to the left and water (an optically denser medium) to the right. The nodal points are displaced toward the denser medium. The ray tracing is as shown in Figure 1-E10. (The lens surfaces are omitted for clarity.)

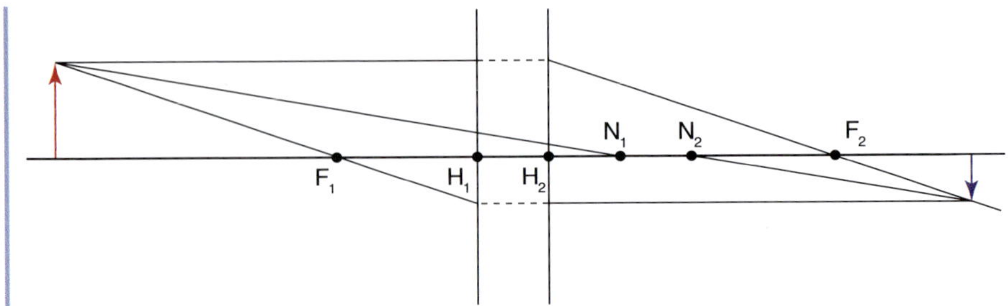

Figure 1-E10 Ray tracing for a general optical system with distinct principal planes and nodal points.

Aberrations

The paraxial theory of image formation discussed earlier is necessarily an idealization of the behavior of real optical systems. The goal of *stigmatic imaging*—recombining the light passing through a finite aperture from an extended object to project all the energy from each object point to a single image point simultaneously—is never perfectly achieved in practice. Even at the best possible focus, light from a single object point is distributed over a small area of the image. Each image point receives light predominantly from one object point but also receives some light from neighboring object points. The image point resembles, but does not duplicate, the object point. Because rays do not focus perfectly stigmatically, the image does not contain as much detail as the original object. This discrepancy is referred to in general as the *aberration* of an optical system.

Point Spread Function

The region over which light from a single object point is spread in a pinhole camera is a *blur circle* (see the section The Camera Obscura: Pinhole Imaging in the Quick-Start Guide). The word *circle* is somewhat misleading, however; even with simple ray tracing through a small circular aperture, the image region is typically an ellipse. Light from any single object point tends to focus to an irregularly shaped smudge. Moreover, within the smudge, light is usually not evenly distributed; some areas are brighter than others. The distribution of light from a single object point in the image is aptly named the *point spread function (PSF)* because it describes how light from a single object point spreads out in the image. For any given source object point, the area under the possible PSF is a constant: it represents the total light energy emitted from the point source. The narrower and more peaked the PSF, the clearer and sharper the image will be.

An image is therefore composed of multiple partially overlapping smudges, 1 smudge for each object point. The PSF is a quantitative description of the smudge and is quite useful because we can deduce all the imaging characteristics of an optical system from the PSF. (The process for extracting image information from the PSF requires advanced mathematics beyond the scope of clinical practice.)

Moreover, the notion of optical power applies to the paraxial region only. There is no such thing as refractive power outside the paraxial region. This is in stark contrast to corneal topographic power maps that assign a "power" to every point on the cornea, even in the periphery. However, corneal power maps define power in 2 ways (axial and tangential), and neither is consistent with the correct definition of refractive power as used in this chapter. In the early 1950s, lens designers developed *wavefront theory*, the appropriate way to analyze the optical properties of imaging systems beyond the paraxial regime, especially aberrations.

Wavefront Theory

Thus far in our discussion of geometric optics, we have employed a number of assumptions as foundational principles to discuss important concepts such as refraction, ray tracing, and more. One other key principle to discuss at this juncture is *Fermat's principle*, which states that light travels between 2 points *only* along the fastest path (Appendix 1-2). Thus, a stigmatic focus can be achieved only when each of the paths from object to image point requires precisely the same amount of time.

We can construct a spherical surface centered on the image point such that all light moving along image rays must cross the arc of that surface simultaneously to achieve a stigmatic focus. This surface is called the *reference sphere* (Fig 1-24).

A geometric *wavefront* is an isochronic (equal-time) surface. We can construct a wavefront anywhere along a group of rays originating from a single object point. All light from a given object point crosses the wavefront simultaneously. If the wavefront that intersects the vertex of the reference sphere is also spherical, then the focus is stigmatic. However, this almost never occurs because a wavefront is in general irregularly shaped. The difference between the wavefront and the reference sphere is the *wavefront aberration* (Fig 1-25).

It is a common misconception that *wavefront* refers in some way to the wave nature of light. Geometric optics ignores the wave nature of light. (See Appendix 2-1 for a brief discussion of the wave nature of light, an aspect of physical optics.) A geometric wavefront is a surface of *equal time*, regardless of whether light is a wave or a particle. The term *isochrone* might be more descriptive, but for historical reasons, the term *wavefront* is entrenched.

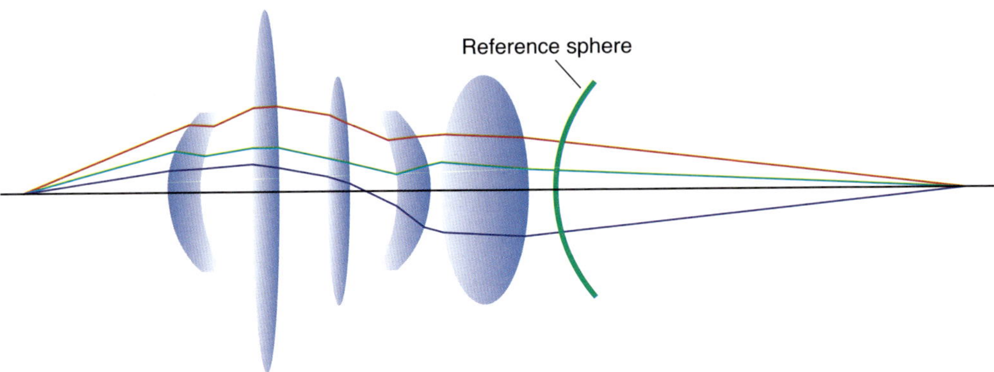

Figure 1-24 The reference sphere, a spherical arc centered on the image point. If all the image rays cross the reference sphere simultaneously, a stigmatic focus results. *(Courtesy of Edmond H. Thall, MD.)*

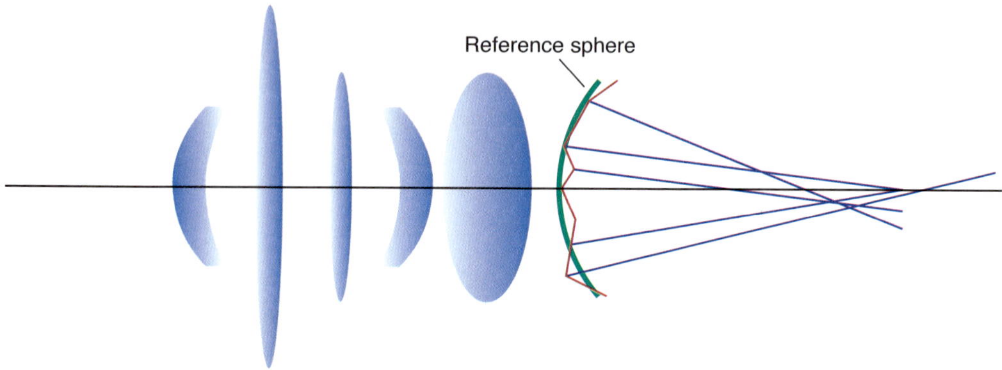

Figure 1-25 The wavefront and wavefront aberration. The actual wavefront is irregularly shaped, and the image is not stigmatic. The difference between the actual wavefront and the reference sphere is the wavefront aberration. *(Courtesy of Edmond H. Thall, MD.)*

The *wavefront aberration* is a smooth but irregularly shaped surface, typically something like the shape of a potato chip or corn flake. The mathematical description of the wavefront aberration may at first seem daunting, but conceptually it is straightforward.

Consider first a toric surface (see the Quick-Start Guide, Astigmatism section). A *toric surface* is the combination of 2 more fundamental surfaces: a sphere and a cylinder. We can represent any toric surface as the sum of a certain amount of sphere and a certain amount of cylinder. The fundamental shapes, sphere and cylinder, never change from one toric surface to another; only the amount of sphere and cylinder (and the cylinder orientation) changes. Sphere and cylinder are the only fundamental shapes necessary to define any toric surface or to express any amount of regular astigmatism.

The same idea applies to wavefront aberration, except that *more than 2 fundamental shapes* are required. Every wavefront aberration is the sum of the same fundamental shapes. The amount of each shape varies from patient to patient, but the fundamental shapes themselves never change.

The most common set of fundamental reference shapes used for this purpose is known as the *Zernike polynomials,* which are mathematical functions defined on a disc-shaped region. The first several Zernike polynomials closely resemble simple combinations of the wavefront aberrations that we commonly encounter with simple optical systems. A detailed discussion of this material is far beyond the scope of this text; a brief qualitative discussion follows.

The most fundamental aberrations were initially described in the nineteenth century by Philipp Ludwig von Seidel. They are known as *Seidel aberrations:* spherical aberration, coma, astigmatism, curvature of field, and distortion (Fig 1-26).

- *Spherical aberration* is a disparity in refraction that affects incoming light rays from a single *axial* object point based on the different distances of the refracted light rays from the center of the lens. Peripheral light rays undergo different amounts of refraction as compared to paraxial light rays.
- *Coma* is a disparity in focal length for rays from a single *off-axis* object point that are refracted at different distances from the center of the lens.

- *Astigmatism* is the disparity in focal length for rays from a single object point that are incident at different meridians of the lens (see the Quick-Start Guide section on astigmatism).
- *Curvature of field* is a disparity in focal length for objects at different distances from the optic axis.
- *Distortion* is a disparity in transverse magnification for objects at different distances from the optic axis.

The low-order Zernike polynomials represent variation from stigmatic imaging very similar to the classic Seidel aberrations. (Figure 1-27 depicts the lowest-order Zernike polynomials.) For example, the first-order Zernike polynomial aberration named *tilt* is, in essence, equivalent to a prismatic deviation.

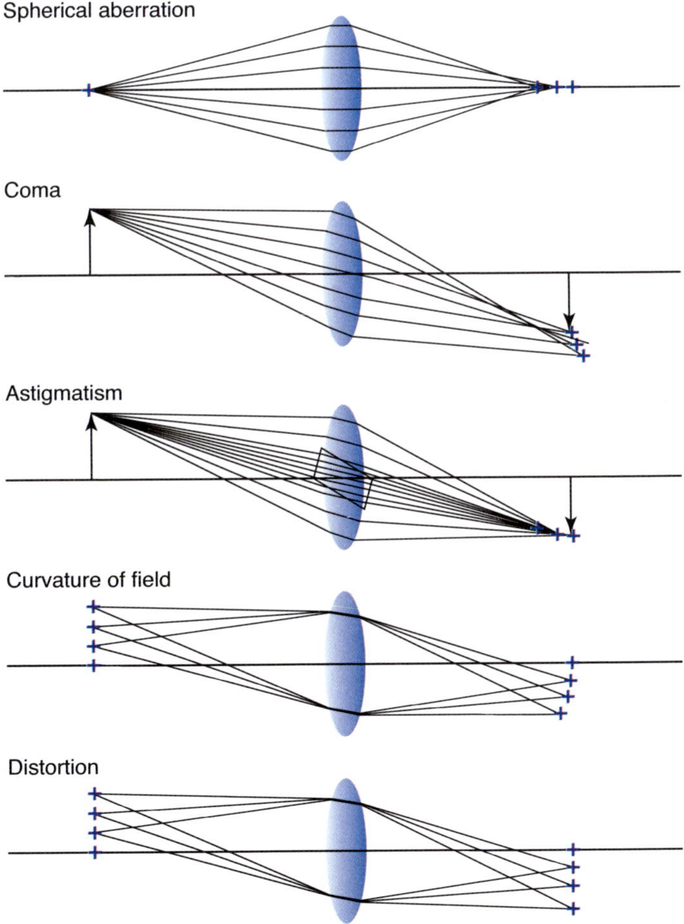

Figure 1-26 Schematic depiction of the classic Seidel aberrations. *(Courtesy of Edmond H. Thall, MD.)*

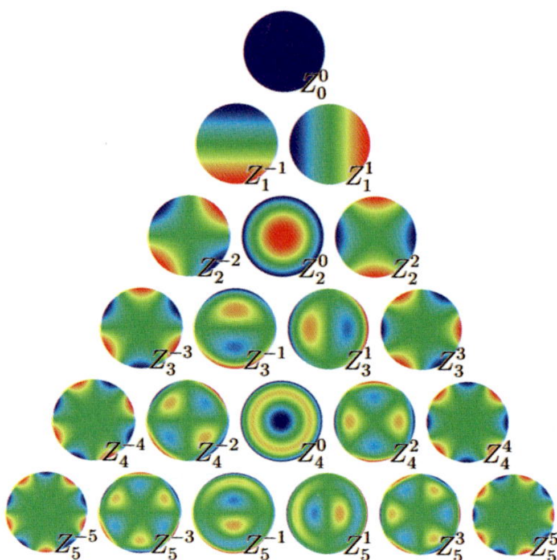

Figure 1-27 Low-order depictions of the first several Zernike polynomials, labeled according to standard notation. *Top row:* "Piston" aberration affects only the phase of light waves and is not ordinarily detectable. *Second row:* "Tilt" corresponds to misdirection of wave propagation, akin to prismatic deviations, shown as vertical or horizontal. *Third row:* The outer functions show astigmatic aberrations; the left function represents oblique astigmatism, and the right function represents vertical astigmatism. The middle function shows variations in focal point with circular symmetry, akin to defocus. *Fourth row:* The middle 2 functions are lobular wavefront errors, akin to the classic coma; the middle-left displays vertical coma, and the middle-right displays horizontal coma. The outer functions represent "trefoil," a 3-fold symmetry sometimes seen as a complication after refractive surgery. The extreme left function represents vertical trefoil, and the extreme right function represents oblique trefoil. *Fifth row:* The extreme left and right functions display oblique and vertical quatrefoil, another higher-order aberration, respectively. The middle-left and middle-right functions display oblique and horizontal secondary astigmatism, respectively. Of significance, the center function displays spherical aberration, which is an extremely important higher-order aberration for consideration during cataract and refractive surgery. *Bottom row:* The middle 2 functions are lobular wavefront errors, akin to the classic coma; the 2 outer-middle functions show variations of trefoil. The extreme left and right functions display pentafoil, another higher-order variation. *(Illustration by Wikipedia user Zom-B via Creative Commons.)*

The second-order Zernike polynomial aberrations are referred to as *defocus,* corresponding to myopia and hyperopia, and *astigmatism,* which corresponds to the potato chip–like waveform surface created by a spherocylindrical lens. The Seidel aberrations are third-order Zernike polynomial aberrations. These include coma, which corresponds to a lobular asymmetry in the waveform surface.

In myopia, the wavefronts are displaced relative to the reference sphere (Fig 1-28). The wavefront is spherical but has a smaller radius than the reference sphere, and the wavefront aberration is parabolic.

While all of the Seidel aberrations have clinical relevance, *spherical aberration* is the most important of them. In positive spherical aberration, rays at the edge of the wavefront focus anteriorly to central (paraxial) rays (Fig 1-29). The wavefront aberration is bowl shaped. The human eye is an "imperfectly perfect" system; for example, spherical aberration has the beneficial effects of increased depth of focus and 3-dimensionality of vision.

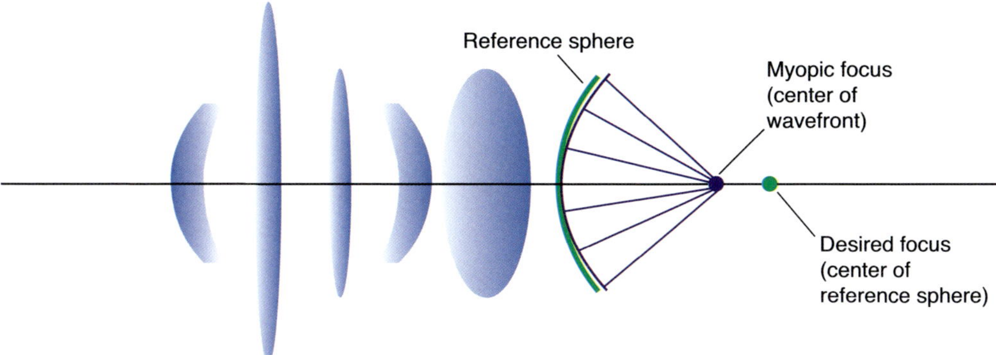

Figure 1-28 Myopia. In pure myopia, the focus is still stigmatic. Therefore, the actual wavefront is also a sphere, but with a smaller radius than the reference sphere. The wavefront aberration has a parabolic shape. *(Courtesy of Edmond H. Thall, MD.)*

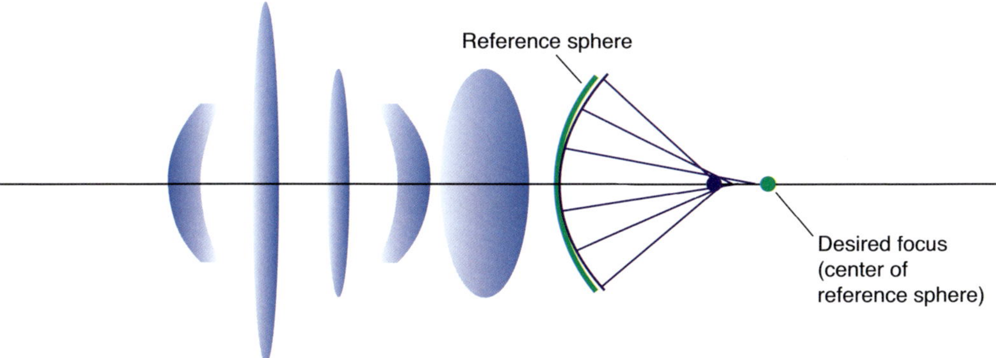

Figure 1-29 Positive spherical aberration. The peripheral rays focus anterior to the paraxial rays. The wavefront aberration has a bowl shape—flat centrally, then strongly curved toward the edge. *(Courtesy of Edmond H. Thall, MD.)*

However, the disadvantages of increased spherical aberration are significant and merit additional discussion.

- Spherical aberration shifts the position of best focus. This aberration is strongly pupil dependent: as the pupil of a patient with positive spherical aberration dilates, the shift in best focus renders the patient more myopic. The condition is known as *night myopia* and can be treated by prescribing spectacles with an extra –0.50 D in the distance correction for use at night or in low light.
- It causes objective decline in visual function, such as reduced contrast sensitivity, especially in low-light conditions.
- It results in subjective decline in visual function, such as glare and halos around point sources of light in low-light conditions.

In current surgical practice, most surgeons will use an aspheric IOL with negative spherical aberration to restore the crystalline lens values, reduce the positive spherical aberration of the eye, and improve the quality of visual acuity after cataract surgery.

Chromatic Aberration

In addition to these "monochromatic" aberrations, images produced by white light may also be degraded by *chromatic aberration,* the spreading apart of colors of white light by a lens system. This effect is caused by dispersion, by which the index of refraction of a material medium may vary with the wavelength of the light passing through it. Just as a prism bends blue light more strongly than it bends red light, in practice, a convex lens will create a *focal point for blue light anterior to the one for red light,* so the eye is typically about 0.50 D more myopic for images formed in blue light than in red light. Clinically, this disparity is the basis for the Lancaster red–green (duochrome) test for accommodative control (not to be confused with the Lancaster red–green test for strabismus, described in BCSC Section 6, *Pediatric Ophthalmology and Strabismus*). See the Quick-Start Guide, Part 2, Refraction.

Astigmatism

The basic properties of toric (spherocylindrical) lenses were introduced in the Quick-Start Guide. Unlike a rotationally symmetric lens (eg, sphere), which produces a point image of a point object, a toric lens always produces 2 linear "images" of a single point. As we have seen, the 2 focal lines are perpendicular to each other—one parallel to the cylinder axis, the other perpendicular to the cylinder axis. The focal lines are found at different distances from the lens, according to the vergence equation for the maximal and minimal powers of the principal meridians of the lens.

EXAMPLE 1-11

(A) A point source is 1 m to the left of a +2.00 +3.00 × 030 toric lens. Where are the images?

The object vergence is −1.00 D. Because this is a spherocylindrical lens, we need to determine how much power is present in each meridian, and we will have to use the vergence equation for each of the 2 meridians. Recall that the +3.00 D of cylinder power has been placed in the 30° axis meridian and will thus exert power at the 120° power meridian only; however, the line formed by light passing through this lens will form at 30°.

For the 30° meridian, the lens will function as a +2.00 D lens and produce a linear image oriented in the 120° meridian. Using the $U + P = V$ equation, $-1 + 2 = +1$. The resulting image will be located 1 m (100 cm) to the right of the lens; this image will be real (V is positive), inverted ($m = U/V = -1$, which is negative), and same size ($|m| = 1$) as the original object.

For the 120° meridian, the lens will function as a +5.00 D lens and produce a linear image oriented in the 30° meridian. Again, using the $U + P = V$ equation, $-1 + 5 = +4$. The resulting image will be located 25 cm to the right of the lens; this image will be real (V is positive), inverted ($m = U/V = -1/4$), and minified ($|m| = 1/4$) compared with the original object.

(B) Suppose that the object point is 25 cm to the left of the same lens. Where are the linear images?

Using the same methods, we get a linear image oriented in the 30° meridian of +1.00 D, or 1 m to the right of the lens. Also, there is a linear image in the 120° meridian with a vergence of −2.00 D, or −50 cm to the left of the lens. In this case, the object point and the linear image in the 30° meridian are real, but the linear image in the 120° meridian is virtual.

(C) Consider a pure cylinder such as +2.00 × 180 and an object 1 m to the left of the lens. Where are the images?

The object vergence is again −1.00 D, and one linear image is −1.00 D + (+2.00 D) = +1.00 D to the right of the lens, real, and oriented along the 180° meridian. The second linear image is −1.00 D + (+0.00 D) = −1.00 D, or 1 meter to the left of the lens, virtual, and oriented in the 90° meridian. Thus, the vertical image is virtual and in the same location as the object.

The notion of a virtual linear image at the object can be confusing, but consider the Maddox rod, which is an array of parallel cylinders of high power. The virtual images these cylinders produce are used to test ocular alignment (Fig 1-E11).

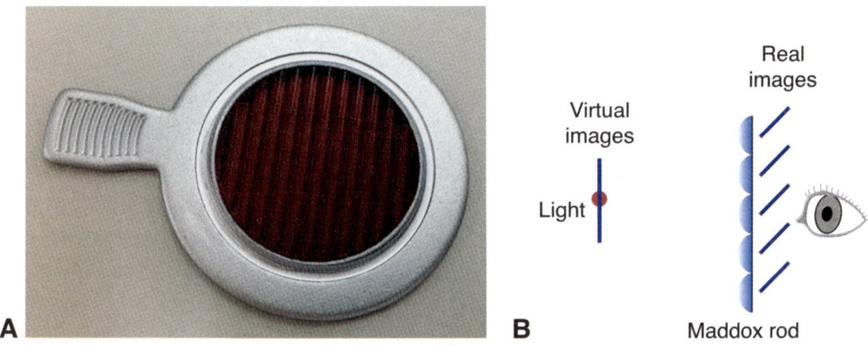

Figure 1-E11 Maddox rod. **A,** The Maddox rod is an array of high-power parallel cylinders. **B,** The cylinders produce real images parallel to, and a few millimeters behind, the cylinders and virtual images perpendicular to the axis through the object. The real images are too close to the eye for the patient to see them. Only the virtual images are visible. *(Part A courtesy of Scott Brodie, MD, PhD; part B courtesy of Edmond H. Thall, MD.)*

The Conoid of Sturm

The geometric figure that is formed by the rays of light leaving an astigmatic lens is called the *conoid of Sturm* (Fig 1-30). Although it is represented in textbooks as a 2-dimensional figure, it is actually a 3-dimensional figure best appreciated as a dynamic image (see Video 1-1). The *circle of least confusion (COLC)* is the circular cross section of the conoid of Sturm that is halfway between the 2 focal lines (in terms of diopters, not linearly). The COLC is also best appreciated as a dynamic image (see Video 1-2). Notice that the COLC in Figure 1-30 is closer to the vertical focal line than to the horizontal one.

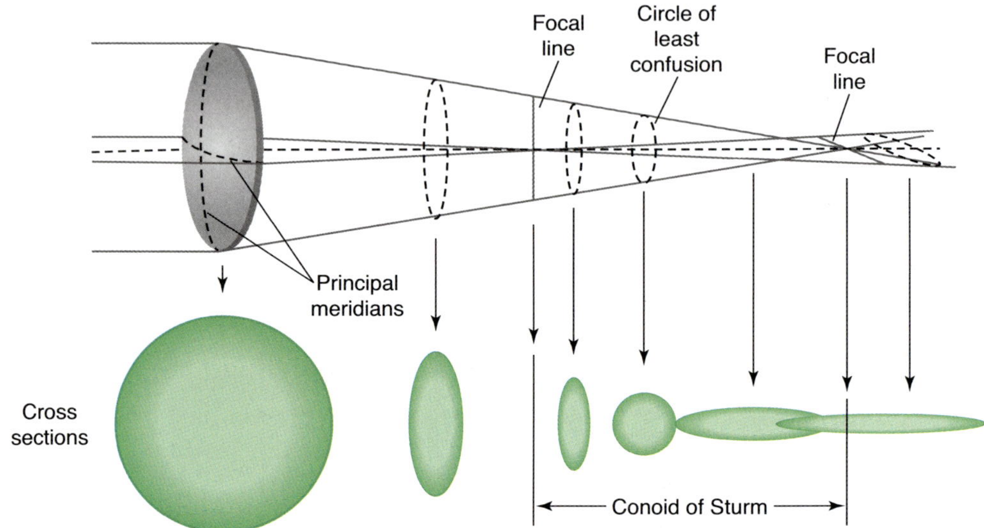

Figure 1-30 Conoid of Sturm, the geometric figure formed by the rays of light leaving an astigmatic lens. The circle of least confusion is the circular cross section of the conoid of Sturm that is halfway (in diopters, not linearly) between the 2 focal lines. *(Reproduced from Guyton DL et al,* Ophthalmic Optics and Clinical Refraction. *Prism Press; 1999.)*

Consider again the spherocylinder of Example 1-11, Part A. There are 2 focal lines separated by 75 cm. The region between these 2 linear foci is the conoid of Sturm. Starting at the linear focus in the 30° meridian 25 cm from the lens and proceeding farther to the right, the focus changes from a line to an ellipse with the long axis in the 30° meridian. Farther to the right, the ellipse becomes a circle, then another ellipse with the long axis in the 120° meridian, and eventually a line in the 120° meridian.

VIDEO 1-1 Conoid of Sturm.
Courtesy of Joshua Young, MD.

VIDEO 1-2 Circle of least confusion.
Courtesy of Joshua Young, MD.

The Spherical Equivalent

The *spherical equivalent (SE)* is the average power of a toric lens. For instance, a +2.00 +3.00 × 010 cylinder has a power of +2.00 D in the 10° meridian and +5.00 D in the 100° meridian. The average is +3.50 D, which is the SE power. If the lens is described in spherocylindrical notation, we calculate the SE as the sum of the sphere and half the cylinder power. For instance, a +2.00 −5.00 × 020 spherocylinder has the SE of −0.50 D. Of note, regardless of whether plus cylinder or minus cylinder notation is used to express the power of a given spherocylindrical lens, the SE is exactly the same.

We can use the SE to calculate the location of the COLC. For example, when the SE is +3.50 D and the object vergence is −1.00 D, the COLC is +2.50 D, or 40 cm to the right of the lens.

The Power Cross

Any spherical, toric (spherocylindrical), or purely cylindrical lens can be represented graphically by a *power cross.* A spherical lens has the same power at every meridian. A toric lens has a different power at every meridian that falls within a range between the maximum and the minimum value. The maximum and minimum powers are always in meridians that are 90° apart. The power cross shows the maximum and minimum powers and their meridians.

A pure cylinder has 0 power along its axis meridian and either highest positive or most negative power perpendicular to its axis *(power meridian).* The rule is that the power meridian of a cylinder is perpendicular to its axis meridian. Light that passes through a spherocylindrical lens will form a line at the axis meridian.

The nomenclature used to describe this is often confusing, especially for trainees, as the axis meridian is conventionally referred to as the *axis,* and the power meridian is sometimes referred to as the *power.* For instance, a +2.00 × 015 cylinder has 0 power in the 15° meridian and +2.00 D power in the 105° meridian (Fig 1-31). When speaking about such a lens—by convention, colloquially, and in everyday clinical practice—some may say, "This lens has 0 power at the 15° axis and +2.00 power at 105°." What is intended is that the axis meridian is 15° and the power meridian is 105°; light that passes through this lens will form a line at 15°.

As discussed in the Quick-Start Guide, a −3.00 +2.00 × 015 toric lens has a −1.00 D power in the 105° meridian and −3.00 D in the 15° meridian (Fig 1-32). Using spherocylinder

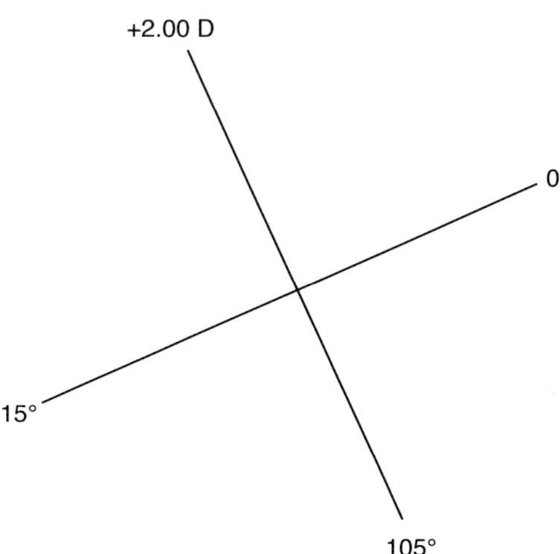

Figure 1-31 Power-cross representation of a +2.00 × 015 cylinder. The power meridian of a cylinder is 90° to its axis meridian. *(Courtesy of Edmond H. Thall, MD.)*

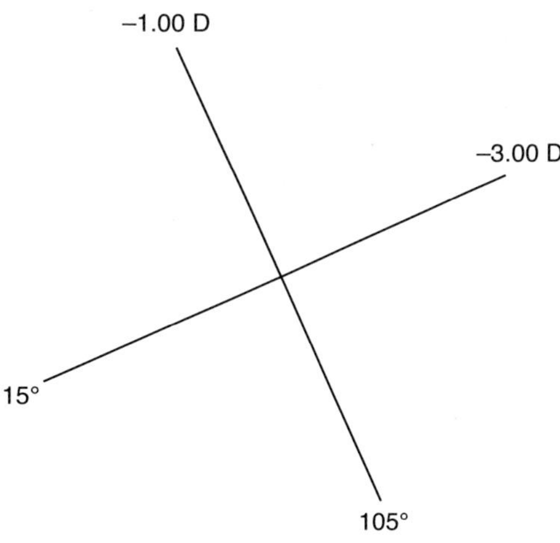

Figure 1-32 Power-cross representation of a −3.00 +2.00 × 015 cylinder. Again, the power of a cylinder is 90° to its axis. *(Courtesy of Edmond H. Thall, MD.)*

notation, we can always represent the same toric lens in 2 ways—a plus cylinder form and a minus cylinder form—which can lead to confusion. To convert from one form to the other (transposition of the spherocylindrical specification):

- The new sphere is the algebraic sum of the old sphere and cylinder.
- The new cylinder has the same value as the old cylinder but with the opposite sign.
- The axis needs to be changed by 90°.

One advantage of the power cross is that any toric lens has only 1 power-cross representation. However, we can use a power cross to combine spherocylinders only when the orientations of their meridians are identical. For instance, what is the result of combining a +2.00 +1.00 × 080 lens with a +3.00 −2.00 × 080 lens? Using a power cross to represent each lens, we can simply add the powers in the corresponding meridians (Fig 1-33).

EXAMPLE 1-12

Use the power-cross representation of astigmatic lenses to show how an astigmatic refractive error can be corrected with a cylindrical lens of the same power as the astigmatic error, placed 90° away from the lens representing the astigmatic error, and combined with a spherical lens of the opposite sign.

Suppose the "excess" power in the eye is equivalent to a cylindrical +1.00 × 180 lens. The power-cross representation of this lens is 0.0 @ 180°, +1.00 @ 90°. Placing a lens with power-cross representation of +1.00 @ 180°, 0.0 @ 90° in front of this eye yields a net excess power of +1.00 @ 180°, +1.00 @ 90°, equivalent to a spherical lens of power +1.00 D. We can correct this net spherical error by using an additional spherical lens of power −1.00 D, for a net correcting lens of −1.00 + 1.00 × 090, because the power of a correcting cylinder is 90° away from the axis of that correcting cylinder.

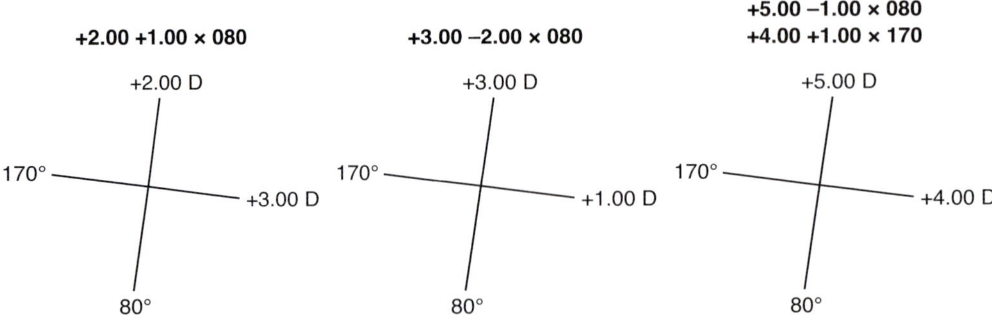

Figure 1-33 Combination of spherocylinders with identical meridians. *(Courtesy of Edmond H. Thall, MD.)*

Section Exercises 1-23 through 1-26

Practice transposition of astigmatic lenses—that is, convert between the plus cylinder and minus cylinder. For example:

$$+1.00 + 2.00 \times 080 = +3.00 - 2.00 \times 170$$

1-23 $+1.00 - 2.00 \times 080$
$-1.00 + 2.00 \times 170$
1-24 $-2.00 - 3.00 \times 010$
$-5.00 + 3.00 \times 100$
1-25 $-2.00 + 1.00 \times 010$
$-1.00 - 1.00 \times 100$
1-26 $-1.00 - 0.75 \times 180$
$-1.75 + 0.75 \times 090$

Power-Versus-Meridian Graph

The (paraxial) power of a spherocylinder varies in every meridian according to the equation

$$P_\theta = P_S + P_C \sin^2 (\theta - \phi)$$

Here, P_θ is the power in the meridian at angle θ from the horizontal (measured counterclockwise, as seen facing the patient), P_S is the power of the spherical component of the spherocylinder, P_C is the power of the cylindrical component, and ϕ is the cylinder axis. For instance, a +3.00 D cylinder with an axis at 020 has a power in the 050 meridian given by

$$P_{050} = +3.00 \text{ D} [\sin^2 (50 - 20)] = +0.75 \text{ D}$$

A power-versus-meridian graph (PVMG) represents the power in every meridian (Fig 1-34). As with a power cross, a toric lens has only 1 PVMG. Whether specified in plus cylinder or minus cylinder form, the PVMG is the same. However, the PVMG is a more complete representation of a spherocylinder because it shows power in all meridians, while a power cross shows power in only 2 meridians. We can use the PVMG to represent the combination of spherocylinders at any axes in a single representation without the need for a separate calculation for cylinders and spheres. We can algebraically add the $\sin^2$ formulas for meridional power of 2 thin spherocylindrical lenses in contact and simplify according to the usual rules for trigonometric functions, regardless of whether the cylinder axes coincide.

Jackson Cross Cylinder

A *Jackson cross cylinder (JCC)* is a spherocylindrical lens with equal but opposite powers in the perpendicular principal meridians. The JCC is conveniently mounted with a handle oriented between the principal meridians in such a way that twirling the handle quickly exchanges the 2 meridians. (See the Quick-Start Guide and Chapter 4.) Exercise 1-27 is an example of a JCC. A JCC may be of any power and always has the SE of 0. Thus, a JCC is any spherocylindrical lens with the SE of 0. We can fabricate such a lens by grinding a cylinder

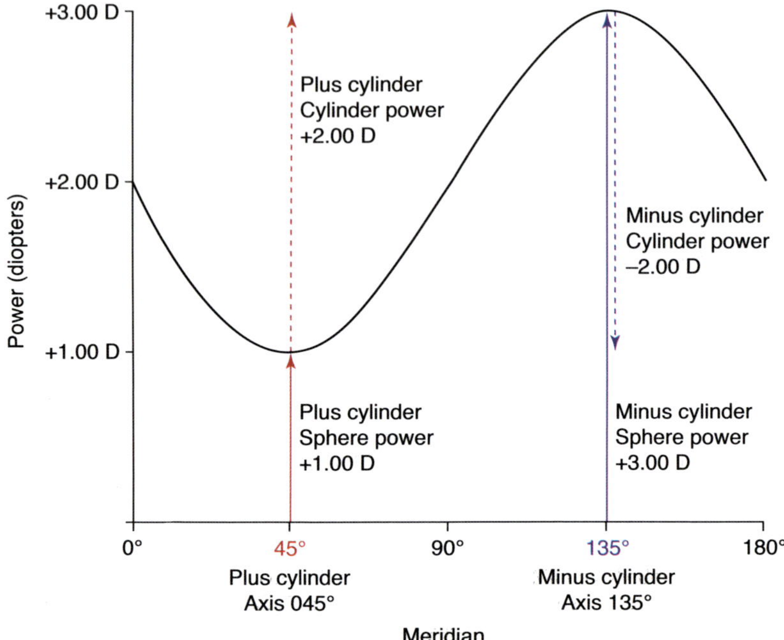

Figure 1-34 Power-versus-meridian graph (PVMG) of a toric lens. There is only 1 PVMG for any toric lens. To read the spherocylinder power in plus cylinder form *(red arrows),* look at the trough (lowest point on the graph). The vertical distance between the trough and the horizontal axis is the sphere power (P_S); the cylinder axis is the meridian of the trough. The (positive) cylinder power is the distance from the trough to the peak (highest point on the graph). For minus cylinder form, the distance of the peak from the horizontal is the P_S; the cylinder axis is the meridian of the peak. The (negative) cylinder power is the distance from the peak to the trough. *(Courtesy of Edmond H. Thall, MD.)*

on 1 surface, paired with a sphere of half the power and opposite sign of the cylinder on the opposite surface.

Section Exercises 1-27 through 1-30

Calculate some spherical equivalents.

1-27 Refraction: −1.00 +2.00 × 180
SE: (−1.00 D) + (2.00 D/2) = 0

This example has the SE of 0 and thus is equivalent to a JCC.

1-28 Refraction: −1.00 +4.00 × 180
SE: (−1.00 D) + (4.00 D/2) = +1.00 D

1-29 Refraction: −1.00 −2.00 × 090
SE: (−1.00 D) + (−2.00 D/2) = −2.00 D

1-30 Refraction: −5.00 −6.00 × 090
SE: (−5.00 D) + (−6.00 D/2) = −8.00 D

Mirrors

The effect of smooth mirrors on the paths of light rays is governed by the *law of reflection.* Sometimes referred to as the law of specular reflection, this law states that the *angle of reflection* between the reflected ray and the surface normal (line perpendicular to the reflecting surface) at the point of reflection equals the *angle of incidence* between the incident ray and the surface normal.

Plane mirrors simply reverse the direction of propagation of light, without altering vergence. This effect is often described as a "reversal of the image space." Images formed by plane mirrors are upright, virtual, the same size as the object, and left–right reversed. Curved mirrors, in addition to reversing the image space, also add or subtract vergence.

For paraxial rays, we can draw a simple geometric construction, akin to the derivation of the vergence equation and the lensmaker's equation, to demonstrate a similar vergence equation for mirrors (Appendix 1-3). We use the following conventions:

$$P = \frac{-2}{r}$$

$$\frac{1}{u} + P = \frac{1}{\text{“}v\text{”}}$$

There are a few key considerations when we use this equation for mirrors:

- We assume that the incident light travels from left to right in the usual way.
- r is the (signed!) radius of curvature of the mirror (in meters), which is twice the value of the focal length. Therefore, the power of a mirror can be calculated as $P = -2/r = -1/f$.
- We can employ the usual sign conventions (a mirror concave to the left has a negative number as its radius, so the power P of such a mirror is a *positive* number; a mirror convex to the left has a positive number as its radius, so the power P is a *negative* number).
- "v" is the distance from the mirror to the image in the *reversed* image space. Rays converging from right to left are considered to have *positive* vergence; rays diverging from right to left are considered to have *negative* vergence. In this book, we use quotation marks around the letter "v" as a reminder that a change in sign convention is necessary when applying the vergence equation to mirrors rather than to lenses.

Notice that the refractive index does *not* appear in these equations—the law of reflection does *not* include a correction for refractive index.

For example, parallel rays moving from left to right, striking a mirror concave to the left (Fig 1-35A), emerge traveling right to left with positive vergence. They converge on the focal point *(f)* of the mirror at half the radius of the mirror *(r)*, to the left of the mirror. Conversely, parallel rays moving from left to right that strike a mirror convex to the left (Fig 1-35B) emerge diverging from right to left, with an apparent focus (a virtual image) at distance $r/2$ to the right of the mirror.

It is often useful to clarify these unusual sign conventions by ray tracing. For mirrors, we recognize 3 special rays: (1) the ray through the center of curvature *(C)* of the mirror

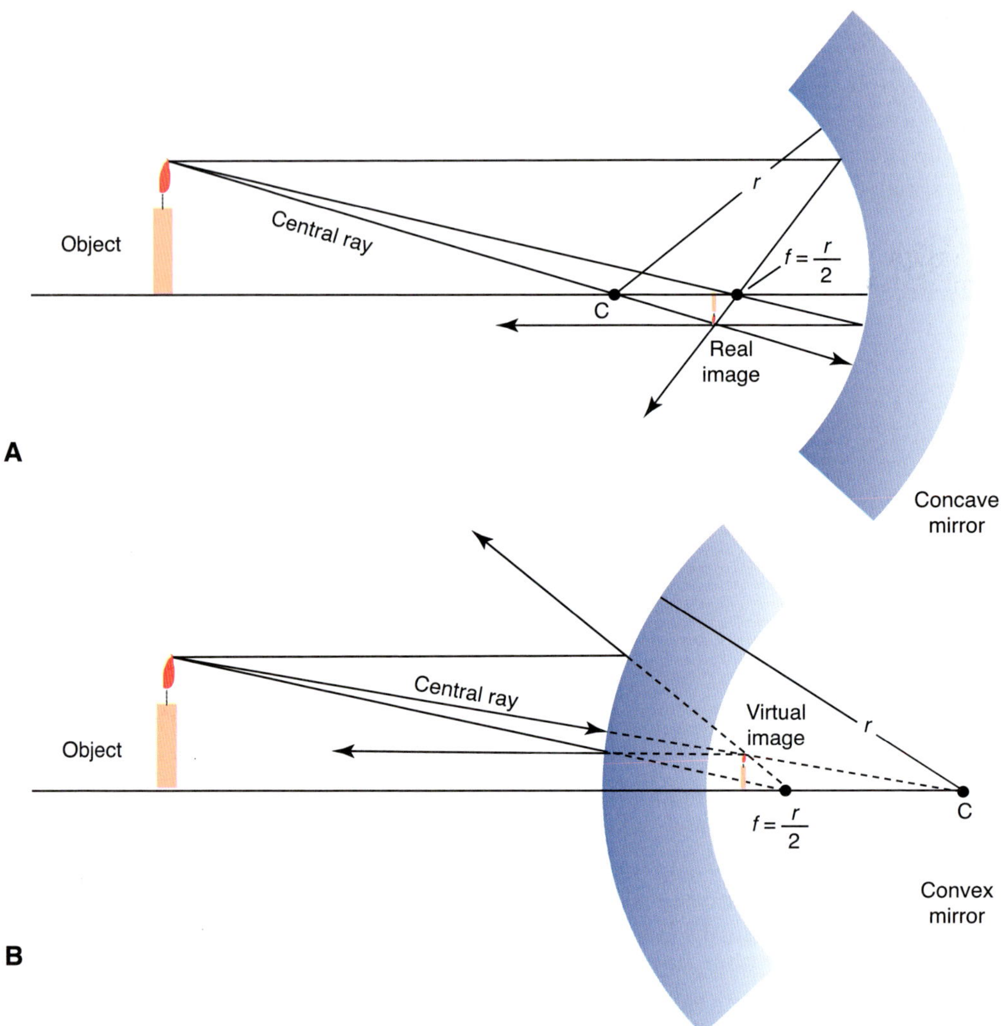

Figure 1-35 Ray tracing for concave **(A)** and convex **(B)** mirrors. The central ray for mirrors differs from the central ray for lenses in that it passes through the center of curvature (C) of the mirror, not through the center of the mirror. *(Illustration developed by Kevin M. Miller, MD, and rendered by C. H. Wooley.)*

(not the vertex on the optic axis, as for lenses) is the undeviated ray; (2) the ray that passes through the focal point is reflected parallel to the optic axis; and (3) the ray that propagates parallel to the optic axis passes through the focal point of the mirror, which is halfway between the mirror surface and the center of curvature.

Convex mirrors will always form virtual, upright, and minified images. Concave mirrors can form a variety of images, depending on where the object is located in relation to the mirror. Of note, only when the object is located to the right of f will the mirror yield an image that is upright, virtual, and magnified. Finally, as the object draws closer to a concave mirror, the magnification will continue to decrease until it is just to the left of the mirror, when the image size will equal object size—similar to a plane mirror.

Only a few examples occur commonly in everyday life: for example, a large-radius concave mirror, such as that used as a cosmetic or shaving mirror, with the source object closer than the focal point (ie, immediately to the right of *f*); and a small-radius convex mirror, such as those used in rearview mirrors on automobiles. In ophthalmic practice, the cornea is used as a small-radius reflecting surface to measure the corneal curvature (keratometry).

EXAMPLE 1-13

Show the ray tracing for a shaving mirror, and compute the image location and magnification.

For a concave mirror to work as a magnifier, suitable as a shaving or cosmetic mirror, the source object (such as your face) must be closer to the mirror than the focal point. Suppose the radius of the mirror is –2.0 m. Using the previously discussed equations, we can determine that the focal point is 1.0 m to the left of the mirror and the power of the mirror is +1.00 D (concave mirror). Suppose we stand 0.5 m to the left of the mirror. We can use the vergence equation: $-1/0.5 + 1.00\ \text{D} = V = -1$. Therefore, $v = -1$ m. The minus sign implies that the image is 1 m to the *right* of the mirror, as the image space is reversed (Fig 1-E13). Thus, the image is twice as far "behind" the mirror as the source was in front of the mirror, and similar triangles yield a magnification factor of +2.0. Similarly, $M_T = U/V = -2/-1 = 2\times$ magnification.

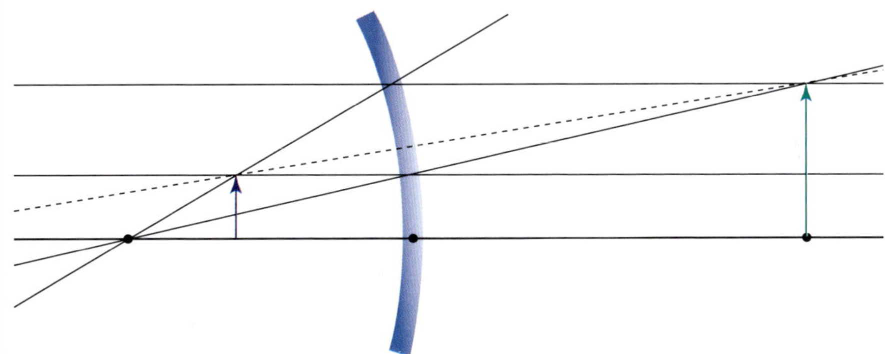

Figure 1-E13 Ray tracing for a concave shaving mirror.

Section Exercise 1-31

Show the ray tracing for the image of a penlight as reflected in the human cornea, as in the Hirschberg test for strabismus (see BCSC Section 6, *Pediatric Ophthalmology and Strabismus*). This diagram is depicted in Figure 1-35B.

Telescopes

Galilean, or terrestrial, *telescopes* consist of a lower-power positive lens (the *objective*) and a higher-power minus lens (the *ocular,* or eyepiece) separated by the difference in their focal lengths. *Keplerian,* or astronomical, *telescopes* consist of a lower-power positive objective lens and a higher-power positive eyepiece separated by the sum of their focal lengths (Fig 1-36). (Technically, the separation of the lenses is $f_1 - f_2$ for both types of telescopes because f_2 is negative for the Keplerian telescope.) We can easily construct both types by using trial lenses. The Galilean telescope produces an upright image; the Keplerian, an inverted image. However, by placing prisms inside the Keplerian telescope, we can achieve an upright image. Most binoculars are Keplerian telescopes with inverting prisms. Many commonly used surgical loupes employ a Galilean telescope construction, though astronomical telescope constructions are also available.

In both types of telescope, an object ray parallel to the optic axis is conjugate to an image ray parallel to the axis. Consequently, the system considered as a whole has no focal points and, thus, is termed an *afocal system.* In addition, considered as a whole, telescopes have no principal planes and no nodal points.

Both types of telescope produce images smaller than the original object: $M_T = -P_1/P_2$. In the examples shown in Figure 1-36, the image is half the size of the object (note the distance between the horizontal entering ray and the horizontal exiting ray). However, the

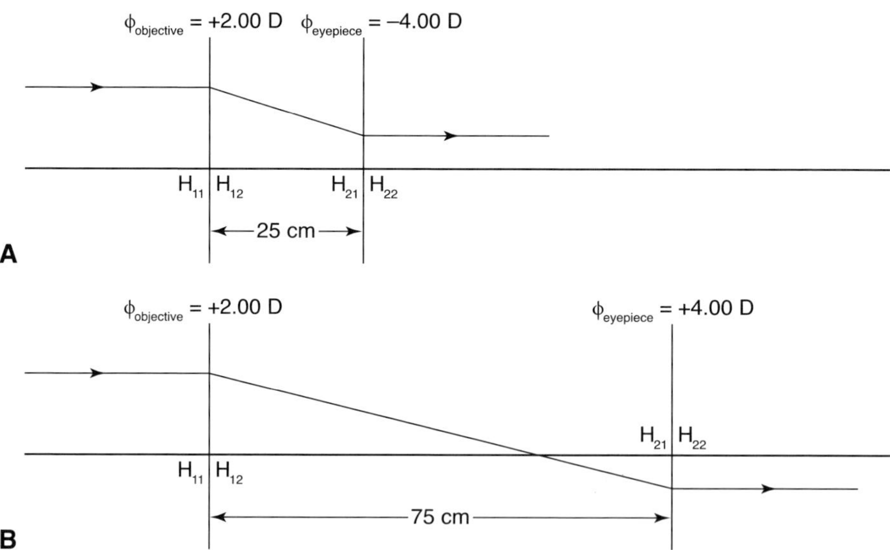

Figure 1-36 Ray tracing for 2 types of telescopes. **A,** A Galilean telescope consists of the objective (a low-power plus lens) and the eyepiece, or ocular (a higher-power minus lens), separated by the difference of their focal lengths. **B,** A Keplerian telescope consists of a low-power plus lens (objective) and a higher-power plus lens (eyepiece). In both cases, an object ray parallel to the axis is conjugate to an image ray parallel to the axis. Consequently, although the individual lenses have focal points, the system as a whole does not. *(Courtesy of Edmond H. Thall, MD.)*

image appears larger because it is much closer to the eye. In those examples, the image appears 4 times closer than the original object. Because the image is half the size of the original object but 4 times closer, the angle the image subtends and the appearance of the image are twice as large as the original object.

In general, we use telescopes to view objects at very great ("astronomical") distances, for which transverse magnification is of little interest. It is more useful to describe the magnification in such a system in terms of the ratio of the angular separation between source objects as seen without the telescope and the angular separation between their images as seen through the telescope. With careful ray tracing, we can show that this ratio, the *angular magnification*, is given by

$$M_a = \frac{-P_{\text{eyepiece}}}{P_{\text{objective}}}$$

Telescopes are sometimes prescribed as visual aids for visually impaired patients (see Chapter 10). The Galilean telescope is generally preferred for visual aids because it is shorter than the Keplerian and produces an upright image. The Keplerian telescope can produce an upright image only by incorporating inverting prisms, which increase the weight of the visual aid. However, Keplerian telescopes gather more light than Galilean telescopes do—a quality that is advantageous in some situations.

The concept of telescopes may also help to explain the magnification experienced by hyperopic and aphakic patients wearing spectacles. If we imagine that the refractive error caused by a minus-powered "error lens" inside the eye of an aphakic patient (−12.50 D) is corrected with +10.00 D spectacles, we can see that this patient is now looking at the world through a Galilean telescope. Using the magnification equation above, we observe that this patient will experience 1.25× magnification and thus may be subjectively unhappy. Similarly, highly myopic patients have a plus-powered "error lens" inside the eye; when these patients are corrected with high-power minus lens spectacles, we have essentially given them a reverse Galilean telescope. These patients may complain of minification issues.

Appendix 1-1

Derivation of the Vergence Equation and the Lensmaker's Equation From Snell's Law

Consider Figure 1-A1. A light ray traveling from left to right (shown in dark green) is incident on a curved refracting surface with radius of curvature r and center of curvature C on the optic axis OC. Suppose the index of refraction to the left of the surface is n_1, to the right of the surface n_2 (shown with $n_2 > n_1$). The incident ray strikes the axis at distance u from the vertex, O, of the refracting surface and meets the surface at a height h from the axis, making an angle, α, with the optic axis. The incident ray makes an angle θ with the surface normal and is then refracted such that it makes, say, a smaller angle, σ, with the surface normal to the right of the refracting surface. The refracted ray (shown in light green) meets the axis at

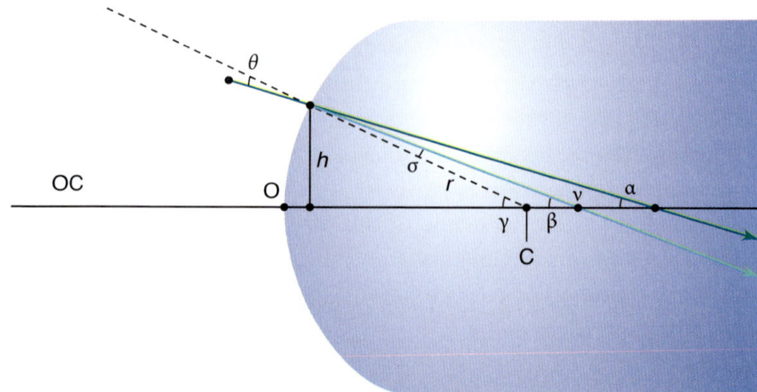

Figure 1-A1 Geometry for deriving the vergence equation and the lensmaker's equation from Snell's law.

a distance ν from the vertex, forming an angle β with the axis. The angle subtended by the height h at the center of the circle is denoted by γ.

In the paraxial regime, angles θ, σ, α, β, and γ are small (that is, h is substantially smaller than r). We use the small-angle approximation from trigonometry: for small angles ϕ,

$$\phi = \sin \phi = \tan \phi$$

With this approximation, Snell's law, $n_1 \sin \theta = n_2 \sin \sigma$, simplifies to

$$n_1\theta = n_2 \sigma \tag{1}$$

Similarly, using the tangent approximation for angles α, β, and γ and, in the same spirit, ignoring the discrepancy between the foot of the perpendicular from the point of incidence and O, we have

$$\alpha = \frac{h}{u}; \beta = \frac{h}{v}; \gamma = \frac{h}{r} \tag{2}$$

Finally, from geometry (the exterior-angle theorem and the fact that opposite angles are equal), we observe that

$$\gamma = \theta + \alpha \text{ and } \gamma = \beta + \sigma$$

so

$$\theta = \gamma - \alpha \text{ and } \sigma = \gamma - \beta \tag{3}$$

From here, it is only algebra: substituting Equation (Eq) 3 into Eq 1 gives

$$n_1(\gamma - \alpha) = n_2(\gamma - \beta)$$

so

$$\gamma(n_2 - n_1) = n_2\beta - n_1\alpha \tag{4}$$

Substituting Eq 2 into Eq 4 gives

$$\left(\frac{h}{r}\right)(n_2 - n_1) = n_2\left(\frac{h}{v}\right) - n_1\left(\frac{h}{u}\right)$$

Clearing the common factor h and rearranging yields

$$\frac{n_1}{u} + \frac{(n_2 - n_1)}{r} = \frac{n_2}{v}$$

Equating $(n_2 - n_1)/r$ with P yields both the vergence equation and the lensmaker's equation at once!

Appendix 1-2

Fermat's Principle

The basic rules of geometric optics (straight-line propagation of light in homogeneous media, the law of reflection, and Snell's law) are readily interpreted as a manifestation of Fermat's principle. This interpretation is frequently stated as the observation that the path of a light ray between 2 fixed points is the path that takes the least time. Thus, in a homogeneous medium, where the shortest path between the 2 points obviously corresponds to the path that takes the least time, it follows that light travels in straight lines.

Similarly, a simple geometric construction confirms that, of all reflecting paths connecting 2 points on the same side of a smooth reflecting surface, the path with the angle of incidence equal to the angle of reflection is the shortest. In this sense, the law of reflection is likewise a manifestation of Fermat's principle (Fig 1-A2A).

The proof of Snell's law is only slightly more difficult. Consider Figure 1-A2B. Among the paths shown between points A and B, the shortest (straight-line) path is not the path of least travel time; we can save time by changing, for example, from Path 3 to Path 2 to reduce the portion of the travel time in glass, where the speed of light is slower than that in air. Eventually, the trade-off works the other way, as in Path 1. We can determine the optimal path by calculating the distance in air and in glass for each possible inflection point and dividing by the speed of light in each medium.

Using the geometry shown in Figure 1-A2C, we denote the distance traveled through a medium 1 and a medium 2 as d_1 and d_2, respectively. Then

$$d_1 = \sqrt{a^2 + x^2} \text{ and } d_2 = \sqrt{b^2 + (l - x)^2}$$

where x is the vertical distance traversed through medium 1 and l is the total vertical distance traversed through both media. We divide by the speed of light in each medium (which is c/n_1 *or* c/n_2, respectively, where c is the speed of light in a vacuum) and add the 2 values to get the total travel time T:

$$T = \sqrt{a^2 + x^2}\left(\frac{n_1}{c}\right) + \sqrt{b^2 + (l - x)^2}\left(\frac{n_2}{c}\right)$$

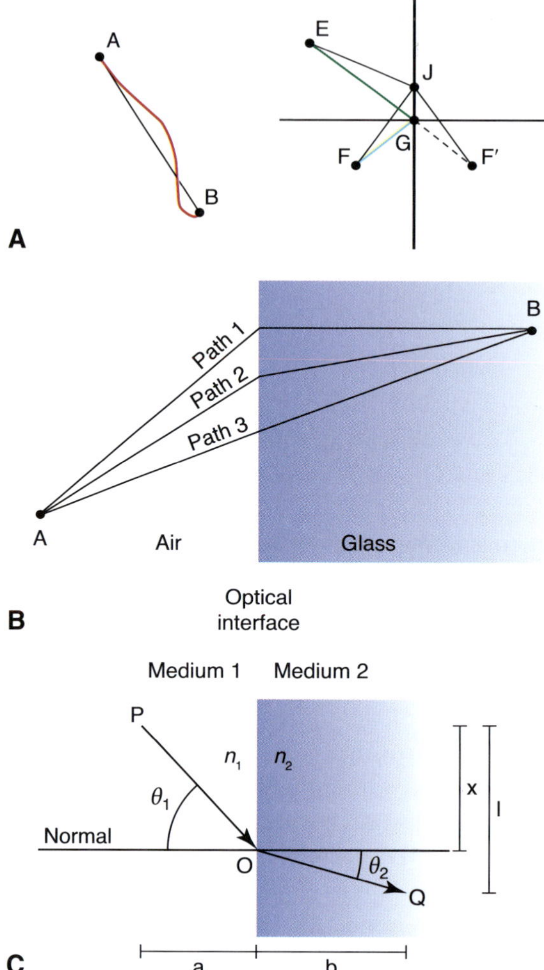

Figure 1-A2 Fermat's principle. **A,** *Left:* The straight path between points A and B is the shortest and thus takes the least time among all possible paths from A to B. *Right:* Light reflecting from point E to point F takes the shortest possible path when the extension of the straight path from E to the mirror reaches the mirror image point F′ along a straight line. That extension locates the point of reflection at G, such that the angle of incidence equals the angle of reflection. Other possible paths, such as that through point J, are longer and take more time. **B,** Because light travels faster through air than through glass, path 3 is not the path of shortest travel time. Path 2 saves time overall by spending less time in glass. **C,** Geometry for demonstration of Snell's law from Fermat's principle.

To minimize the total transit time, we seek the value of x for which the *derivative* of the transit time, dT/dx, is equal to 0. Dredging up our knowledge of freshman calculus (and canceling the common factor of c), we obtain

$$\frac{n_1 x}{\sqrt{a^2+x^2}} - \frac{n_2(1-x)}{\sqrt{b^2+(l-x)^2}} = 0$$

But careful inspection of Figure 1-A2C indicates that the fractions in this equation are in fact the sines of the angles of incidence and refraction, respectively—that is,

$$n_1 \sin \theta_1 = n_2 \sin \theta_2$$

which is Snell's law.

Appendix 1-3

Derivation of the Vergence Equation for Mirrors

Consider Figure 1-A3. The incident ray (shown in dark green) moves from left to right and would intersect the optic axis at u if the ray did not first intersect the mirror (here drawn convex to the left, with radius of curvature r) at height h above the optic axis. The direction of the reflected ray (shown in light green) is determined by the law of reflection, so the angle $\gamma/2$ between the incident ray and the mirror's surface normal (drawn as a dashed line) equals the angle $\gamma/2$ between the surface normal and the reflected ray. The reflected ray travels from right to left, but if extended, it would intersect the optic axis at ν. The angles between the optic axis and the reflected ray, radius of curvature to the point of reflection, and incident ray are denoted α, θ, and β, respectively.

In this case, the direction of the reflected ray is determined by the law of reflection instead of Snell's law. We have:

$$\alpha = \gamma + \beta \tag{1}$$

$$\alpha = \theta + \frac{\gamma}{2}$$

$$\gamma = 2\alpha - 2\theta \tag{2}$$

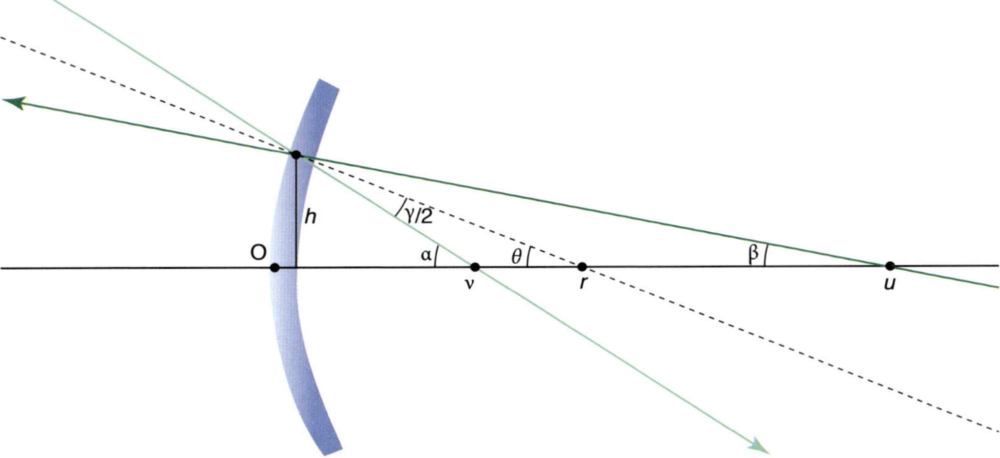

Figure 1-A3 Geometry for deriving the vergence equation for mirrors from the law of reflection. *(Illustration developed by Scott E. Brodie, MD, PhD.)*

Inserting Eq 2 into Eq 1 gives

$$\alpha = 2\alpha - 2\theta + \beta$$

so

$$\alpha = 2\theta - \beta$$

Using the small-angle approximations for α, β, and θ (as in Appendix 1-1), we have

$$\frac{h}{v} = 2\frac{h}{r} - \frac{h}{u}$$

Canceling the common factor h and rearranging gives

$$\frac{1}{u} - \frac{2}{r} = -\frac{1}{v}$$

By identifying $P = -2/r$ as the power of the mirror and interpreting the minus sign on the right side of the equation as indicating a vergence of "1/v" in the "reversed" image space, we obtain the vergence equation for mirrors.

Appendix 1-4

Dynamic Ray Tracing

Image formation by simple lenses can be readily simulated by means of dynamic geometry software. Four examples of this are accessible via the QR code below. The "One Point" drawings illustrate a point source object imaged by convex and concave lenses. Dragging the "source object" dots demonstrates the effects on image size and location of moving the source object. The "Locus" drawings illustrate the imaging of a circular source object. Clicking on the arrow at the lower left animates the drawing and shows, in particular, the disparity between transverse and axial magnification. Compare with Figures 1-14, 1-15, and 1-21.

CHAPTER 2

Physical Optics

This chapter includes a related video. Go to www.aao.org/bcscvideo_section03 or scan the QR code in the text to access this content.

Highlights

- Quantum electrodynamics (QED) explains all the properties of light we know, resolving the wave–particle confusion.
- For physical phenomena at the macroscopic level, such as polarization, interference, coherence, and diffraction, it suffices to consider the wavelike behavior of light.
- We differentiate between radiometric and photometric measures of light; photometry can be considered a subtype of radiometry that adjusts for the variable spectral response of the human eye.
- To understand lasers and their therapeutic interaction with tissue, it becomes crucial to consider the quantum behavior of light.
- Therapeutic and nontherapeutic damage to the eye caused by light is primarily dependent on the wavelength as well as the irradiance and duration of light exposure.

Glossary

Coherence A measure of the uniformity and homogeneity of a beam of light. Coherence governs the ability of light to produce interference phenomena.

Diffraction The spreading of light beyond the edges of a small aperture or "bending around the corners" of an obstruction into a region where—using strictly geometric optics reasoning—we would not expect to see it. This phenomenon sets a limit on the resolution that can be achieved in any optical instrument. With a circular aperture such as the pupil, for example, the image of a point source of light formed on the retina—the point spread function (PSF)—in the absence of aberrations takes the form of alternating bright and dark rings surrounding a bright central spot, the Airy disc, rather than a point.

Geometric scattering Scattering of light by particles that occurs if the particle size is very large compared to the wavelength of incident light. The interaction of light with the particle is usually sufficiently described by the laws of geometric optics (refraction and reflection). The formation of a rainbow, for example, is sufficiently described by refraction and reflection by raindrops.

Interference Interference reveals the correlation between light waves and occurs when 2 light waves are brought together (superposition of waves), reinforcing each other and resulting in a wave of greater amplitude (ie, *constructive* or additive *interference*), or subtracting from each other and resulting in a wave of lower amplitude (ie, *destructive* or subtractive *interference*).

Laser Acronym for Light Amplification by Stimulated Emission of Radiation. A device which produces highly monochromatic, highly coherent beams of light.

Mie scattering Scattering of light produced by particles whose size is the same order of magnitude as the wavelength of incident light. Mie scattering caused by water droplets contributes to the white appearance of clouds. Similarly, Mie scattering caused by a cataract accounts for the whitish appearance of the lens under slit-lamp examination.

Photometry A measurement of the human visual system's psychophysical response to light. Basically, photometry can be considered a subtype of radiometry that adjusts for the varying sensitivity of the eye to different wavelengths in the visible spectrum.

Polarization Light is said to be polarized when the orientation of the electric field, as it oscillates perpendicularly to the direction of propagation, is not random. The polarization state can be pictorially represented by the path that the tip of the electric-field vector traces with time as viewed along the propagation axis while one looks toward the source, and can be linear, circular, or elliptical.

Quantum electrodynamics (QED) The quantum theory of the interaction of light and matter that resolves the wave–particle confusion. The theory describes most of the phenomena of the physical world—including all observed phenomena of light—except for gravitational and nuclear phenomena.

Radiometry Refers to the direct measurement of light in any portion of the electromagnetic spectrum. In contrast to photometric measurements, radiometric measurements weight equally the energy transmitted at every wavelength of the electromagnetic spectrum.

Rayleigh scattering Wavelength-dependent scattering that occurs when light interacts with particles much smaller than the wavelength of the light. The blue appearance of the sky during daytime and its reddish appearance during sunrise or sunset is due to Rayleigh scattering by atmospheric gas molecules. The bluish appearance of the cornea and lens (particularly noticeable in young eyes) under slit-lamp examination is also due to Rayleigh scattering by stromal collagen and lenticular fiber cells.

Wave-particle confusion The ambiguity of the behavior of light as observed at different scales: at large scales, light exhibits wave properties, such as polarization and interference. At smaller scales, light behaves as a stream of particles, transferring momentum and transferring energy in discrete quanta.

Introduction

The discussion of *geometric optics* in Chapter 1 disregards the wavelength and photon character of light. It uses the artificial construct of light rays to show how light behaves on a large scale, compared with the dimensions of interest.

Physical optics goes beyond ray tracings and vergence calculations and deals with the properties of light on smaller scales, providing explanations for many of the phenomena of the physical world, such as *polarization, interference, coherence,* and *diffraction,* for which the ray approximation of geometric optics is insufficient.

What Is Light?

Visible Light

In ophthalmic optics, the term *light* generally refers to visible light, which is just a very narrow portion of a long scale, analogous to a musical scale, in which there are "notes" both higher and lower than we can perceive (Fig 2-1). The visual perception of these notes—specified by *frequency* (ν) and *wavelength* (λ) along the "scale" of light *(the electromagnetic*

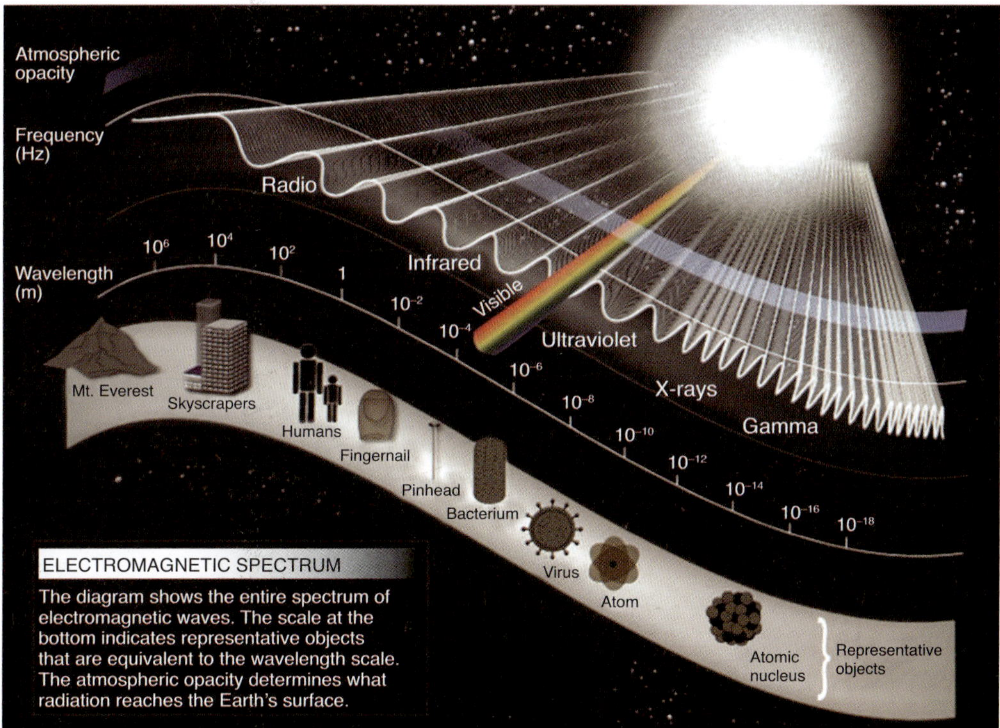

Figure 2-1 The electromagnetic (EM) spectrum. The spectrum is divided into several regions according to the wavelength or frequency of light. Note that visible light is just a very narrow portion of the entire EM spectrum. *(Courtesy of NASA.)*

spectrum) and related to each other via the "speed of light" ($c = \nu\,\lambda \approx 3 \times 10^8$ m/s in a vacuum)—is what we call (spectral) *color.*

Although the visible spectrum is normally considered to run from 400–700 nm, the boundaries are not precise. Under certain conditions, such as with sufficiently intense light, the eye's sensitivity extends into the infrared and ultraviolet (UV) regions. As another example, in aphakia, without the UV absorption of the natural lens, the retina can detect wavelengths well below 400 nm.

Wave or Particle?

The earliest comprehensive theories on the nature of light were advanced around the turn of the 17th century. In 1690, Christiaan Huygens put forward a *wave theory* of light, demonstrating how light waves might superimpose (interfere) to form a wavefront, similar to water waves (Fig 2-2), and travel in a straight line (in accordance with the ray approximation of geometric optics). As such, Huygens's wave theory covered little of what we would call physical optics today and was soon overshadowed by Isaac Newton's particle viewpoint. Newton suggested that light was made of particles—he called them "corpuscles." The *particle theory* of light took precedence and was accepted essentially unchallenged for over a century.

In the early 19th century, Thomas Young's double-slit experiment appeared to prove the wavelike behavior of light, via the observation of bright and dark bands (fringes) upon illumination of a barrier with 2 narrow openings, very similar to the interference pattern that results from the superposition of water waves. Later that century, James Clerk Maxwell formulated light entirely as a wave; that is, as the propagation of electromagnetic waves (Fig 2-3) according to his Maxwell equations. Thus, for many years after Newton, as interference, diffraction, and other phenomena were readily explained by waves, the wave model became the dominant theory of the nature of light.

However, it is now clear that light also exhibits properties of particles, as seen in experiments with instruments that are sensitive enough to detect very weak light. An example of such an instrument is a photomultiplier, which produces "clicks" when light is shined on it. According to the wave theory, these clicks should become less loud as the intensity of the impinging light is decreased. In reality, these clicks remain equally loud but decrease in frequency. Thus, light can be thought of as something like raindrops, with each little "drop" being called a photon.

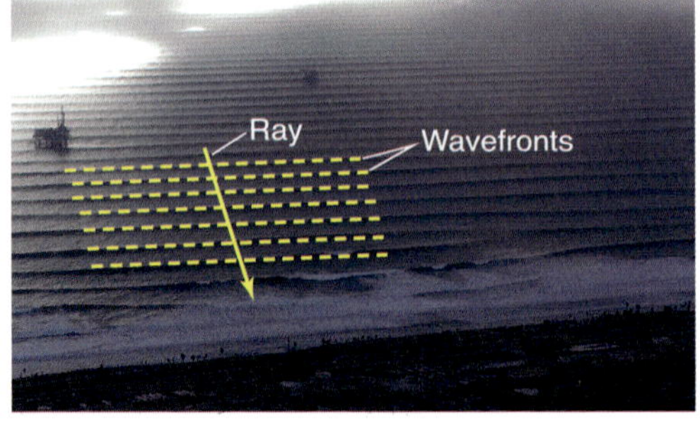

Figure 2-2 Construct of wavefronts, representing the wave crests (namely the locations for which the wave is maximum at a given time), illustrated in the example of water waves. Note that wavefronts are perpendicular to the ray direction. *(Photograph by Sang Pak; developed by Kristina Irsch, PhD.)*

In the early 20th century, Albert Einstein postulated light as the sum of individual packets (quanta) of energy, and thus was born the word *photon* and the quantum theory of light (Fig 2-4). This influenced the formation of the concept of a *wave–particle duality* of light, which was not a very satisfactory theory, but rather represented a state of confusion as to exactly which model to use in each circumstance. Maxwell's theory of electromagnetism (which fails to explain the observations with very dim light falling on photomultipliers) had to be modified to conform with the concepts of *quantum mechanics* (essentially a description of the motion of electrons in matter).

A new theory—*quantum electrodynamics (QED)*—the quantum theory of the interaction of light and matter, developed by a number of physicists in 1929 and clarified by Richard Feynman and 2 other physicists, Julian Schwinger and Sin-Itiro Tomonaga, in 1948, unites Maxwell's equations of electricity and magnetism with quantum mechanics. QED,

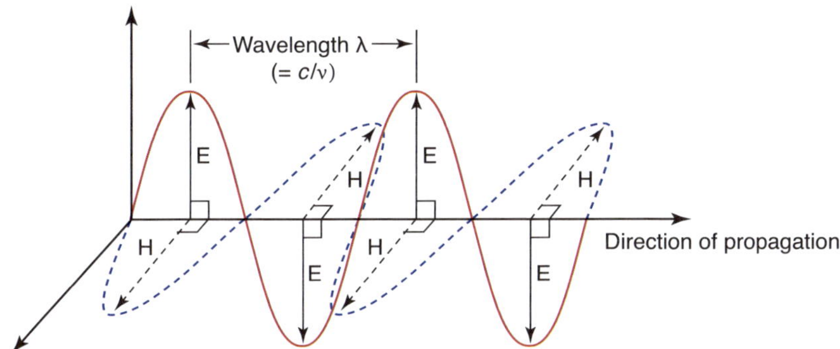

Figure 2-3 Electromagnetic wave theory. According to EM wave theory, light may be described as a transverse EM wave, whose oscillating electric (E) and magnetic (H) fields are perpendicular both to each other as well as to the direction that the light travels. The wavelength (λ) and frequency (ν) of light are related to each other via the "speed of light" ($c = \nu\lambda \approx 3 \times 10^8$ m/s in vacuum). *(Illustration by Kristina Irsch, PhD.)*

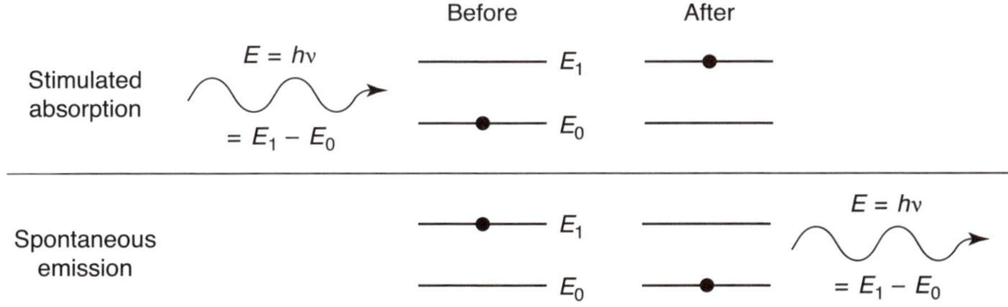

Figure 2-4 Quantum theory. According to quantum theory, electrons in atoms (or molecules) exist in nonradiating states, with each state being associated with a specific energy level. In a process called stimulated absorption, an electron moves between its lowest energy (ground) state (E_0) and an excited state (E_1) after picking up (absorbing) a photon or quantum of energy ($E = E_1 - E_0 = h\nu$). Similarly, a photon is given off (emitted) when an electron moves from a higher energy state to a lower one (spontaneous emission). *h* is the Planck constant. *(Reproduced with permission from Steinert RF, Puliafito CA.* The Nd:YAG Laser in Ophthalmology: Principles and Clinical Applications of Photodisruption. *Saunders; 1985. Redrawn by C. H. Wooley and modified by Kristina Irsch, PhD.)*

which states that light is made of particles, thereby resolves the wave–particle confusion—not in the ordinary sense of providing equations that can be used to predict exactly what will happen in any given experiment, but rather by providing tools with which one is able to calculate the probability of an outcome event.

Thus, contrary to what is taught in many ophthalmology and ophthalmic optics textbooks, there is one theory that explains all the properties of light we know: QED. Note that for most purposes, it suffices to consider the wavelike behavior of light (see Fig 2-3) for phenomena at the macroscopic level and the simple quantum-view of the light (see Fig 2-4) at the microscopic level, as will be illustrated in this chapter.

Feynman RP. *QED: The Strange Theory of Light and Matter.* Princeton University Press; 2014.

Quantum Electrodynamics: Unifying Theory of Light

Quantum electrodynamics describes most of the phenomena of the physical world, except for gravitational and nuclear phenomena. All these phenomena can be deduced from 3 basic actions, each of which occurs with a certain probability that can be calculated using the tools of the theory: (1) a photon goes from point to point, (2) an electron goes from point to point, and (3) an electron emits (or absorbs) a photon. Qualitatively, the theory boils down to photons, which make up the light, going from one electron to another, and electrons, which make up matter, picking up and giving off photons while moving about.

Refraction and Reflection

Both refraction (transmission) and reflection are the result of the interaction of light and matter, that is, of photons with electrons in the atoms and molecules inside the refractive and/or reflective media.

Chapter 1 explains that light changes speed and direction when moving from one medium to another. However, the individual photons do not move more slowly inside the material. Slowing of the light is caused by the electrons throughout the material scattering the photons, and the degree to which there is scattering is called the refractive index for that particular medium. Similarly, light is not reflected off a surface. In reality, the photons are scattered by the electrons in the material, the net result of which is the same as if the photons hit and were reflected at the surface.

This is what essentially happens during refraction and reflection: a photon arrives from the outside, hits an electron, and is picked up by the electron *(absorption);* some time later, the electron emits a new photon. This dance of photons and electrons is called *scattering* of light. Thus, in refracted and reflected light, the photon that emerges from the process is not the same photon as the one that went in. Hence, the behavior of light in classical optics reflects the net result rather than the actual path of the photon, providing a convenient "straight-line" approximation to describe the phenomena we are familiar with.

Scattering

The scattering of light by an electron in an atom is the phenomenon that accounts for reflection and transmission (refraction) in a medium. Light scattering, among other factors, is also responsible for the visible appearance or perception of color and may be divided into 3 regimes—*Rayleigh scattering, Mie scattering,* and *geometric scattering*—according to the dimensions of the scattering medium compared with the wavelength of the incident light. Note that the Tyndall effect, a term commonly used in ophthalmology and chemistry for scattering of light by colloidal suspensions, does not describe a separate scattering regime, but rather the effect of the light beam becoming visible. For example, normally you cannot see a beam of light in water or the aqueous humor. Shining a flashlight beam in a glass of water after adding a few drops of milk is an excellent demonstration of the Tyndall effect. The milk proteins will stay suspended in the water (a colloid suspension), making the beam visible. Similarly, if we can see the beam of light in the aqueous humor during slit-lamp examination, this is an indication of inflammation; in other words, an indication resulting from the presence of suspended protein in the aqueous.

Rayleigh scattering

Rayleigh scattering occurs when light interacts with particles *much smaller* than the wavelength of the light. The degree of this form of scattering varies strongly with wavelength, more precisely, inversely to its fourth power. Therefore, the probability that light will scatter is much higher for shorter wavelengths (higher frequencies), such as blue light, than for longer wavelengths (lower frequencies), such as red light.

The effect of Rayleigh scattering of sunlight on gas molecules that make up the Earth's atmosphere is what produces the blue appearance of the sky during daytime and its reddish appearance during sunrise or sunset. This is because during daytime, when the sun is overhead, the highly scattered wavelengths from the blue end of the spectrum that are emitted by the sun reach your eye from all directions, whereas the weakly scattered redder wavelengths miss your line of sight when you look at the sky away from the direction of the sun. At sunrise and sunset, with the sun at the horizon, it is the weakly scattered wavelengths from the red end of the spectrum that can still be seen, passing through the atmosphere toward your eyes almost undeviated, while the blue light that is scattered misses your line of sight. This can be appreciated and re-created at home, with the help of a flashlight and a transparent bowl containing some water and a few drops of milk. With direct viewing of the flashlight beam, and with the light traveling through the diameter of the bowl, a red or orange glow can be perceived. If, on the other hand, the light is shined from above, a blue glow can be observed.

Stromal collagen and lenticular fiber cells cause Rayleigh scattering of incident light, which is responsible for the bluish appearance of the cornea and lens (particularly noticeable in young eyes) under slit-lamp examination.

Mie scattering

Mie scattering is produced by particles whose size is the *same order of magnitude* as the wavelength of incident light. Unlike Rayleigh scattering, this form of scattering, on average, does not vary strongly with wavelength and tends to be stronger in the forward direction (ie, a direction that is within 90° of the direction of propagation) than in any other direction.

Mie scattering contributes to the white appearance of clouds. This is because the water droplets that make up the cloud are of comparable size to the visible wavelengths, so that the probability of being scattered is about identical for the different wavelengths (or frequencies) in the white sunlight, and the clouds therefore appear to be white.

In the eye, age-related increase in scattering is mostly associated with an increase in Mie scattering by cataract formation, which adds a strong forward, but less wavelength-dependent, component to the Rayleigh scattering (the predominant scattering component in healthy young eyes). Mie scattering caused by a cataract accounts for the whitish appearance of the lens under slit-lamp examination. The increase in forward scattering is what results in decreased contrast of the patient's retinal image, and hence increased glare sensitivity. Similarly, Mie scattering on microvacuoles is responsible for degraded visual quality associated with the formation of glistenings in intraocular lenses.

Geometric scattering

If the particle size is much larger than the wavelength of incident light, the interaction of light with the particle is usually sufficiently described by the laws of geometric optics (refraction and reflection). For example, refraction and reflection are sufficient to explain the formation of a rainbow. This is because raindrops are larger than water droplets in clouds and can be considered as merely refracting and reflecting the white sunlight from their surfaces. This nicely illustrates how at the macroscopic level the quantum behavior of light can be conveniently disregarded.

Phenomena of Light

Although QED can account for all observed phenomena of light, several macroscopic phenomena of light, such as polarization, coherence, and interference, can completely, and more easily, be explained by Maxwell's classical theory of electromagnetic waves. In this context, light may therefore be described as a transverse electromagnetic wave whose oscillating electric and magnetic fields are perpendicular both to each other as well as to the direction that the light travels (see Fig 2-3).

Polarization

Fundamentals

As light travels within homogeneous and isotropic media, the magnetic field is always perpendicular and proportional to the electric field. It is thus convenient to focus on only one of them when considering polarization, typically the electric field. The orientation of the electric field, as it oscillates perpendicularly to the direction of propagation, defines the state of polarization. Note that the electric-field vector, which is shown oriented in a single plane in Figure 2-3, typically changes rapidly and randomly, resulting in randomly polarized light that is said to be *unpolarized.* When the movement of the electric-field vector is not random, the light is said to be polarized. Pictorially, the polarization state can be represented by the path that the tip of the electric-field vector traces with time as viewed along the propagation axis, looking toward the source (Lissajous figures). Figure 2-3 depicts *linearly polarized light,* with the electric-field vector being constrained to a single plane; when viewed head-on, it traces a single line. In *circularly polarized light,* the electric-field vector rotates, tracing a corkscrew pattern as the light propagates (Video 2-1). Viewed head-on, the pattern mapped out by the tip of the electric-field vector is a circle. In *elliptically polarized light,* which represents a more general case of circular polarization, the electric-field vector rotates and at the same time changes its amplitude as the light propagates, tracing an ellipse instead of a circle when viewed head-on.

VIDEO 2-1 Circularly polarized electromagnetic wave.
Animation developed by Kristina Irsch, PhD; based on graphics from Dave3457/Wikimedia Commons (public domain).

Polarized light can be produced in a number of ways. One way to produce completely or *partially polarized light* is by reflection. Partial polarization, as the name implies, is a mixture of unpolarized and polarized light (linear, circular, or elliptical). Fresnel showed that the polarized component of reflected light tends to be linear, parallel to the interface. Reflected light is completely polarized if the angle of incidence equals the *Brewster angle:*

$$\text{Brewster Angle} = \tan^{-1}\frac{n_t}{n_i}$$

where n_t and n_i are the refractive indices of the transmitted and incident media, respectively. At the Brewster angle, all the *reflected* light is linearly polarized, but not all the linearly incident light is reflected. Consequently, the *transmitted* light is a mixture of linearly and randomly polarized (commonly referred to as "unpolarized") light—that is, it is partially polarized.

Applications and clinical relevance

Ophthalmic applications of polarization are numerous, some of which are discussed briefly here. Polarizing sunglasses are sometimes useful for reducing glare from reflected sunlight. Reflected light is somewhat polarized parallel to the reflecting surface, and in most environments, reflecting objects tend to be horizontal. In boating, for example, sunlight reflected from the water surface is partially polarized, usually horizontally, as is light reflected from a road surface or from the hood of a car. Even the sky acts as a partial polarizer by means of the scattering properties of air molecules. Accordingly, sunglasses incorporate vertically oriented linear polarizers (polarizing filters) to block the horizontally polarized component of reflected light.

Several stereopsis tests incorporate the use of linear polarizers. The well-known Stereo Fly test, for example, displays 2 slightly displaced images that linearly polarize light in perpendicular meridians. The person being assessed wears glasses containing linear polarizers, also at right angles to each other; each eye sees just 1 of the images. Thus, a single 3-dimensional (3D) image is perceived by someone with normal 3D or stereoscopic vision.

Interference and Coherence

Fundamentals

Figure 2-5 illustrates the basic concept of interference by means of Young's double-slit experiment, discussed earlier. Upon illumination of a single slit or pinhole aperture, spherical wavefronts emanate; this is similar to what can be observed when water waves encounter a

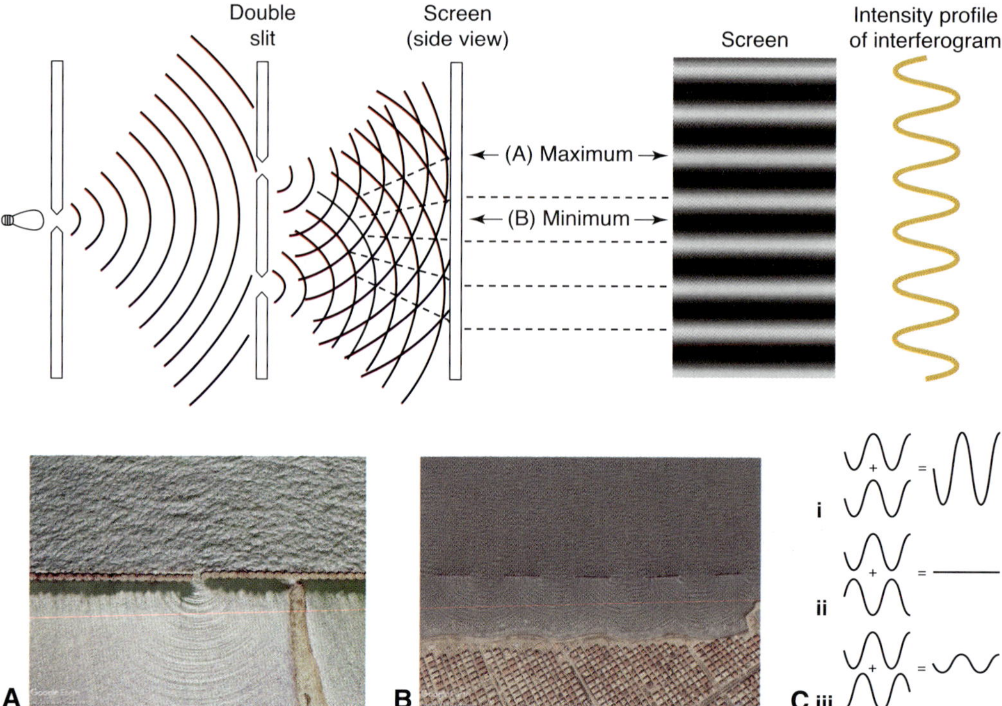

Figure 2-5 Pictorial explanation of interference via Young's double-slit experiment. Upon illumination of a single-slit or pinhole aperture, spherical wavefronts emanate, similar to water waves encountering a barrier with an opening **(A).** The wavefronts (curved lines) then strike a double-slit from which new wavefronts emerge, which are then superimposed on a screen, creating an interference pattern of a series of bright and dark bands (fringes), similar to what can be observed from the superposition of water waves **(B). C,** Superposition of waves of identical frequency and amplitude produces stable interference patterns. **i,** Waves overlap "in phase"—peaks (wave crests) coincide with peaks and troughs with troughs—producing a resultant wave of twice the amplitude. **ii,** Waves overlap "out of phase"—the peak of one wave coincides with the trough of the other—and the waves cancel. **iii,** Waves partially overlap—neither completely in nor out of phase—producing a wave of intermediate amplitude (between zero and twice the amplitude). *(Main illustration by Jonathan Clark; modified by Kristina Irsch, PhD. Part A from Google, IndianaMap framework data. Part B from Google, Maxar Technologies. Part C illustration developed by Edmond H. Thall, MD, and redrawn by C. H. Wooley.)*

barrier with a narrow opening (see Fig 2-5A). These wavefronts then strike a barrier with 2 narrow openings or a double slit, from which new wavefronts emerge; these are then brought together (superimposed) on a screen. If light of a single color (ie, monochromatic light) is used, a series of alternating bright and dark bands (fringes) is created. This interference pattern is very similar to what can be observed from the superposition of water waves (see Fig 2-5B) and reveals the interaction between the waves.

As shown in Figure 2-5C, the light waves may either reinforce each other, resulting in a wave of greater amplitude (ie, *constructive* or additive *interference*), or subtract from each other, resulting in a wave of lower amplitude (ie, *destructive* or subtractive *interference*). Note that the curved lines (wavefronts) represent the crests of the waves at a particular instant. Where the crests coincide (ie, the waves overlap "in phase"; eg, at i), a resultant wave of twice the amplitude is produced and brightness (intensity) on the screen is maximized. Note that intensity is a measure proportional to the square of the amplitude; with the amplitude of the wave doubled, the detected intensity is hence quadrupled. Where the crest of one wave coincides with the trough of the other wave (ie, the waves overlap "out of phase"; eg, at ii), the waves cancel each other and intensity is minimized. Where the waves partially overlap (ie, neither completely in nor out of phase; eg, at iii), a resultant wave between zero and twice the amplitude is produced and intensity on the screen is intermediate.

Another way to generate such interference patterns or interferograms is via a Michelson interferometer. In Michelson interferometry, as depicted in its basic configuration in Figure 2-6, light is first separated into 2 parts by a partially reflecting mirror or beam splitter. Each half-wave then propagates to a different mirror (50% of the light is reflected toward mirror 1 and the other 50% is transmitted to mirror 2) and, upon reflection from either mirror, is recombined with the other half-wave at the same beam splitter. Rather than the resultant interference-fringe pattern with areas of increased and decreased brightness being displayed by a screen or a camera, generally a detector is used to register interference effects by measuring the intensity level at the center of the interferogram.

The reader should be aware, however, that certain conditions have to be met in order to observe such interference phenomena. Not all sources of light generate visible interference-fringe patterns or detectable interference signals. A key ingredient missing from our basic discussion of interference thus far is coherence, which describes the ability of light to produce interference phenomena. If it generates a fringe pattern with areas of complete constructive and destructive interference, the light is considered to be fully

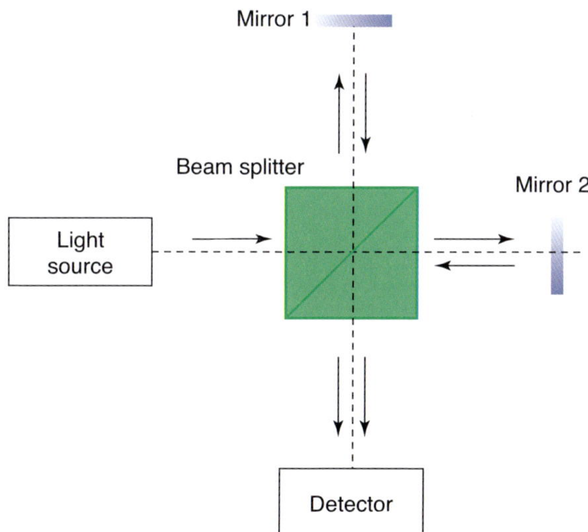

Figure 2-6 Basic concept of interferometry. Light is separated into 2 parts by a beam splitter; one half-wave is reflected toward mirror 1 and the other half is transmitted toward mirror 2. Upon reflection from either mirror, both parts recombine at the same beam splitter and are superimposed on a detector, which registers the resulting interference effects by measuring a signal of increased or decreased intensity, representing constructive and destructive interference of the waves, respectively. *(Illustration developed by Kristina Irsch, PhD.)*

coherent; if no fringe pattern is observable, it is considered incoherent. Light is considered partially coherent if a fringe pattern is still detectable, with less than "perfect" areas of constructive and destructive interference.

The visibility of interference effects thus provides a measure of the amount of coherence, which mathematically relates to the correlation of the light wave at different points in time or space. Hence, one generally differentiates between *temporal coherence* and *spatial coherence.* The latter refers to the similarity of wavefronts at different points in space, while the former describes the regularity of their spacing in time, or, in other words, how monochromatic the light is. More precisely, temporal coherence is the correlation of the light wave (at a single location) at different moments in time; spatial coherence is defined as the light wave correlation at the same moment in time, at different locations in space.

The basic concepts of coherence are illustrated in Figure 2-7. A white light source produces incoherent light, emitting wavefronts of diverse colors (wavelengths) and shapes. However, if incoherent light is passed through a pinhole aperture (spatial filter), *spatial coherence* of the light is improved; that is, the resulting wavefronts are more regularly arranged. If spatially coherent light is passed through a narrowband filter, which selects a limited band of wavelengths (we will discuss later how these filters work), *temporal coherence* of the light is also improved—that is, the resulting wavefronts have the same wavelength—thereby making the light more nearly monochromatic. Laser light is highly spatially and temporally coherent. However, as shown here, coherent light can be produced even without a laser, but at the expense of discarding a large amount of the light.

Similarly, the first pinhole aperture depicted in Young's double-slit experiment (see Fig 2-5) serves to create spatially coherent wavefronts. In fact, the double-slit experiment is a demonstration of spatial coherence and enables the measurement of the ability of light to interfere with a spatially shifted version of itself. Interference fringes are detectable on the final screen only when the double-slit area (defined by the separation between the 2 narrow openings) falls within the (spatial) coherence area of the incident light.

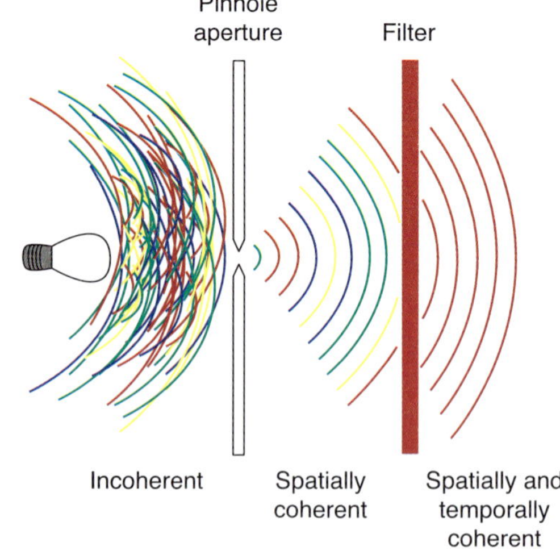

Figure 2-7 Pictorial explanation of coherence. A white-light source produces incoherent light, emitting wavefronts of diverse wavelengths and shapes. If incoherent light is passed through a pinhole aperture (spatial filter), spatial coherence is improved; that is, the resulting wavefronts are more regularly arranged in space. If spatially coherent light is passed through a narrowband filter, selecting a limited band of wavelengths, temporal coherence is improved; that is, the resulting wavefronts also have the same wavelength. *(Illustration developed by Kristina Irsch, PhD.)*

Conversely, Michelson interferometry provides a measure of temporal coherence of light, namely the light's ability to interfere with a time-delayed version of itself. By adjusting the position of one of the interferometer's mirrors, referred to as the reference mirror (eg, mirror 1 in Fig 2-6), the path of the light in the so-called reference arm is altered by a known distance, generating a path–length difference, Δz, with the other arm. The other arm is called the sample arm, as it may contain a sample with a reflecting surface in place of the mirror, as illustrated in Figure 2-8. Interference effects are detectable only for path–length differences, that is, the differences in optical distances traveled by the light in the sample and reference arm ($\Delta z = z_R - z_S$), matching to within the light's coherence length, l_C. The interference signal disappears for path–length differences above the coherence length of the light source, with only a diffuse spot of light remaining on the detector. In other words, *coherence length* is the maximum path–length difference for good visibility of interference fringes. Likewise, the time it takes light to travel a distance equal to the coherence length is called *coherence time*. These concepts of coherence length and coherence time are essential to the understanding of the basic principle of optical coherence tomography (OCT; see Chapter 9).

Both coherence time and coherence length are inversely proportional to the *spectral bandwidth* of the light source (ie, the frequency or wavelength range over which sources

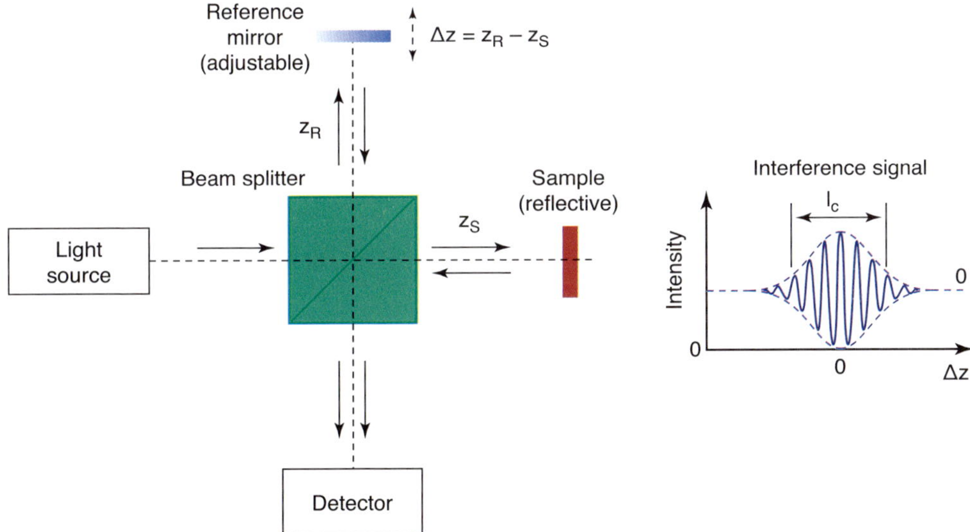

Figure 2-8 Demonstration of temporal coherence via Michelson interferometry. By adjusting the reference mirror position, the ability of light to interfere with a time-delayed version of itself can be measured. After being split into 2 parts, the wave that has traveled an unknown time and distance (z_S) from a sample is compared (interfered) with the wave that has traveled a known time and distance (z_R) from the reference mirror. An interference signal is detected only when the path–length difference, Δz, which is the difference in optical distances traveled by the light in both the sample and reference paths ($\Delta z = z_R - z_S$), is smaller than or equal to the coherence length of the light (l_C). For path–length differences above the coherence length, the interference signal disappears and only a diffuse spot of light remains on the detector. *(Illustration developed by Kristina Irsch, PhD.)*

emit light). This is illustrated in Figure 2-9 and means that a source with a narrow spectral bandwidth (light of nearly a single wavelength or that is wholly monochromatic; eg, laser light) has a high temporal coherence (ie, long coherence time), whereas a source with a broad bandwidth (light of multiple wavelengths; eg, white light) has a low temporal coherence (ie, short coherence time).

Hence, when a narrowband (or highly temporally coherent) source is used to perform interferometry (eg, laser interferometry), interference fringes will occur over a long range of path–length differences (Fig 2-10). In low-coherence interferometry, that is, when a broadband light source is used, on the other hand, interference occurs only when the time traveled by the light in the reference and sample arms is nearly equal within the short coherence length of the source. Low-coherence interferometry therefore enables greater sensitivity in separating out reflections, especially from a sample with multiple, closely spaced reflecting surfaces (Fig 2-11), and forms the basis of OCT (see Chapter 9).

Applications and clinical relevance

One familiar application of interference in ophthalmic optics is the use of *antireflection coatings* on spectacle lenses (Fig 2-12). To decrease unwanted reflections from the surfaces of spectacle lenses, a thin film of a transparent material with a refractive index that is different from that of the lens is deposited on the lens surface, so that some light will be reflected from the back surface and an equal amount will be reflected at the front surface of the thin film. These reflected waves—if the thickness of this deposited film is chosen

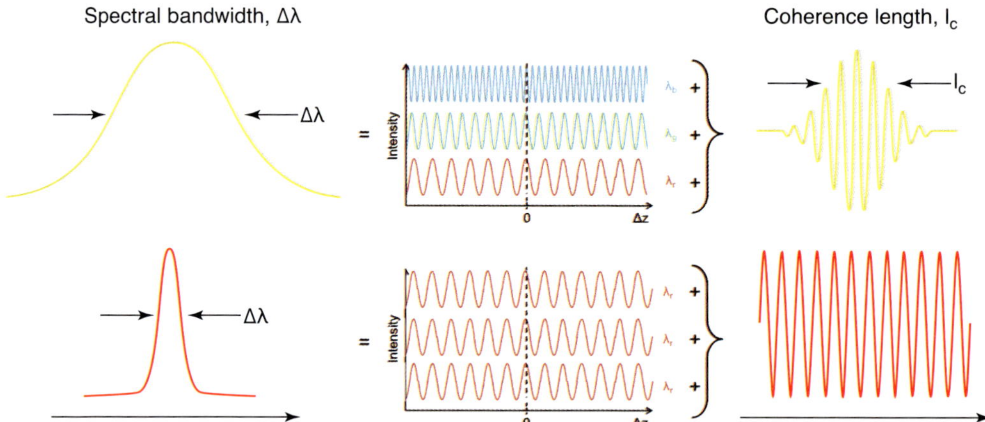

Figure 2-9 Inverse relationship between spectral bandwidth (Δλ) of a light source and its coherence length *(l_C)*. A light source with a broad bandwidth has a short coherence length (upper panel) because it is composed of multiple wavelengths (eg, white light). The emitted polychromatic waves, as illustrated in the example of 3 distinct colors (blue, green, red), are all in-phase (with their crests coinciding) only when the optical path–length difference (Δz) is zero. The composite interference signal that results from the superposition of the waves therefore is localized around $\Delta z = 0$. A light source with a narrow spectral bandwidth, on the other hand, has a long coherence length *(lower panel)* because it emits nearly a single wavelength or wholly monochromatic light (eg, laser light). The emitted monochromatic waves, as depicted in the example of red light, are all in-phase not only at $\Delta z = 0$. When superimposed, they thus generate a nonlocalized and repetitive interference signal. *(Illustration developed by Kristina Irsch, PhD.)*

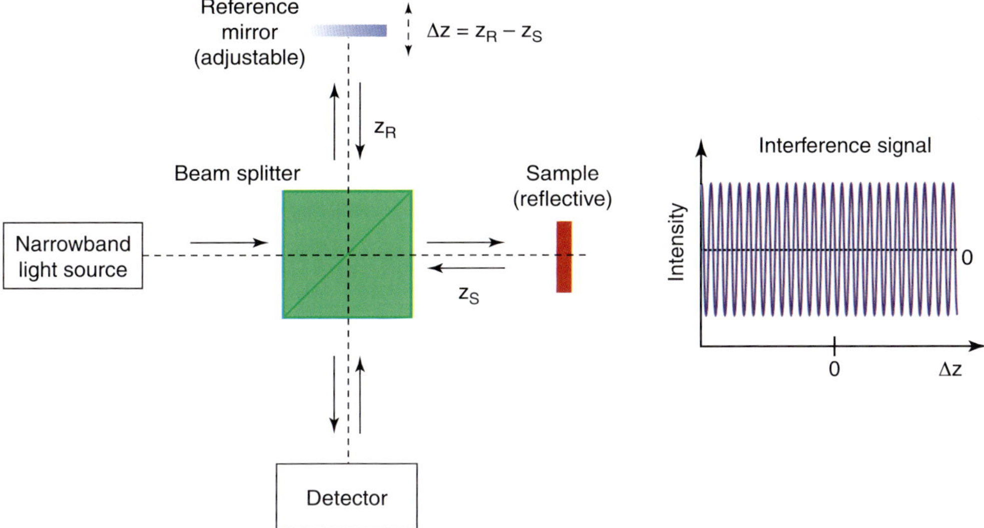

Figure 2-10 Concept of laser interferometry. Due to the long coherence length of the narrowband light source, interference effects are detectable over a long range of path–length differences, Δz, between the light traveled in the reference and sample arms (ie, the wave reflected from the reference mirror and the sample, respectively). In other words, with alteration of the reference mirror position, z_R, the detector registers an interference signal even when the mirror position is not close to the reflecting surface of the sample, z_S. *(Illustration developed by Kristina Irsch, PhD.)*

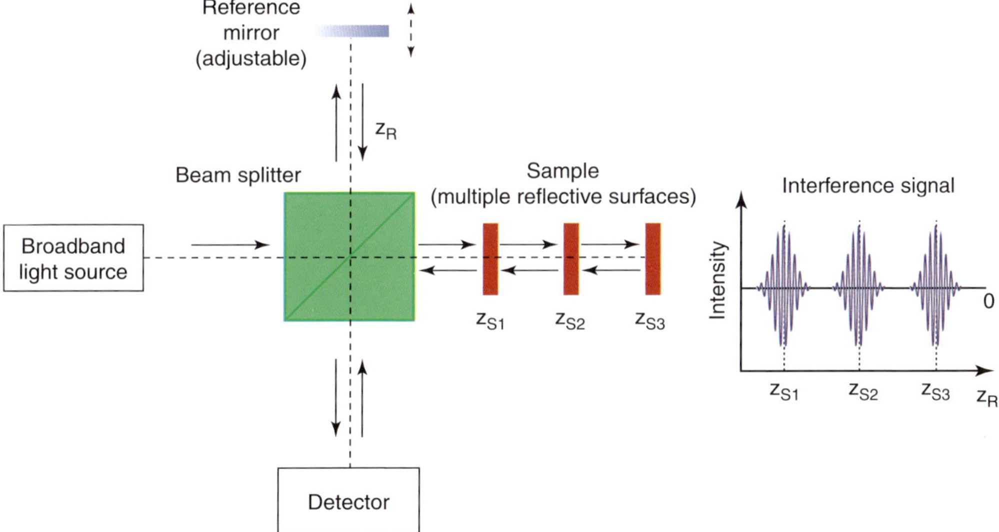

Figure 2-11 Concept of low-coherence interferometry. Due to the short coherence length of the broadband light source, interference effects are detectable only when the optical distance traveled by the light in the reference arm is nearly equal to that of the light traveled in the sample arm. In other words, with alteration of the reference mirror position, z_R, the detector registers an interference signal only when the mirror position is nearly equidistant to one of the sample's reflecting surfaces (z_{S1}, z_{S2}, z_{S3}). *(Illustration developed by Kristina Irsch, PhD.)*

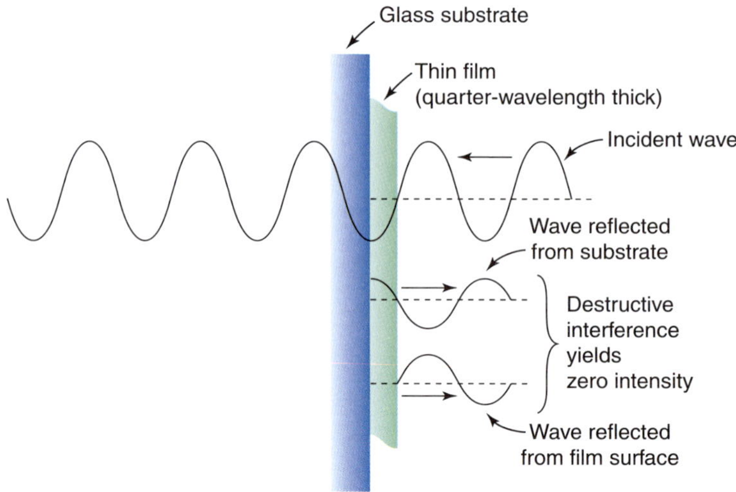

Figure 2-12 Antireflection coating on a spectacle lens. The thickness of the thin film deposition is chosen such that it is one-quarter of a specified wavelength of light, which results in complete destructive interference and therefore eliminates the reflections. *(Redrawn by C. H. Wooley.)*

such that it is one-quarter of a specified wavelength of light—will be one-half wavelength out of phase, resulting in complete destructive interference and therefore eliminating the reflections.

The use of *narrowband interference filters,* such as in fluorescein and indocyanine green angiography, as well as autofluorescence imaging (discussed in Chapter 9), is another application of interference in ophthalmology. To produce very sharp boundaries and separate excitation from fluorescent light, a thin film of a transparent material is deposited on a glass substrate, similar to the previous example but in this case with a thickness that is a multiple of the desired wavelength and surfaces that are partially reflecting. Multiple reflections of light with the desired wavelength, from the front and back surfaces of this deposited film, will exit in phase and reinforce each other, whereas light of other wavelengths will exit out of phase and the wavelengths will cancel each other (Fig 2-13). Modern narrowband filters exist that consist of several thin layers of transparent materials that allow only light of wavelengths within a few nanometers to be transmitted and block everything else.

Diffraction

Fundamentals

If we try to pass light through a very small hole, we will realize that it actually does not go in a straight line, but rather spreads out (see Fig 2-5A). This apparent "spreading out beyond the edges" of an aperture or "bending around the corners" of an obstruction, into a region where—using strictly geometric optics—we would not expect to see it, is referred to as *diffraction.* Diffraction may be thought of as light, when encountering an obstacle, scattering

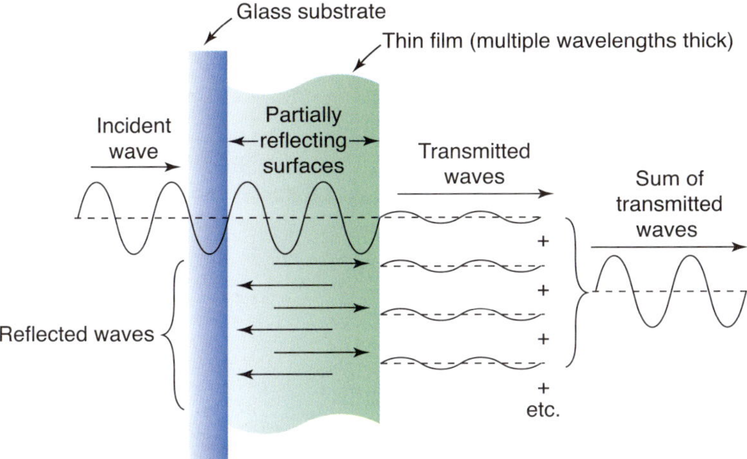

Figure 2-13 Interference filter. Multiple reflections from the front and back surfaces of the deposited film (which has a thickness that is a multiple of the desired wavelength) exit in phase and reinforce each other, whereas light of other wavelengths exits out of phase and the wavelengths cancel each other. *(Redrawn by C. H. Wooley.)*

off in different directions at the edges. What really happens, of course, is that light interacts with the electrons in the material, most noticeably with the electrons at the edges.

While a more detailed description of diffraction is beyond the scope of this text, we can appreciate that once light scatters off in different directions, it usually interferes with other parts of the diffracted light. Hence, in classical wave theory, the phenomenon of diffraction of light, as it passes beyond an obstacle of comparable size to its wavelength, is generally described as due to the interference of the light emerging from the aperture or obstacle.

For apertures, the consequence of these interference effects created by diffraction is that there is a limit to the resolution that can be achieved in any optical instrument; this immediately brings us to applications and clinical relevance in ophthalmology.

Applications and clinical relevance

All apertures produce diffraction to some extent, even an opening as large as the pupil of an eye. Thus, we are constantly aware of its effects in ophthalmology.

With a circular aperture, such as the pupil, in the absence of aberrations, the image of a point source of light formed on the retina—the point spread function (PSF)—takes the form of alternating bright and dark rings surrounding a bright central spot, the Airy disc (Fig 2-14), rather than a point. This pattern is the consequence of diffraction and its associated interference effects. The latter are apparent by the concentric bright and dark rings that are analogous to the fringes observed in Young's double-slit experiment (see Fig 2-5). Most of the energy is concentrated in the central disk, so the outer rings are usually ignored. The diameter of the Airy disc is given by the equation

$$\text{Airy Disc Diameter} \approx 2.44\lambda \frac{f}{D}$$

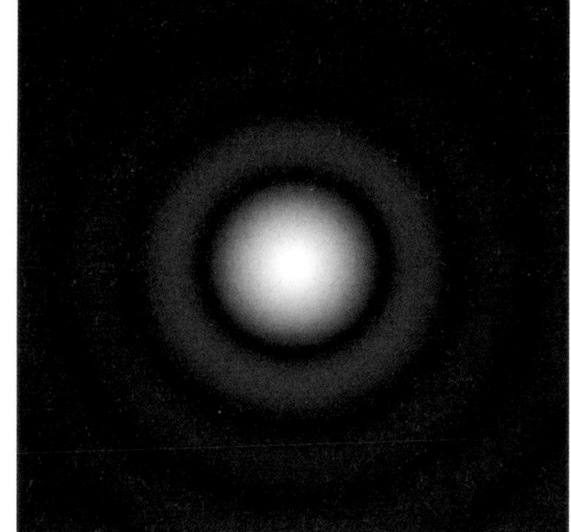

Figure 2-14 Diffraction pattern produced by a small circular aperture. The central bright spot is called an Airy disc. *(From Wikimedia Commons, public domain. https://commons.wikimedia.org/wiki/File:Airy-pattern.svg)*

where D is the diameter of the aperture (pupil) and f is the focal length—the distance from the aperture to the diffracted image. This equation illustrates that longer wavelengths (eg, red light) have a larger Airy disc than shorter wavelengths (eg, blue light) and therefore diffract more. Similarly, diffraction *increases* as the pupil size *decreases.*

Under photopic lighting conditions, the pupil of the human eye is around 2–3 mm in diameter. With pupil sizes smaller than that (in a person with emmetropia), diffraction effects become visually significant, that is, they limit visual acuity. For an eye with a 3-mm-diameter pupil (and f-number, that is f/D, of about 5), for example, and a 555-nm light source, corresponding to the maximum photopic sensitivity of the retina (see the section Measures of Light), the Airy disc diameter is approximately 7.4 μm, encompassing the outer segments of roughly 11 photoreceptors. The smallest resolvable detail is approximately equal to the Airy disc radius. An Airy disc of 3.7 μm radius corresponds roughly to 20/15 visual acuity.

Thus, in theory, the larger the pupil size, the smaller the Airy disc and therefore the better the visual acuity or the higher the resolution of an image on the retina. However, in practice (as discussed in Chapter 9), higher-order aberrations occur at larger pupil sizes. While there are ways to correct for wavefront aberrations (adaptive optics, discussed in Chapter 9), we cannot suppress diffraction. Diffraction sets an absolute limit on the best resolution obtainable with any optical system, including the eye, and is represented by the Airy disc pattern (see Fig 2-14).

Diffraction can also be used to advantage in ophthalmic optics in the creation of diffractive-optics multifocal lenses or extended depth of focus intraocular lenses. For example, etching a specially designed pattern of closely spaced circular steps on one of the surfaces of a contact lens or intraocular lens can cause light to diffract such that the resulting interference effects of the diffracted light create a second focal point for the lens, allowing somewhat clear vision at near, with the overall curvature of the lens simultaneously providing distance focus.

Measures of Light

For many clinicians, the measurement of light is one of the most confusing topics in the field of clinical optics. This section attempts to clarify the subject.

As we learned previously, light is a range of electromagnetic radiant energy, comprising the range of wavelengths to which the eye is ordinarily sensitive—about 400–700 nm. The measurement of light thus naturally derives from more general methods for the measurement of electromagnetic radiant energy—specifically, from general methods to measure the *transfer* of energy by electromagnetic radiation.

Power is the rate at which energy is transformed or transferred from one form to another. It is measured in units of work (or energy) per unit time, typically joules per second (J/s) or watts (W). The watt is used to describe various forms of energy transfer, including but not limited to those that take place in mechanical devices, electrical power lines, and heat generation.

Radiometry

Measurements of the power transferred by means of electromagnetic radiation are typically described with derived units in accordance with the above scheme (Table 2-1). In principle, the fundamental measurement tool for this purpose is the blackbody radiometer. This is an object (frequently realized in the form of a hollow cavity) that absorbs radiant electromagnetic radiation at all wavelengths with equal efficiency. The amount of energy absorbed is determined by measuring the increase in the temperature of the blackbody, converting heat to energy according to the laws of thermodynamics and knowledge of the heat capacity of the detector, and dividing by the length of time the radiometer is exposed to the radiation.

In practice, care must be taken to account for the geometry of the detector and of the source of radiation. The simplest case for the latter is a point source that radiates equally in all directions. It would be difficult to surround such a point source with a detector, which would simultaneously absorb the output in every direction. As a result, the detector would typically intercept the radiation over only a small area. Assuming the radiation output to be uniform in every direction, it would thus be appropriate to normalize the measurement by dividing the energy transfer intercepted by the detector by the solid angle it subtends (in essence, the area of the detector divided by the distance from the point source). This description of the energy output from a point source in watts per steradian (W/sr) is referred to as its *radiant intensity.* With the total solid angle of the space surrounding a point being 4π steradians, multiplying this quantity by 4π would yield the energy output of the point source in watts.

If, on the other hand, the radiation source is an extended planar object, rather than a point source, the appropriate description of its energy output would be in terms of watts per unit area, say W/m^2. This description of the energy output is referred to as the *radiant exitance* of the extended source. If one prefers to measure the rate at which radiant energy impinges on an extended object, the appropriate units are again W/m^2, but in this context, the energy transfer is referred to as *irradiance.*

Note that *intensity*, depending on the context or the background of the person using the term, can have alternative meanings. In optics (and in particular, laser physics), it

Table 2-1 Comparison of Radiometric and Photometric Units

Radiometric Quantity	SI Unit	Photometric Quantity	SI Unit
Radiant energy, Q_e	Joule (J) = watt second (W · s)	Luminous energy, Q_v	Lumen second (lm · s)
Fluence, H_e (Energy density)	Joules per meter² (J/m²) = (W · s/m²), joules per centimeter² (J/cm²)	Luminous exposure, H_v	Lumen second per meter² (lm · s/m²)
Radiant flux, Φ_e (Power)	Watt (W) = joules per second (J/s)	Luminous flux, Φ_v	Lumen (lm) = candela steradian (cd · sr)
Radiant intensity, I_e	Watts per steradian (W/sr)	Luminous intensity, I_v	Candela (cd) = lumen per steradian (lm/sr)
Irradiance, E_e (Radiant exitance power density)	Watts per meter² (W/m²), watts per centimeter² (W/cm²)	Illuminance, E_v (Luminous exitance)	Lux (lx) = (cd · sr/m²) = (lm/m²)
Radiance, L_e	Watts per meter² per steradian (W/m²·sr)	Luminance, L_v	Nit (cd/m²) = (lm/m²·sr)

generally refers to *power density* (ie, radiometric irradiance) and most commonly is expressed in watts per square centimeter (W/cm²). Similarly in this context, and as you will notice during the discussion of lasers later in this chapter, *energy density (fluence)* is most commonly expressed in joules per square centimeter (J/cm²).

Further note that *radiance* refers to the radiant intensity per unit area, and thus is expressed in units of W/m²·sr.

Photometry

In contrast to the radiometric measurements, which weight equally the energy transmitted at every wavelength of the electromagnetic spectrum, *photometry* takes into account the variable spectral response of the human eye. It is based on empirical measurements of the relative sensitivity of human vision to light of the various wavelengths, resulting in a weighting curve that is referred to as the *spectral luminous efficiency function,* usually denoted by $V(\lambda)$ or V_λ. The photometric measurement of the radiant energy output or input in a system is the summation (or, better, integral) of the energy transfer at each wavelength multiplied by the value of V_λ for that wavelength.

The photometric equivalent of the measurement of the total radiant output of a point source is the *lumen (lm),* the V_λ-weighted version of the watt. This quantity is referred to as the *luminous flux.* For example, the output of an ordinary incandescent or light-emitting diode (LED) light bulb (which can be regarded for most purposes as a point source) is now often indicated in lumens. A 60-W incandescent bulb might typically have a light output of 800 lumens. (In contrast, an 800-lumen LED bulb might consume only 12 W of power.)

The photometric equivalent of the measurement of the radiant output of a point source per unit of solid angle is the *candela (cd),* or lm/sr. This quantity is referred to as the *luminous intensity* of the point source. For historical reasons, the candela is the primary SI (metric system) unit for the measurement of light, intended to approximate the light output of the standard wax candles that were originally used for this purpose. One candela is defined as the luminous intensity of a source emitting monochromatic radiation at a frequency of 540 THz and a radiant intensity of 1/683 W/sr. Note that 540 THz corresponds to approximately 555 nm ($= c \times 10^9 / \nu = 3 \times 10^8 \times 10^9 / 540 \times 10^{12}$), the wavelength to which the human eye is most sensitive under light-adapted or photopic lighting conditions, and that 1/683 was chosen to make 1 cd equal to the old unit, the "candle," which was based on the actual luminous intensity of a wax candle flame.

The photometric equivalent of the measurement of the radiant output of an extended planar source is the lm/m^2. This quantity is referred to as the *luminous exitance.* Similarly, the photometric equivalent of the measurement of the radiant energy incident on an extended planar surface is also measured in lm/m^2. This quantity is known as the *illuminance.* As a unit for illuminance, the lm/m^2 is known as the *lux.* Conversely, *luminance* refers to the luminous intensity per unit area and is thus expressed in units of $cd/m^2 = lm/sr \cdot m^2$. This last unit is also referred to as the *nit.* To further help develop a "feel" for photometric units, Table 2-2 lists photometric values associated with visual functions.

Note that the spectral luminous efficiency function depends in practice on the state of light-adaptation or dark-adaptation of the eye. Most measurements are made under light-adapted conditions and use the light-adapted (or photopic) efficiency function. Under dark-adapted (scotopic) conditions, the efficiency function shifts toward shorter wavelengths (the Purkinje shift), reflecting the difference between the absorption spectrum of rhodopsin (the visual pigment in retinal rods) and the summed absorption spectra of the 3 visual pigments in the retinal cones. The scotopic spectral luminance efficiency function is often referred to as $V'(\lambda)$ or V'_λ. It has a maximum at 507 nm, whereas the photopic efficiency function has a maximum at 555 nm. In precise work, the choice of luminance efficiency function should be specified.

Table 2-2 Luminance Levels Associated With Various Visual Functions

Visual Function	Luminance (nits)
Best acuity	1000
Cone threshold	10^{-4}
Damage	10^8
Limit of rod sensitivity	10^{-7}
Mesopic range	10^{-4}–10
Photopic range	10–10^8
Rod saturation	10
Scotopic range	10^{-7}–10^{-4}

Conversion Between Radiometric and Photometric Outputs

So, now that we have defined the radiometric and photometric measures of light, how do we convert from one to the other? In other words, if a light source has a known radiometric output, can we determine its corresponding photometric output? Yes, if we know the spectral properties of the lamp, that is, the radiometric output at each wavelength. The output at each wavelength is multiplied by the sensitivity of the eye to that wavelength as well as by the conversion factor that is given by the definition of the candela (according to which there are 683 lumens per watt for 555-nm light), and the results are summed to obtain the total response of the eye to light from that source.

For example, if a light source has a known output in watts, how much is its output in lumens? If we assume a monochromatic light source, such as a 650-nm (red) laser pointer with a photometric power of 5 mW, the photoptic weighting factor is 0.096, and therefore the corresponding luminous flux is $0.096 \times 0.005 \text{ W} \times 683 \text{ lm/W} = 0.33 \text{ lm}$. If we had a green (532 nm) laser pointer, this value would rise to $0.828 \times 0.005 \text{ W} \times 683 \text{ lm/W} = 2.83 \text{ lm}$.

Light Sources: Lasers

The classical theory of electromagnetic waves successfully explains "macroscopic" light phenomena, but fails to explain phenomena at the atomic and molecular levels. Quantum theory, as illustrated in Figure 2-4, can explain such phenomena. For the following considerations, it therefore becomes crucial to consider the quantum behavior of light.

According to quantum theory, electrons in atoms (or molecules) exist in *nonradiating* states; each state is associated with a specific energy level. The energy states possible for an atom differ from element to element, and those for a molecule differ from compound to compound. Each element or compound has a unique distribution of energy states. When an electron drops from a higher energy state to a lower one, the difference in energy *(E)* is radiated as a packet, called a photon, with a characteristic frequency (ν) given by

$$E = h\nu$$

where h is the Planck constant. Similarly, an electron can jump to a higher energy state by absorbing a photon, with the resulting energy absorption equal to the energy difference between states (see Fig 2-4).

Fundamentals

When an electron absorbs a photon and jumps to a higher energy level (*stimulated absorption*; see Fig 2-4), usually it quickly drops back to the original level and emits a photon identical in frequency to the one it absorbed (*spontaneous emission*; see Fig 2-4).

However, atoms of some elements have 2 energy levels that are close together. When a photon is absorbed, the electron jumps to the higher energy level. Instead of dropping back to the original level, the electron first transitions to a slightly lower level without emitting visible energy. Next, it drops to the initial energy level and emits a photon. The emitted photon has less energy than the stimulating, absorbed photon and, therefore, a lower frequency, or longer wavelength (and different perceived color). This phenomenon, called *fluorescence,* occurs only in materials possessing close spacing between energy levels. Its clinical utility derives from the essential feature that the absorbed and emitted photons have different wavelengths and is the basis of fluorescein angiography and macular autofluorescence (discussed in Chapter 9).

A photon of appropriate frequency passing near an electron in a metastable state may stimulate the electron immediately to drop to a lower state and radiate an identical photon (Fig 2-15). Such *stimulated emission* is the basis of the light emission in lasers. In fact, the word *laser* originated as an acronym for Light Amplification by Stimulated Emission of Radiation.

Lasers use an *active medium* with an appropriate metastable state. Energy is introduced into the active medium in a variety of ways. For example, *optical pumping* uses a bright incoherent light source to excite a large number of electrons into the metastable state. The active medium is inside a *resonator cavity*, which typically has a fully reflecting mirror on one end and a partially reflecting one on the other; this design causes light to make numerous passes through the active medium, producing more and more photons, by stimulated emission, with each pass (Fig 2-16).

Contrary to common belief, lasers are not very efficient light sources. Compared with the amount of energy required to power a laser, the amount of energy produced is modest. The light produced, however, has unique and useful characteristics. Laser light has a very narrow bandwidth (ie, it is nearly a single wavelength or monochromatic) and, consequently, it has high temporal coherence. The coherence length is relatively long—about half the length of the resonator cavity—typically a few centimeters. Lasers are the most intense sources of monochromatic light available.

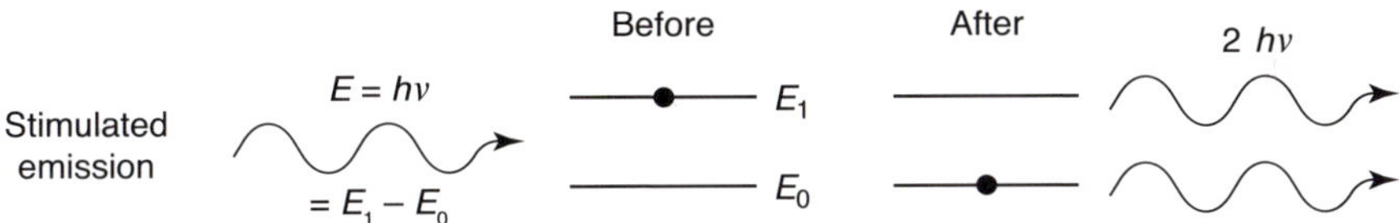

Figure 2-15 In a process called stimulated emission, which is the basis of light emission in lasers, a photon of appropriate frequency passing near an electron in an excited state may stimulate the electron to drop to a lower state and emit an identical photon. *(Reproduced with permission from Steinert RF, Puliafito CA.* The Nd:YAG Laser in Ophthalmology: Principles and Clinical Applications of Photodisruption. *Saunders; 1985. Redrawn by C. H. Wooley.)*

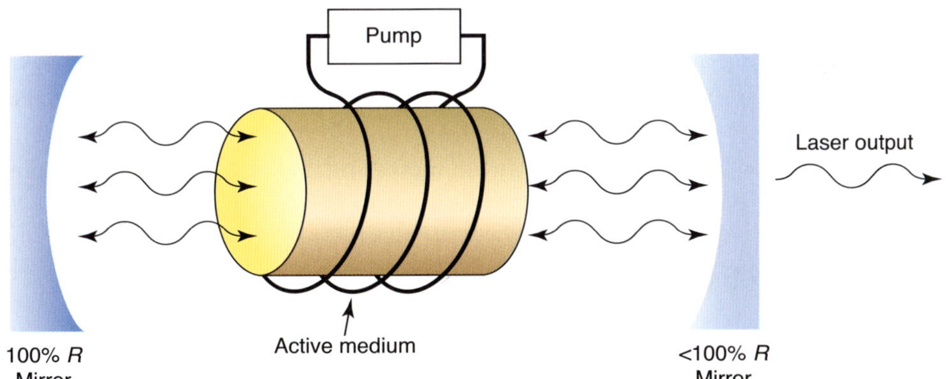

Figure 2-16 Simple schematic of a laser. The active medium within the resonator cavity formed by the mirrors and the pump, which raises a majority of electrons to elevated states (population inversion) in the active medium. One mirror is fully reflective (100% *R*), whereas the other is partially transparent (<100% *R*). As drawn, the mirror is 66% reflective, and the average light wave makes 3 round-trips through the active medium before being emitted. *(Reproduced with permission from Steinert RF, Puliafito CA.* The Nd:YAG Laser in Ophthalmology: Principles and Clinical Applications of Photodisruption. *Saunders; 1985. Redrawn by Jonathan Clark.)*

Although the total energy in laser light may be slight, it can be focused on a very small area to produce a very high energy density (ie, energy that is transferred per square centimeter, or fluence; see Table 2-1). Laser light is also highly directional and, depending on the design of the resonator, may also be polarized.

Lasers are usually named after their active media. A medium can be a gas (argon, krypton, carbon dioxide, argon with fluoride [excimer], or helium with neon), a liquid (dye), a solid (an active element supported by a crystal, such as neodymium: yttrium-aluminum-garnet [Nd:YAG], neodymium: glass [Nd:Glass], and titanium: sapphire [Ti:Sapphire]), or a semiconductor (diode).

Lasers may operate continuously (eg, an argon laser for photocoagulation), commonly referred to as *continuous wave,* or in pulses (eg, a Nd:YAG laser for capsulotomy, or an Nd:Glass laser for corneal flap creation). Mode-locking and Q-switching are 2 common methods of producing a *pulsed* output. The details of such pulse-shaping mechanisms are beyond the scope of this chapter. Note, however, that while *Q-switching* allows for the production of short pulses (mainly on the order of nanoseconds, ie, 10^{-9} s), it is *mode-locking* that can produce *ultrashort pulses,* with a duration on the order of picoseconds (ie, 10^{-12} s) or femtoseconds (ie, 10^{-15} s), depending on the properties of the laser. In fact, the pulse duration is mainly dependent on the spectral bandwidth of the laser medium; the larger its spectral bandwidth, the shorter the pulse that can be realized. Thus, ultrashort laser pulses are not monochromatic, and for the generation of femtosecond pulses, a laser with a large spectral bandwidth is required. For a Ti:Sapphire laser with a 128-THz spectral bandwidth, for example, the shortest pulse that can be created would be around 3.4 femtoseconds (ie, 10^{-15} s). Note, hence, what is commonly referred to as femtosecond laser does not constitute a different laser type but rather special pulse-shaping mechanisms that are employed to produce femtosecond pulses from the laser medium. Solid-state lasers, such as Nd:Glass lasers, offer relatively broad spectral bandwidths, necessary for femtosecond pulse generation, and are used in a wide range of evolving ophthalmic applications, as discussed in the following sections.

We have learned that power is the amount of energy delivered in a given time period. A watt is 1 joule of energy delivered over 1 second. The same joule delivered over a nanosecond has a power of 1 billion watts; over a picosecond, 1 trillion watts; and over a femtosecond, 1 quadrillion watts. Pulsing is a way of increasing the power of a laser's output by delivering a modest amount of energy over a very short period.

Therapeutic Laser–Tissue Interactions

The fundamental process of any therapeutic laser application is the energy transfer to the tissue via absorption of light, which is a function of the nature of the tissue (its distribution of energy states) as well as the wavelength (photon energy) of the light. Therapeutic laser–tissue interactions may be divided into 5 different types (Table 2-3), each of which will be discussed in detail: *photochemical interaction, thermal interaction, photoablation, plasma-induced ablation,* and *photodisruption.* These mechanisms are primarily determined by the power density (irradiance) of the laser light and its interaction time (laser pulse duration) with the tissue. All therapeutic laser–tissue interaction mechanisms share a common characteristic, in that all meaningful energy densities (the energy that is transferred to the tissue—fluence) vary typically between 1 and 1000 J/cm^2 (Fig 2-17).

Niemz MK. *Laser-Tissue Interactions: Fundamentals and Applications.* 4th ed. Springer; 2019.

Photochemical interaction

Photochemical interaction, sometimes referred to as *photoactivation,* takes place at long exposure times, ranging from seconds to continuous, and very low power densities or irradiances (typically 1 W/cm^2). This type of interaction is based on the use of a photosensitizing dye (eg, rose bengal, riboflavin, or verteporfin), which serves as a chemical (electron reaction) catalyst. Laser irradiation, at a wavelength coupled to the specific dye

Table 2-3 Laser–Tissue Interaction Types and Associated Mechanisms

Interaction Type	Mechanism
Photochemical interaction	Photocatalysis
Thermal interaction	Increase in temperature
Photoablation	UV dissociation
Plasma-induced ablation	Plasma ionization
Photodisruption	Shock-wave generation

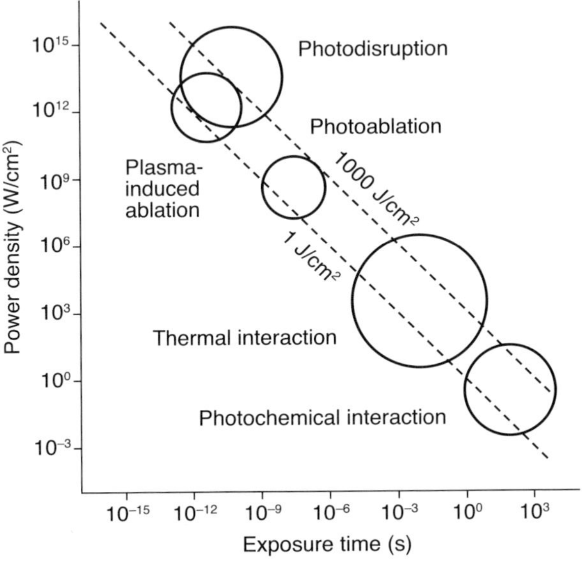

Figure 2-17 According to the laser light's power density (irradiance) and exposure time (pulse duration), laser–tissue interactions may be divided into 5 different types: photochemical interaction, thermal interaction, photoablation, plasma-induced ablation, and photodisruption. All meaningful energy densities (transferred energy to the tissue) vary typically between 1 and 1000 J/cm^2 for therapeutic laser–tissue interactions. *(Reprinted/adapted with permission from Springer Nature: Interaction Mechanisms in* Laser–Tissue Interactions: Fundamentals and Applications. *3rd enlarged ed., by Markolf H. Niemz. Copyright 2007.)*

used, causes a photochemical reaction only within tissues in which the dye is present and when irradiated.

This is, for example, used in photodynamic therapy (PDT), in which a photosensitizing agent is injected into the circulation. The blood vessels are then treated with laser irradiation to activate the photosensitizer. A chemical reaction occurs, resulting in thrombosis and closure of the blood vessels. Other than retinal PDT in age-related macular degeneration (AMD), a specific example of this (though it is rarely used) is the treatment of a vascularized cornea with rose bengal and green argon laser irradiation to thrombose blood vessels and thereby reduce the chance of rejection of a subsequent graft. Another ophthalmic application is the use of UVA light after application of riboflavin onto the corneal surface to promote corneal crosslinking in the treatment of keratoconus.

Thermal interaction

At somewhat shorter exposure times—ranging from microseconds to a minute—and higher power densities—ranging from 10 W/cm^2 to 10^6 W/cm^2—diverse thermal effects at different temperatures may be distinguished (Table 2-4 and Fig 2-18). This type of interaction is based on the generation of heat (molecular motion) by the absorption of light.

Photocoagulation, which is associated with protein and collagen denaturation, is the most commonly used thermal laser–tissue interaction in ophthalmic surgery. Natural chromophores or dyes within the tissue absorb light and convert it to heat, which causes denaturation. Their absorption strongly depends on the wavelength of incident

Table 2-4 Occurrence of Thermal Effects at Different Temperatures

Temperature (°C)	Biological Effect
37	—
>42	Hyperthermia
>60	Coagulation (denaturation of proteins and collagen)
100	Vaporization
>100	Carbonization
>300	Melting

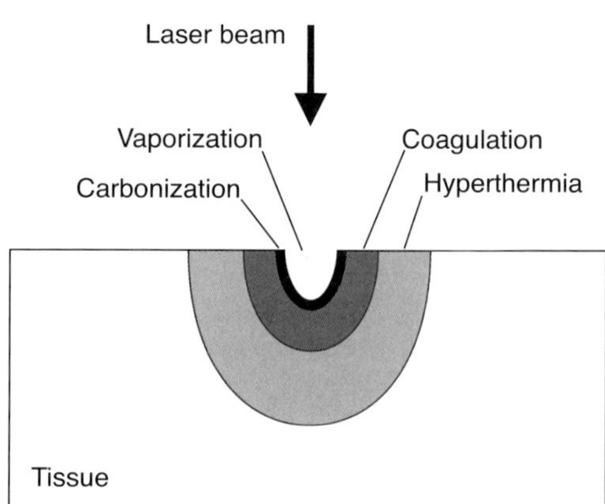

Figure 2-18 Thermal interaction effects inside biological tissue. *(Reprinted/adapted with permission from Springer Nature: Interaction Mechanisms in* Laser–Tissue Interactions: Fundamentals and Applications. *3rd enlarged ed., by Markolf H. Niemz. Copyright 2007.)*

light. Thus, laser light of appropriate wavelength must be selected to target specific ocular structures. The main natural chromophores within ocular tissues that are targeted during photocoagulation are hemoglobin (eg, in blood vessels) and melanin (eg, in the iris or deep retinal layers), which strongly absorb wavelengths from about 400–580 nm. Laser wavelengths longer than 500 nm are generally the preferred choice, in particular for treatment near or in the macula, as light between 450 nm and 500 nm is strongly absorbed by the yellow xanthophyll pigments in the macula. Formerly, large argon gas–filled tubes were used to create green laser beams (513 nm), but newer solid-state devices can emit these wavelengths, such as frequency-doubled Nd:YAG (ie, one-half of the fundamental 1064-nm wavelength of the Nd:YAG laser, thus 532 nm), or more compact diode lasers.

The most common ophthalmic applications of photocoagulation include laser coagulation to prevent retinal detachments, photocoagulation of retinal vessel disease, panretinal photocoagulation in diabetic retinopathy, transpupillary thermotherapy for malignant choroidal melanoma and choroidal neovascularization in AMD, laser trabeculoplasty for open-angle glaucoma, and laser iridotomy for closed-angle glaucoma.

Photocoagulation has also been used for photothermal shrinkage of stromal collagen, known as *laser thermo-keratoplasty (LTK),* in the treatment of hyperopia. The cornea does not absorb enough visible light, even highly concentrated light, to produce a significant temperature increase. However, the cornea is opaque to some infrared wavelengths; thus an infrared laser (eg, holmium: yttrium aluminum garnet [Ho:YAG]) is used in LTK.

Photoablation

If we deliver photons in a short-enough time, so that no heat is transferred, and with sufficient energy—typically in the 5–7 electron voltage (1 eV ~ 1.602×10^{-19} J) range—then we can directly split molecules, that is, break their covalent chemical bonds. Excimer lasers, which generate photons with wavelengths in the UV range (eg, a 193-nm argon fluoride excimer laser), are ideally suited for photoablation. This results in ejection of fragments and very clean ablation without necrosis or thermal damage to adjacent tissue. We can think of this type of interaction as "vaporization" without the surrounding thermal effects from Figure 2-18. Typical threshold values for this type of interaction are irradiances of 10^7–10^8 W/cm^2 and pulses in the nanosecond range. Photoablation is used in the cornea, which absorbs UV light below ~315 nm, for refractive surgery of the cornea such as photorefractive keratectomy (PRK) and laser in situ keratomileusis (LASIK).

Plasma-induced ablation

Under even higher concentrated peak irradiances (but ideally low-pulse energies, compared to photodisruption; see Fig 2-17), typically 10^{11}–10^{13} W/cm^2, and shorter exposure times, in the picosecond and femtosecond range, we can not only break molecules (as during photoablation), but even strip electrons from (ionize) their atoms and accelerate them ("optical breakdown"). The accelerated electrons, in turn, can collide with and ionize further atoms, as illustrated in Figure 2-19. This process is called *cascade ionization* and leads to a *plasma formation,* a highly ionized state. It enables a very clean and well-defined removal of tissue without any evidence of thermal or mechanical damage. This type of interaction also makes it possible to transfer energy to transparent media without the

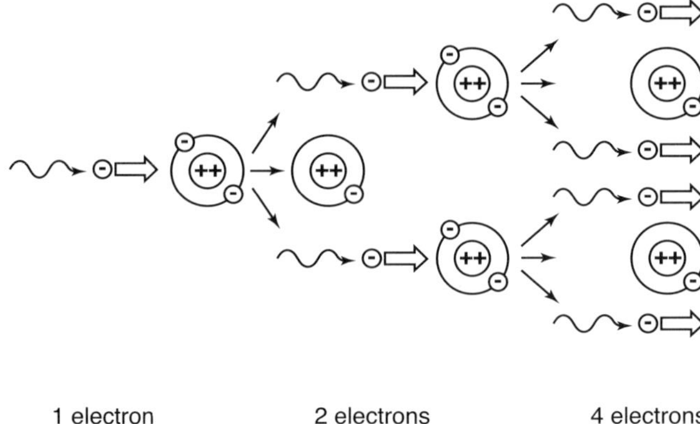

Figure 2-19 Cascade ionization (in which electrons are stripped from their atoms) leading to plasma formation, a highly ionized state. *(Reprinted/adapted with permission from Springer Nature: Interaction Mechanisms in* Laser–Tissue Interactions: Fundamentals and Applications. *3rd enlarged ed., by Markolf H. Niemz. Copyright 2007.)*

use of UV lasers by creating a plasma that is capable of absorbing non–UV laser photons. Especially in ophthalmology, transparent tissue such as the cornea, which is essentially transparent to wavelengths from ~315–1400 nm, can be treated with non-UV lasers by using plasma-induced ablation.

Note that there are secondary mechanical side effects, such as the generation of a shock wave (ie, plasma electrons are not confined to the focal volume of the laser beam) and cavitation bubbles, but they do not define the global effect upon the tissue in the plasma-induced ablation process. This kind of ablation is primarily caused by plasma ionization itself (the dissociation of molecules and atoms), which is distinct from the more mechanical interaction process called *photodisruption.* Plasma-induced ablation is what is generally attempted with emerging methods of corneal refractive surgery that use Nd:Glass (femtosecond) lasers. The most common application of Nd:Glass lasers in corneal refractive surgery is the formation of the corneal flap (for LASIK). Other procedures include intrastromal ablation or cutting, such as femtosecond lenticule extraction (FLEx) or small-incision lenticule extraction (SMILE).

Photodisruption

At higher pulse energies (typically 1–1000 J/cm^2), and thus higher plasma energies, mechanical side effects become more significant and might even determine the global effect upon the tissue, in which case we refer to the interaction process as photodisruption.

The most important ophthalmic application of this photodisruptive interaction is posterior capsulotomy using the Nd:YAG laser. During a photodisruption procedure, it is the mechanical (acoustic) wave and not the laser light itself (as with plasma-induced ablation) that breaks the capsule. Since both interaction mechanisms—plasma-induced ablation as well as photodisruption—rely on plasma generation and graphically overlap (see Fig 2-17), it is not always easy to distinguish between these 2 processes. In fact, most literature sources attribute all tissue effects evoked by ultrashort laser pulses to photodisruption. However, during photodisruption, the tissue primarily is split by *mechanical forces,* with shock-wave and cavitation effects propagating into adjacent tissue, thus limiting the localizability of the interaction zone. In contrast, plasma-induced ablation is spatially confined to the breakdown region and laser focal spot, with the tissue primarily being removed by *plasma ionization itself.* The primary distinguishing parameter between the 2 interaction processes is energy density (see Fig 2-17).

Why ultrashort laser pulses or the use of femtosecond lasers?

Per the definition of power (energy per second), the shorter the pulse duration, the higher the power that can be delivered at a given energy. In other words, picosecond or femtosecond (ultrashort) pulses permit the generation of high peak powers with considerably lower pulse energies than nanosecond pulses.

Another consequence of this is that, for ultrashort pulses, especially in the femtosecond range, considerably lower pulse energies are needed to achieve optical breakdown (plasma generation), and therefore purely plasma-induced ablation can be observed. For nanosecond pulses, on the other hand, as illustrated in Figure 2-20, the threshold energy density for optical breakdown is higher, so purely plasma-induced ablation is not observed, but it is always associated with photodisruption. Since disruptive effects can damage adjacent tissue, ultrashort laser pulses are generally preferred (depending on the application).

Note that for a laser with high-energy pulses (photodisruption regime), which causes disruptive effects that propagate beyond its focal spot, lower repetition rates are needed; in contrast, for a laser with low-energy pulses (plasma-induced ablation regime), higher repetition rates are necessary and produce smoother surface cuts without increasing the time of the procedure (Fig 2-21). Femtosecond-laser technology has evolved significantly since

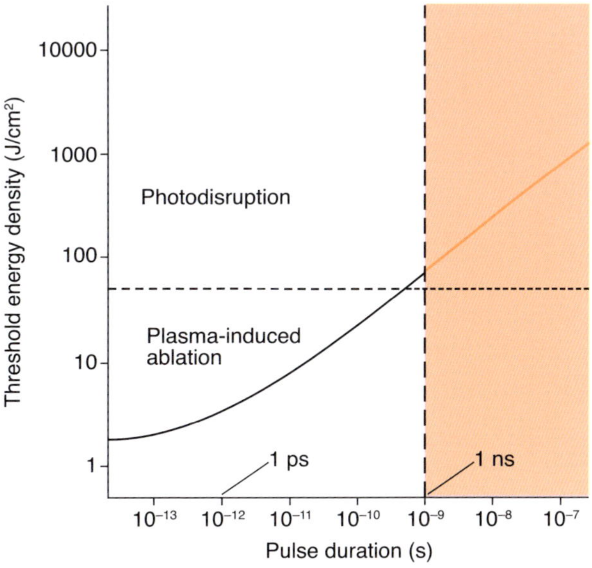

Figure 2-20 Distinction of plasma-induced ablation and photodisruption according to applied energy density. Note that for nanosecond pluses, purely plasma-induced ablation is not observed but is always associated with disruptive effects, even at the very threshold for optical breakdown *(dashed line). (Reprinted/adapted with permission from Springer Nature: Interaction Mechanisms in* Laser–Tissue Interactions: Fundamentals and Applications. *3rd enlarged ed., by Markolf H. Niemz. Copyright 2007.)*

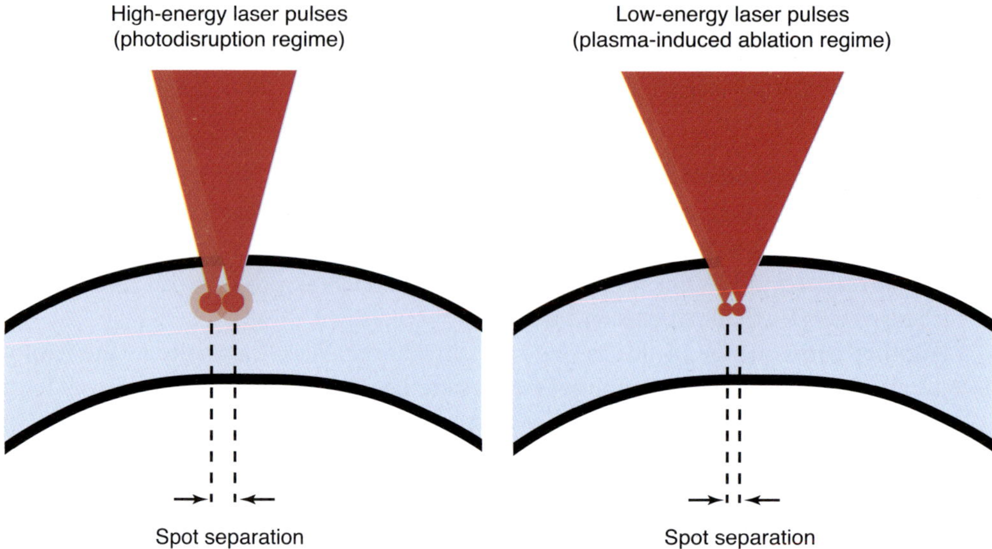

Figure 2-21 Repetition rate versus energy density. *(Left)* For high-energy laser pulses (photodisruption regime), which cause disruptive effects that propagate beyond the laser's focal spot, lower repetition rates are needed, whereas *(right)* for low-energy pulses (plasma-induced ablation regime), higher repetition rates are necessary. Note that the latter will produce smoother surface cuts without increasing the time needed for the procedure. *(Illustration developed by Kristina Irsch, PhD.)*

its introduction, with commercial Nd:Glass laser systems now operating with repetition rates in the MHz regime; this reduces energy per pulse and facilitates penetrating corneal or intrastromal incisions with high precision.

Light Hazards

As with any therapeutic light application, nontherapeutic damage to the eye caused by light is primarily dependent on the wavelength as well as the irradiance and duration of light exposure.

For example, the sun itself produces a power density (irradiance) of about 10 W/cm^2, which will rise to 170 W/cm^2 if that sunlight is focused and falls well within the range of thermal interaction (see Fig 2-17); in fact, retinal photocoagulation was first performed by focusing sunlight onto the retina. Similarly, prolonged irradiation or cumulative exposure from the operating microscope or indirect ophthalmoscope through a focusing lens, in particular on an eye with a dilated pupil, may be harmful to the eye. For instance, there is some evidence that cases of cystoid macular edema after cataract extraction are related to microscope illumination.

The anterior segment of the eye is essentially transparent to wavelengths from about 400–1400 nm and opaque to light outside that wavelength range, thereby reducing and protecting the subsequent ocular media from direct exposure to UV as well as infrared (IR) light. This is thanks to the crystalline lens essentially blocking UVA light (315–400 nm) and the cornea essentially blocking UVB (280–315 nm) light, UVC (280 nm and below) light, as well as IR-B and IR-C (1400 nm to 1 mm) radiation. The filtering properties of anterior-segment components are inherently related to their absorptive capabilities, UV radiation causes breakdown of the absorptive molecules in the cornea and lens, and IR radiation causes a temperature rise and subsequent denaturation of protein in the cornea. Therefore, the anterior segment is not only susceptible to injury from UV irradiation, from which photokeratitis (from short-term exposure to UVB and UVC) and cataract (from long-term cumulative exposure) may result, but also to thermal injury from IR radiation. Damage from thermal injury may be caused by any light above 400 nm.

In the retina, natural chromophores, including melanin, hemoglobin, and xanthophyll, as previously discussed, strongly absorb wavelengths from about 400–580 nm. This makes the retina susceptible to photochemical injury in that region, especially from blue light. Note that in an aphakic eye, this susceptibility to damage extends to below 400 (to about 315 nm) without the UVA absorption capability of the natural lens, and is the basis for incorporating UV-blocking and blue-blocking chromophores in some intraocular lenses. The retina is also susceptible to thermal injury from optical radiation occurring from the visible to near-infrared wavelengths of 400–1400 nm.

Appendix 2-1

Reconciliation of Geometric Optics and Physical Optics

We have seen how the basic principles of geometric optics are consequences of Fermat's principle. In turn, Fermat's principle can be understood as a consequence of the wave properties of light. Although a rigorous derivation is beyond the scope of this volume, a heuristic description of the concepts can be instructive.

A beam of light propagates as a wave, oscillating perpendicular to the direction of travel. Two such waves that coincide will interfere with one another. This interference is constructive or destructive, according to whether the peaks and troughs of the waves coincide (see Fig 2-5C). If 2 coincident waves of light emanate from a common source, their peaks and troughs coincide whenever the travel time of the 2 waves is identical. In this case, the full strength of the light waves is evident. Conversely, if the travel times of 2 coincident waves differ such that the arrival of their peaks and troughs differ by exactly half a wavelength, the waves cancel each other perfectly, and no light appears to be transmitted.

When small variations in the light path occur, possible paths for which the travel time is essentially unchanged will thus contribute strongly to the resultant image, whereas those paths that vary more strongly in travel time will essentially cancel out. Paths for which small variations (often referred to as "perturbations") of the light path have little effect on travel time are referred to as *extremal* paths. The most familiar of these are the paths of shortest travel time, such as the straight-line paths of light through uniform media. The formal derivation of these observations is the concern of the mathematical subject known as the "calculus of variations," which is beyond the scope of this book.

In rare instances, paths other than those of shortest travel time may also be extremal and are also permitted by the wave properties of light. One important example occurs in fiber-optic light-guides, which are fabricated with a gradient in the refractive index such that the "densest" material is at the center of each fiber. The path down the center of the fiber takes the longest time of all possible nearby light paths, steering the light down the center of each fiber.

Chapter Exercises

Questions

2.1. Which theory provides the most comprehensive description of light?
  a. wave theory
  b. particle theory
  c. ray theory
  d. quantum electrodynamics

2.2. The Airy disc image on the retina is larger in which circumstance?
  a. The wavelength of light is shortened.
  b. The focal length of the eye is shorter.
  c. The pupil size decreases.
  d. Macular degeneration is present.

2.3. Corneal haze secondary to corneal edema is primarily caused by which light phenomena?
  a. reflection
  b. light scattering
  c. refraction
  d. diffraction

2.4. Which light phenomenon is the underlying basis of optical coherence tomography?
  a. diffraction
  b. interference
  c. fluorescence
  d. polarization

2.5. Which laser–tissue interaction is the basis of laser in situ keratomileusis (LASIK)?
  a. photodisruption
  b. photochemical interaction
  c. plasma-induced ablation
  d. photoablation

2.6. In aphakia, the susceptibility to photochemical injury to the retina is which of the following?
  a. decreased without the focusing capability of the natural lens
  b. unchanged
  c. increased without the ultraviolet absorption of the natural lens
  d. not an issue

Answers

2.1. **d.** In general, it suffices to consider the wavelike behavior of light for phenomena at the macroscopic level and the simple quantum-view of light at the microscopic level. However, the quantum theory of the interaction of light and matter—quantum electrodynamics—explains all the properties of light we know, resolving the wave-particle confusion.

2.2. **c.** The Airy disc is the central portion of a pattern of light and dark rings formed when light from a point source passes through a circular aperture and is diffracted. The size of the Airy disc increases with smaller pupil size (especially pupil diameter < 2.5 mm), longer wavelengths of light, and longer focal lengths. Retinal conditions such as macular degeneration have no effect on the size of the Airy disc.

2.3. **b.** Light scattering occurs when small particles suspended in a transparent medium interfere with the transmittance of light and cause photons to deviate from a straight path. Short wavelengths of light are scattered more strongly than are longer wavelengths. Larger particles scatter light more intensely than do smaller particles. In a healthy cornea, the tightly arranged and regularly spaced collagen molecules minimize the effects of scattering. When a cornea becomes edematous, excess fluid in the stroma disrupts the regular collagen structure, causing light scattering.

2.4. **b.** Optical coherence tomography (OCT) is an echo technique similar to ultrasound imaging, but uses infrared light instead of sound. The much higher speed of light, compared with that of sound, makes infeasible the direct electronic measurement of the shorter "echo" times it takes light to travel from different structures at axial distances within the eye. Interferometry enables us to overcome this difficulty. More precisely, OCT uses interference of broadband or tunable coherent light to generate optical sections of the retina and cornea.

2.5. **d.** Laser in situ keratomileusis (LASIK) and photorefractive keratectomy (PRK), common refractive surgeries of the cornea, are based on photoablation with excimer lasers that generate photons with wavelengths in the ultraviolet (UV) range that are absorbed within the corneal tissue.

2.6. **c.** In the retina, natural chromophores strongly absorb wavelengths from about 400–580 nm, which makes the retina susceptible to photochemical injury in that region, especially from blue light. This susceptibility to damage is increased in an aphakic eye; without the UVA absorption capability of the natural lens, wavelengths of between about 315 nm and 400 nm may also be absorbed. Because of this, UV-blocking and blue-blocking chromophores are incorporated in some intraocular lenses.

CHAPTER 3

Optics of the Human Eye

Highlights

- The major challenges to understanding the optics of the human eye lie in the complexities and "imperfections" of some of the eye's optical elements.
- Important axes to take note of include the "line of sight," the pupillary axis, and the optical axis; important angles to remember are the angle alpha (α), the angle kappa (κ), and the angle lambda (λ).
- The development of myopia is a complex interaction of multiple genetic and environmental factors.
- As the lens loses elasticity from the aging process, the accommodative response wanes, a condition called *presbyopia* (from Greek: "old eyes"), even though the amount of ciliary muscle contraction (or accommodative effort) is virtually unchanged.

Glossary

Accommodation The faculty of the eye to increase the optical power of the lens—may be used to focus on near objects, or to self-correct hyperopic refractive errors.

Against-the-rule astigmatism Astigmatism with the greatest refractive power in the horizontal meridian.

Ametropia Any refractive error—any deviation from emmetropia.

Angle alpha (α) In an ideal eye with centered optics, the angle between the optical axis and the visual axis.

Angle kappa (κ) In an ideal eye with centered optics, the angle between the pupillary axis and the visual axis.

Angle lambda (λ) In an actual eye, the angle between the pupillary axis and the line of sight.

Aniseikonia Disparity in the size of the retinal images formed in the 2 eyes of a patient.

Anisometropia Different refractive errors in the 2 eyes of a patient.

Astigmatism A refractive error in which the power of the eye varies in different meridians.

Contrast sensitivity The ability to detect small spatial variations in the luminance of a visual stimulus; quantitatively, the reciprocal of the contrast threshold.

Contrast sensitivity function The relationship between the contrast threshold of a grating target and its spatial frequency (spacing between the bars of the grating).

Contrast threshold The minimum contrast at which a target is detectable.

Emmetropia The refractive state of an eye, which, with relaxed accommodation, focuses objects at optical infinity on the fovea.

Entrance pupil The image of the anatomical pupil as seen through the cornea.

Gullstrand model eye A detailed schematic eye model developed by Allvar Gullstrand.

Hyperopia A refractive error in which objects at infinity are focused behind the retina, with relaxed accommodation.

Irregular astigmatism A refractive error in which the astigmatism varies significantly across the optical aperture of the eye.

Line of sight The line from the fixation point to the center of the entrance pupil of the eye.

Modulation transfer function A function that describes the relationship between the contrast of a visual stimulus and the contrast of the image of the stimulus on the retina, as a function of spatial frequency.

Myopia A refractive error in which objects at infinity are focused in front of the retina, with relaxed accommodation.

Optical axis In an ideal eye with centered optics, the extension of the rotational axis of symmetry of the crystalline lens through the optical center of the cornea.

Optotype A standardized letter or other character, typically defined by features that subtend one-fifth of the height of the character, such as the horizontal bars and the spaces between them, of the letter E.

Pinhole visual acuity Measurement of visual acuity as perceived through an occluder with pinhole apertures that reduce the impact of refractive error.

Presbyopia The loss of accommodation with increasing age.

Pupillary axis The line from the center of curvature of the cornea that passes through the midpoint of the entrance pupil, perpendicular to the corneal surface.

Reduced schematic eye A simplified schematic eye model with a single refracting surface at the corneal apex.

Regular astigmatism A refractive error in which the astigmatism is approximately constant across the optical aperture of the eye.

Snellen visual acuity The ability to identify small letters or other optotypes (presented at high contrast).

Spatial frequency The number of stripes or cycles of a periodic test target per degree of visual angle.

Visual axis In an ideal eye with centered optics, the hypothetical (broken) line that connects the fixation point with the fovea, and passes through the nodal points. Often casually identified as the line of sight.

With-the-rule astigmatism Astigmatism with the greatest refractive power in the vertical meridian.

Introduction

This chapter presents conceptual tools to aid in understanding the optics of the human eye. In addition, it covers the various methods used to measure the eye's ability to "see" and reviews the types of refractive errors of the eye. Treatment of refractive errors is discussed in Chapters 4, 5, and 6 of this volume.

Schematic Eyes

The major challenges to understanding the optics of the human eye lie in the complexities and "imperfections" of some of the eye's optical elements. Simplifications and approximations make models easier to understand but limit their ability to explain all the subtleties of the eye's optical system. As an example, the anterior surface of the cornea is frequently assumed to be spherical, but the actual anterior surface tends to flatten toward the limbus. Also, the center of the crystalline lens is usually decentered with respect to the cornea and the visual axis of the eye.

Many mathematical models of the eye's optical system are based on careful anatomical measurements and approximations. The model developed by Gullstrand (Fig 3-1, Table 3-1), a Swedish professor of ophthalmology, so closely approximated the human eye that he was awarded a Nobel Prize in 1911. Although very useful, this model is cumbersome for most clinical calculations and is often simplified further.

EXAMPLE 3-1

What is the depth of the anterior chamber of the Gullstrand model eye? As shown in Figure 3-1 and Table 3-1, the distance from the apex of the cornea to the front surface of the lens is 3.6 mm, while the thickness of the cornea is 0.5 mm, so the depth of the anterior chamber is 3.1 mm.

Because the principal points of the cornea and lens are fairly close to each other, a single intermediate point can substitute for them. Note that the principal points of the cornea lie at the front of the cornea, with the second principal point farther from the corneal

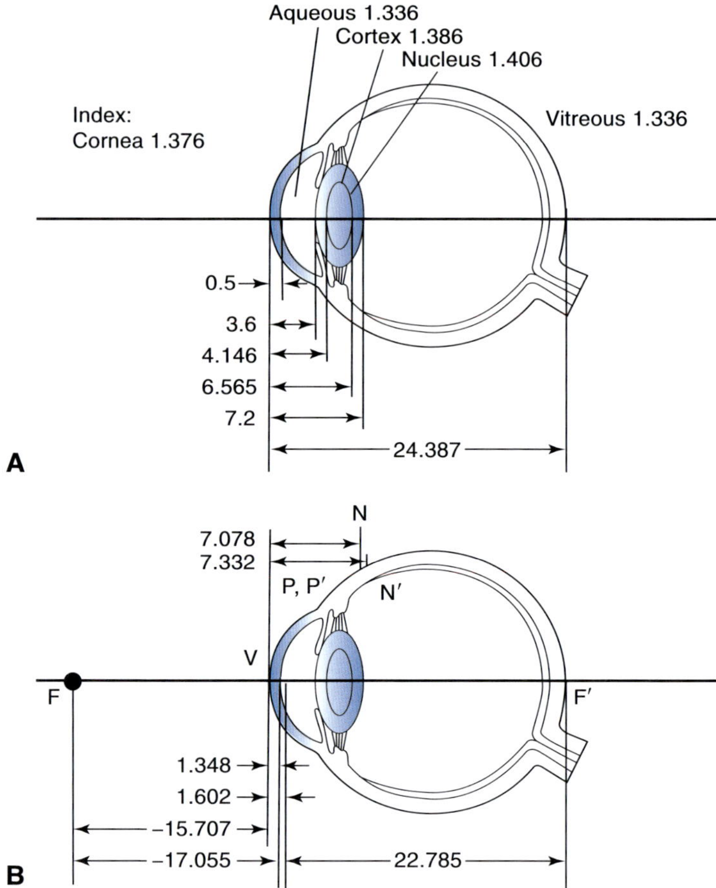

Figure 3-1 Optical constants of the Gullstrand eye. All values in millimeters. **A,** Refractive indices of the media and positions of the refracting surfaces. **B,** Positions of the principal points, which are used for optical calculations. *(Illustration by C. H. Wooley.)*

apex than the first. In a similar fashion, the nodal points of the cornea and lens can be combined into a single nodal point located 17.0 mm in front of the retina. Thus, we can treat the eye as if it were a single refracting element, an ideal spherical surface separating 2 media of different refractive indices: 1.000 for air and 1.333 for the eye (Fig 3-2). This simplified model is known as the *reduced schematic eye.*

Using this reduced schematic eye, we can calculate the retinal image size of an object in space (such as a Snellen letter). This calculation utilizes the simplified nodal point, through which light rays entering or leaving the eye pass undeviated. The geometric principle of similar triangles can be used for the calculation of retinal image size if the following information is given: (1) the actual height of a Snellen letter on the eye chart, (2) the distance from the eye chart to the eye, and (3) the distance from the nodal point to the retina. The formula for this calculation is as follows:

$$\frac{\text{Retinal Image Height}}{\text{Snellen Letter Height}} = \frac{\text{Nodal Point to Retina Distance}}{\text{Chart to Eye Distance}}$$

Table 3-1 The Schematic Eye

	Accommodation Relaxed[a]	Maximum Accommodation[a]
Refractive index		
Cornea	1.376	1.376
Aqueous humor and vitreous body	1.336	1.336
Lens	1.386	1.386
Equivalent core lens	1.406	1.406
Position		
Anterior surface of cornea	0	0
Posterior surface of cornea	0.5	0.5
Anterior surface of lens	3.6	3.2
Anterior surface of equivalent core lens	4.146	3.8725
Posterior surface of equivalent core lens	6.565	6.5275
Posterior surface of lens	7.2	7.2
Radius of curvature		
Anterior surface of cornea	7.7	7.7
Posterior surface of cornea	6.8	6.8
Anterior surface of lens	10.0	5.33
Anterior surface of equivalent core lens	7.911	2.655
Posterior surface of equivalent core lens	–5.76	–2.655
Posterior surface of lens	–6.0	–5.33
Refracting power (diopters)		
Anterior surface of cornea	48.83	48.83
Posterior surface of cornea	–5.88	–5.88
Anterior surface of lens	5.0	9.375
Core lens	5.985	14.96
Posterior surface of lens	8.33	9.375
Corneal system (diopters)		
Refracting power	43.05	43.05
Position of first principal point	–0.0496	–0.0496
Position of second principal point	–0.0506	–0.0506
First focal length	–23.227	–23.227
Second focal length	31.031	31.031
Lens system (diopters)		
Refracting power	19.11	33.06
Position of first principal point	5.678	5.145
Position of second principal point	5.808	5.255
Focal length	69.908	40.416
Complete optical system of eye (diopters)		
Refracting power	58.64	70.57
Position of first principal point, P	1.348	1.772
Position of second principal point, P′	1.602	2.086
Position of first focal point, F	–15.707	–12.397
Position of second focal point, F′	24.387	21.016
First focal length	–17.055	–14.169
Second focal length	22.785	18.930
Position of first nodal point, N	7.078	NA[a]
Position of second nodal point, N′	7.332	NA
Position of fovea centralis	24.0	24.0
Axial refraction	–1.0	–9.6

NA = not applicable.

[a]All values in millimeters unless otherwise noted.

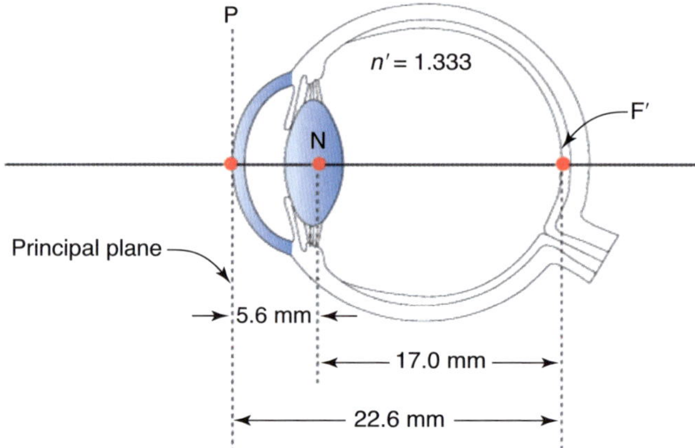

Figure 3-2 Dimensions of the reduced schematic eye, defined by the anterior corneal surface (P), the simplified nodal point of the eye (N), and the fovea (F′). The distance from the simplified nodal point to the fovea is 17.0 mm, and the distance from the anterior corneal surface to the nodal point is 5.6 mm. The refractive index for air is taken to be 1.000, and the simplified refractive index for the eye *(n′)* is 1.333. The refractive power of this reduced schematic eye is 60.00 D, with its principal plane at the front surface of the cornea. *(Illustration by C. H. Wooley.)*

Although in principle the distance from the eye chart should be measured to the nodal point, it is much easier to measure the distance to the surface of the cornea. The difference between these measurements is 5.6 mm, which is usually insignificant. For example, if the distance between the nodal point and the retina is 17.0 mm, the distance between the eye chart and the eye is 20 ft (6000 mm), and the height of a Snellen letter is 60 mm, then the resulting image size on the retina is 0.17 mm.

Katz M, Kruger PB. The human eye as an optical system. In: Tasman W, Jaeger EA, eds. *Duane's Clinical Ophthalmology* [CD-ROM]. Vol 1. Lippincott Williams & Wilkins; 2013:chap 33.

Important Axes of the Eye

Thus far in this volume, we have discussed "centered" optical systems, in which successive refractive elements share a common axis of symmetry, referred to as the "optical axis." Unfortunately, this situation poorly approximates the real eye. Even to the extent that one can approximately identify a common axis for the eye's optical elements, this axis rarely passes through the fovea. Thus, the direction of gaze seldom coincides with the optical axis. This disparity is important in the estimation of alignment of the eyes and in the centration of optical interventions such as corneal refractive surgery and centration of intraocular lenses.

For the purposes of measuring ocular alignment, it is convenient to envision a direction of gaze for each eye, often referred to as the "visual axis" or "line of sight." This connects the fixation target with the fovea. (In precise analysis, the "visual axis" is envisioned as the hypothetical broken line that connects the fixation target with the fovea and passes through the nodal points—even this concept requires that the optical elements constitute a centered optical system, as misaligned compound optics do not possess nodal points.) The "line of sight" may be taken more precisely as the line connecting the fixation target with the center of the entrance pupil (the image of the anatomic pupil seen through the cornea). Neither the optical axis nor the visual axis can be identified clinically.

On the other hand, it is convenient to estimate the orientation of the globe by sighting the reflection of a small light source in the cornea. The "pupillary axis" can readily be determined as the line extending forward from the center of curvature of the cornea, through the center of the entrance pupil, and perpendicular to the cornea. This is the direction from which the corneal light reflex appears centered in the entrance pupil. The angle between the pupillary axis and the visual axis is commonly designated as the "angle kappa." It is considered positive if the line of sight is nasal to the pupillary axis, as is commonly the case (Figure 3-3).

For the purposes of centration of refractive procedures or intraocular lens placement, the angle between the pupillary axis and the line of sight is designated as the "angle lambda," in contrast to the (hypothetical) angle kappa between the pupillary axis and the visual axis. The (hypothetical) angle between the optical axis and the visual axis is designated as the "angle alpha."

Uozato H, Guyton DL. Centering corneal surgical procedures. *Am J Ophthalmol.* 1987;103 (3 Pt 1):264–275.

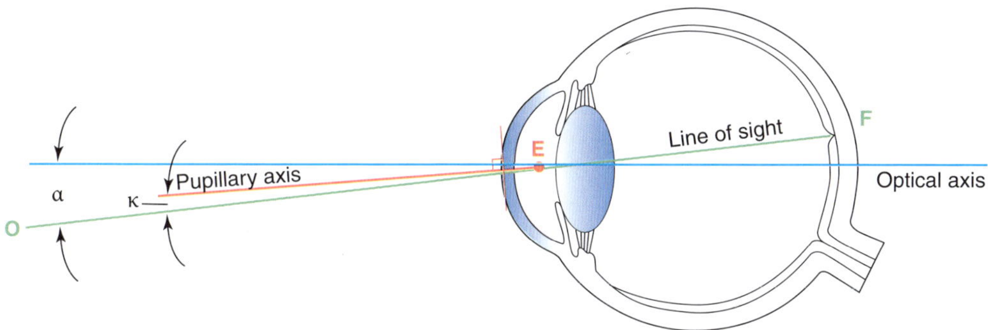

Figure 3-3 Idealized rendition of the important axes and angles of the eye. The pupillary axis *(red line)* is the line perpendicular to the corneal surface and passes through the midpoint of the entrance pupil (E). The line of sight *(green line)* is shown as the line connecting the fixation target (O) and the fovea (F). The optical axis *(blue line)* is the line through the optical centers of the cornea and the lens; it cannot be observed clinically. If all the optical elements of the human eye were in perfect alignment, these lines would overlap; however, the fovea is normally displaced from its expected position. The angle between the pupillary axis and the visual axis *(leader line)* is called the angle kappa (κ) and is considered positive when the fovea is located temporally, as is the usual case. Conditions that cause temporal dragging of the retina, such as retinopathy of prematurity, can lead to a large positive angle kappa. Clinically, this will present as pseudoexotropia. A large positive angle kappa may also mask a small-angle esotropia, which can be detected by the cover-uncover test. Angle alpha (α) is the angle between the optical axis and visual axis and is considered positive when the visual axis lies on the nasal side of the optical axis, as is normally the case. It cannot be observed clinically. *(Courtesy of Neal H. Atebara, MD. Revised illustration based on a drawing by C. H. Wooley.)*

Pupil Size and Its Effect on Visual Resolution

The size of the blur circle on the retina generally increases as the size of the pupil increases. If a pinhole aperture is placed immediately in front of an eye, it acts as an artificial pupil, and the size of the blur circle is reduced correspondingly (Fig 3-4).

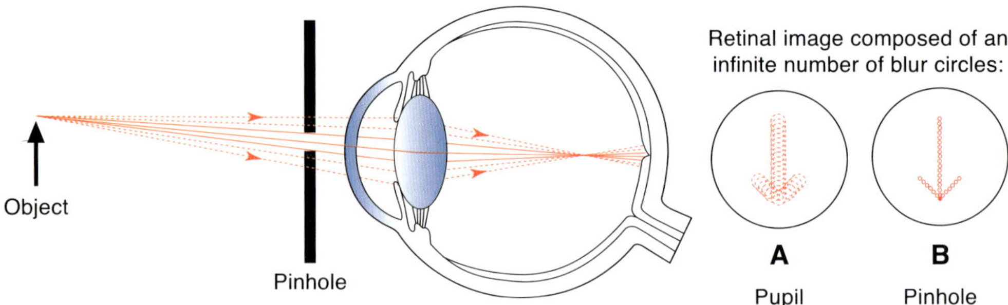

Figure 3-4 Light rays from each point on an object *(upright arrow)* form a blur circle on the retina of a myopic eye. The retinal image is the composite of all blur circles, the size of each being proportional to the diameter of the pupil (A) and the amount of defocus. If a pinhole is held in front of the eye, the size of each blur circle is decreased; as a result, the overall retinal image is sharpened (B). *(Courtesy of Neal H. Atebara, MD. Revised illustration based on a drawing by C. H. Wooley.)*

The pinhole is used clinically to measure *pinhole visual acuity.* If visual acuity improves when measured through a pinhole aperture, a refractive error is usually present. The most useful pinhole diameter for general clinical purposes (refractive errors between –5.00 D and +5.00 D) is 1.2 mm. If the pinhole aperture is made smaller, the blurring effects of diffraction around the edges of the aperture overwhelm the image-sharpening effects of the smaller aperture. For refractive errors greater than 5.00 D, the clinician needs to use a lens that corrects most of the refractive error in addition to the pinhole.

After the best refractive correction has been determined, the pinhole can also be used with a dilated pupil. If visual acuity improves, optical irregularities, such as corneal and lenticular light scattering or irregular astigmatism, are likely to be present, given that the pinhole serves to restrict light to a relatively small area of the eye's optics. (This technique also can be used to identify optical causes of *monocular diplopia.*) If visual acuity worsens, macular disease must be considered, as a diseased macula is often unable to adapt to the reduced amount of light that enters through the pinhole.

Because of the refractive effects of the cornea, the entrance pupil is about 13%–15% larger than the actual pupil and displaced somewhat anterior to the plane of the iris. This explains why the anterior chamber is actually deeper than it looks.

CLINICAL PROBLEM 3-1

Why do persons with uncorrected myopia squint?
To obtain a pinhole effect (or rather a stenopeic slit effect). Better visual acuity results from smaller blur circles (or even smaller blur "slits").

Does pupil size affect the measured near point of accommodation?
Yes. With smaller pupil size, the eye's depth of focus increases, and objects closer than the actual near point of the eye remain in better focus.

Why are patients less likely to need their glasses in bright light?
One reason is that the bright light causes the pupil to constrict, allowing the defocused image to be less blurred on the retina.

EXAMPLE 3-2

Estimate the location of the entrance pupil, that is, the image of the anatomical pupil as seen through the cornea. (Assume the anatomical pupil lies in the same plane as the lens apex.) Using the Gullstrand model eye, the distance from the *second* principal plane of the cornea to the lens apex in millimeters is $0.0506 + 3.6 = 3.6506$ mm. (Because the source object [the iris] is *behind* the refracting surfaces [cornea], the usual roles of the first and second principal planes are reversed.) As the corneal system's power is 43.05 D, the vergence equation gives $-1.336/0.0036506 + 43.05 = 1/x$, where 1.336 is the refractive index of the aqueous and vitreous body, and x is the distance from the *first* principal plane to the image of the pupil (as seen by an external observer in air). This gives $1/x = -322.92$ D, or $x = -3.097$ mm. Thus, the entrance pupil and the external observer's view of the iris are about 0.55 mm closer to the observer than the anatomical pupil and the true iris plane.

Visual Acuity

Clinicians often think of visual acuity primarily in terms of Snellen acuity, but visual perception is a far more complex process than is encapsulated by this single measurement. Indeed, there are many ways to measure visual function. The following are definitions of terms used in the measurement of visual function:

- *Minimum legible threshold:* the point at which a patient's visual ability cannot further distinguish progressively smaller letters or forms from one another; Snellen visual acuity is the most common method of determining this threshold
- *Minimum visible threshold:* the minimum contrast of a target at which the patient can distinguish the target from the background
- *Minimum separable threshold:* the smallest visual angle formed by the eye and 2 separate objects at which a patient can distinguish them individually
- *Vernier acuity:* the smallest detectable amount of misalignment of 2 line segments

Snellen visual acuity is measured with test letters or similar targets (optotypes) constructed such that each optotype as a whole is 5 times larger than the individual strokes or gaps that make up the optotype (eg, the horizontal lines, and the spaces between them, of the letter E, or the gap that differentiates a circle from the letter C). Letters of different sizes are designated by the distance at which the letter subtends an angle of 5 arcmin (Fig 3-5). The Snellen chart is designed to measure visual acuity in angular terms. However, the traditional convention does not specify visual acuity in angular measure; instead, it uses a notation in which the numerator is the *testing distance* (in feet or meters) and the denominator is the *distance at which a letter subtends the standard visual angle of 5 arcmin.* Thus, on the 20/20 line (6/6 in meters), the letters subtend an angle of 5 arcmin when viewed at 20 ft. In examination rooms with shorter distances than 20 ft (6 m), mirrors can be used to increase the viewing distance. On the 20/40 (6/12) line, the letters subtend an angle of 10 arcmin when viewed at 20 ft, or 5 arcmin when viewed at 40 ft. The "40" in

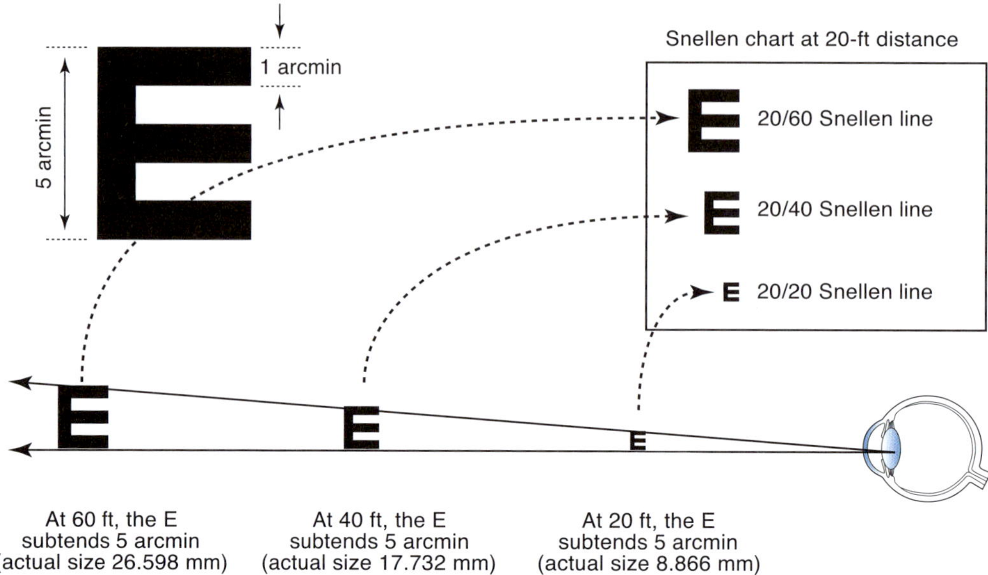

Figure 3-5 Snellen letters are constructed such that they subtend an angle of 5 arcmin when located at the distance specified by the denominator. For example, if a Snellen E is about 26 mm in height, it subtends 5 arcmin at 60 ft. Correspondingly, a 26-mm letter occupies the 20/60 line of the Snellen chart at the standard testing distance of 20 ft. *(Courtesy of Neal H. Atebara, MD. Revised illustration based on a drawing by C. H. Wooley.)*

the 20/40 letter (or the "12" in the 6/12 letter) refers to the viewing distance at which this letter subtends the "normal" visual angle of 5 arcmin. Table 3-2 lists conversions of visual acuity measurements for the various methods in use—the Snellen fraction, decimal notation (Visus), visual angle in minutes of arc, and *base-10 logarithm of the minimum angle of resolution* (logMAR). LogMAR is useful for averaging the results of multiple measurements of Snellen visual acuity.

Though widely accepted, common Snellen eye charts are not perfect. The letters on different Snellen lines are not necessarily related to one another by size in any regular geometric or logarithmic sense. For example, the increase in letter size from the 20/20 line to the 20/25 line (an increase of 25%) differs from the increase from the 20/25 line to the 20/30 line (an increase of 20%). In addition, certain letters (such as C, D, O, and G) are inherently harder to recognize or to distinguish than others (such as A and J), partly because there are more letters of the alphabet with which they can be confused. For these reasons, alternative visual acuity charts have been developed and popularized in high-quality clinical trials (eg, the Early Treatment Diabetic Retinopathy Study [ETDRS] and Bailey-Lovie charts) (Fig 3-6). These charts feature careful choices of optotypes, uniform proportional (logarithmic) progression of optotype size from line to line, and the same number of optotypes on each line. See Appendix 3-1 for details.

Computer-based acuity devices that display optotypes on a monitor screen have also become popular because they allow presentation of a random assortment of optotypes

Table 3-2 Visual Acuity Conversion Chart

Snellen Fraction					
Feet	Meters	4-Meter Standard	Decimal Notation (Visus)	Visual Angle Minute of Arc	LogMAR (Minimum Angle of Resolution)
20/10	6/3	4/2	2.00	0.50	–0.30
20/15	6/4.5	4/3	1.33	0.75	–0.12
20/20	**6/6**	**4/4**	**1.00**	**1.00**	**0.00**
20/25	6/7.5	4/5	0.80	1.25	0.10
20/30	6/9	4/6	0.67	1.50	0.18
20/40	6/12	4/8	0.50	2.00	0.30
20/50	6/15	4/10	0.40	2.50	0.40
20/60	6/18	4/12	0.33	3.00	0.48
20/80	6/24	4/16	0.25	4.00	0.60
20/100	6/30	4/20	0.20	5.00	0.70
20/120	6/36	4/24	0.17	6.00	0.78
20/150	6/45	4/30	0.13	7.50	0.88
20/200	6/60	4/40	0.10	10.00	1.00
20/400	6/120	4/80	0.05	20.00	1.30

and scrambling of letters, thereby eliminating problems associated with memorization by patients. The original Snellen eye chart used letters of an ordinary typeface and of various sizes. However, it is preferable to choose optotypes from simpler typefaces that better present identifying features as 20% of the overall letter height and to restrict the choice of letters to a subset of the alphabet that is as uniform in distinguishability as possible. A standard set of letters in a simple, sans-serif font, known as the *Sloan letters* (C, D, H, K, N, O, R, S, V, and Z) is commonly used. (Note that the letter E is not a Sloan letter.) The original ETDRS charts featured Sloan letter optotypes. ETDRS-type charts are now available with many alternative optotype sets, including the Landolt C, HOTV, tumbling E, as well as numerals and picture optotypes such as the LEA symbols (Fig 3-6B–E). Alternative optotypes are available for patients with special needs: the tumbling E and Landolt C optotypes are suitable for preliterate patients, and the 4-letter HOTV test can be used with a reference sample to allow patients to point to the optotypes they see, even if they cannot name the letters. Picture charts are often useful for small children. The carefully calibrated LEA symbols (circle, square, house, apple) are far preferable to the older, traditional picture set (hand, horse, telephone, bird, birthday cake), because the LEA symbols blur into indistinguishable circles with decreasing acuity, whereas the traditional pictures can often be recognized even after the smallest details can no longer be resolved.

Levi DM. Visual acuity. In: Levin LA, Nilsson SFE, Ver Hoeve J, Wu SM, eds. *Adler's Physiology of the Eye.* 11th ed. Elsevier; 2011.

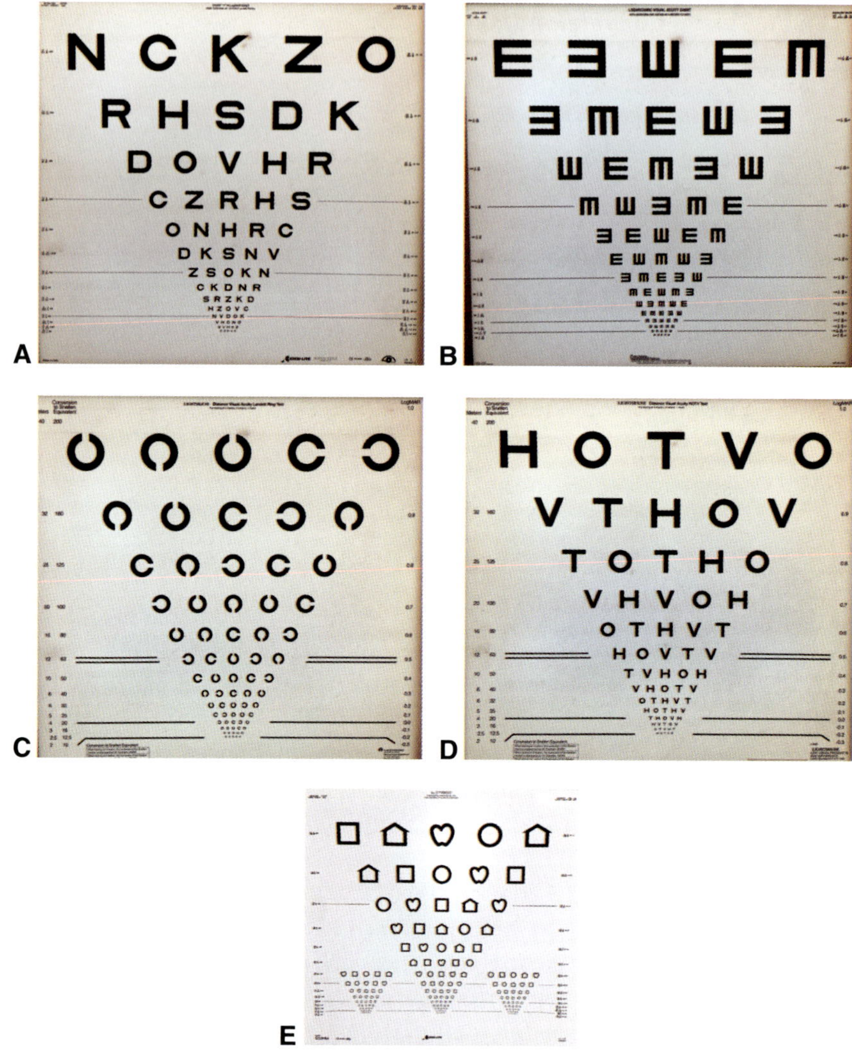

Figure 3-6 Modified Early Treatment Diabetic Retinopathy Study (ETDRS)–type eyecharts with alternative optotypes. **A,** Visual acuity chart intended for use at 13 ft (4 m) but can also be used at 20 ft (6 m) or 5 ft (1.5 m) with appropriate scaling. The optotypes are Sloan letters. **B,** Tumbling E optotypes. **C,** Landolt C optotypes. **D,** HOTV optotypes. **E,** LEA optotypes. *(Parts A–D courtesy of Singapore National Eye Center. Part E courtesy of Vicki Chen, MD.)*

Contrast Sensitivity and the Contrast Sensitivity Function

Another important dimension in the measurement of visual function is contrast sensitivity—the sensitivity of an observer to differences in luminance between an object and the background. In general, the higher the contrast, the easier an optotype is to decipher. Over a broad range, the visual system is relatively insensitive to the absolute brightness of a visual stimulus, but is much more attuned to the contrast between adjacent surfaces. For example, the dark ink on a printed page reflects about 10% of the incident light. In comparison, the white paper background has a reflectance of perhaps 90%, regardless of the level of absolute illumination. Thus, when reading under bright sunlight, we still appreciate the printed text as black, even though the absolute brightness of the reflected light is greater than that reflected from white paper in dim illumination, as in twilight. If the brightness of an object (I_{min}) and the brightness of its background (I_{max}) are known, the following formula can be used to measure the degree of contrast between the object and its background:

$$\text{Contrast} = \frac{I_{max} - I_{min}}{I_{max} + I_{min}}$$

Thus, for typical printed matter, the contrast is about 80% (90% – 10%)/(90% + 10%). Snellen visual acuity is commonly tested with illuminated or projected charts that *approximate* 100% contrast. Therefore, when we measure Snellen visual acuity, we are measuring, at approximately 100% contrast, the smallest optotype that the visual system can recognize. In everyday life, however, 100% contrast is rarely encountered, and most visual tasks must be performed in lower-contrast conditions.

To take contrast sensitivity into account when measuring visual function, we can use the *modulation transfer function (MTF).* Consider a target in which the light intensity varies from some peak value to zero in a sinusoidal fashion. The contrast is 100%, but instead of looking like a bar graph, it looks like a bar graph with softened edges. The number of light bands per unit length or per unit angle is called the *spatial frequency* and is closely related to Snellen acuity. For example, the 20/20 E optotype is composed of bands of light and dark, in which each band is 1 arcmin. Thus, for a target at 100% contrast, 20/20 Snellen acuity corresponds roughly to 30 cycles per degree of resolution when expressed in spatial frequency notation. The relationship between spatial frequency and the contrast sensitivity at each spatial frequency constitutes the MTF.

In clinical practice, the ophthalmologist presents a patient with targets of various spatial frequencies and peak contrasts. A plot is then made of the minimum resolvable contrast target that can be seen for each spatial frequency. The minimum resolvable contrast is the *contrast threshold.* The reciprocal of the contrast threshold is defined as the *contrast sensitivity,* and the manner in which contrast sensitivity changes as a function of the spatial frequency of the targets is called the *contrast sensitivity function (CSF)* (Fig 3-7). Figure 3-8 shows a typical contrast sensitivity curve obtained with sinusoidal gratings. Contrast sensitivity can also be tested with optotypes of variable contrast (eg, the Pelli-Robson or Regan charts), which may be easier for patients to use. It is important to perform contrast sensitivity testing with the best possible optical correction in place. In addition, luminance must be kept constant when CSF is tested, because mean luminance affects the shape of the normal CSF curve. In low luminance, the low spatial frequency fall-off disappears and the peak shifts toward the lower frequencies. In brighter light, there is little change in the shape of the normal CSF curve through a range of luminance for the higher spatial frequencies. Generally, contrast sensitivity is measured at normal room illumination, which is approximately 30–70 lux.

Figure 3-7 Campbell-Robson contrast sensitivity grating. In this example, the contrast diminishes from bottom to top, and the spatial frequency of the pattern increases from left to right. The pattern appears to have a hump in the middle, at the frequencies for which the human eye is most sensitive to contrast. *(Courtesy of Brian Wandell, PhD.)*

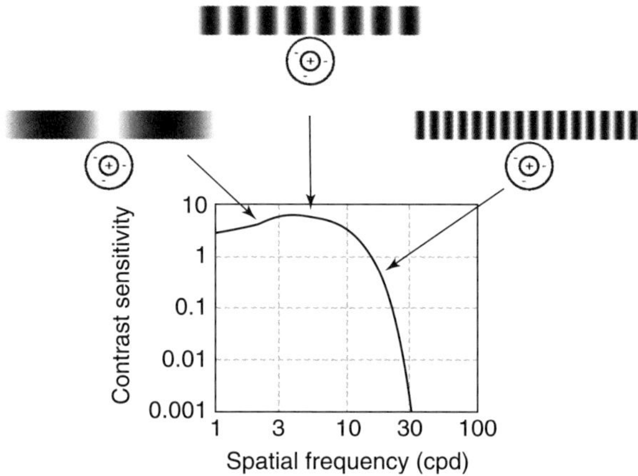

Figure 3-8 An example of a contrast sensitivity curve. The ability to discern various contrast sensitivities as spatial frequency is tested and plotted on this chart. *(Used with permission from Brian Wandall, PhD.)*

Various physiologic and pathologic conditions of the eye affect contrast sensitivity. Any corneal pathology that causes distortion or edema can affect contrast sensitivity. Lens changes, particularly incipient cataracts, may significantly decrease CSF, even with normal Snellen visual acuity. Retinal pathology may affect contrast sensitivity more (as with retinitis pigmentosa or central serous retinopathy) or less (certain macular degenerations) than it does Snellen visual acuity. Glaucoma may produce a significant loss in the midrange of spatial frequencies. Optic neuritis may also be associated with a notch-type pattern of sensitivity loss. Amblyopia is associated with a generalized attenuation of the curve. Pupil size also has an effect on contrast sensitivity. With miotic pupils, diffraction reduces contrast sensitivity; with large pupils, optical aberrations may interfere with performance.

Impairments in perception of contrast may be disqualifying in certain occupational situations, such as driving heavy vehicles. Recognition of these difficulties is often valuable in understanding the concerns of patients, who may have difficulty with certain visual tasks notwithstanding good Snellen acuity as measured with the standard high-contrast eye charts.

Refractive States of the Eyes

In considering the refractive state of the eye, we can use either of the following approaches:

1. The *focal point* concept: The location of the image formed by an object at optical infinity through a nonaccomodating eye determines the eye's refractive state. Objects that focus at points anterior or posterior to the retina form blurred images on the retina, whereas objects that focus on the retina form sharp images.
2. The *far point* concept: The far point is the point in space that is conjugate to the fovea of the nonaccommodating eye; that is, the far point is where the fovea would be imaged if the light rays were reversed and the fovea became the object.

Emmetropia is the refractive state in which parallel rays of light from a distant object are brought to focus on the retina in the nonaccommodating eye (Fig 3-9A). The far point of the emmetropic eye is at infinity, and infinity is *conjugate* with the retina (Fig 3-9B). *Ametropia* refers to the absence of emmetropia and can be classified by presumptive etiology as *axial* or *refractive.* In *axial ametropia,* the eyeball is either unusually long *(myopia)* or short *(hyperopia).* In *refractive ametropia,* the length of the eye is statistically normal, but the refractive power of the eye (cornea and/or lens) is abnormal, being either excessive (myopia) or deficient (hyperopia). *Aphakia* is an example of extreme refractive hyperopia unless the eye was highly myopic (>20.00 D) before lens removal. An ametropic eye requires either a diverging or a converging lens to image a distant object on the retina.

Ametropias may also be classified by the nature of the mismatch between the optical power and length of the eye. In myopia, the eye possesses too much optical power for its axial length, and (with accommodation relaxed) light rays from an object at infinity converge too soon and thus focus in front of the retina (Fig 3-10A). This results in a defocused image on the retina; the far point of the eye is located in front of the eye, between the cornea and optical infinity (Fig 3-10B). In hyperopia, the eye does not possess enough optical power for its axial length, and (with accommodation relaxed) an object at infinity comes to a focus behind the retina, again producing a defocused image on the retina (Fig 3-11A); the far point of the eye (actually a virtual point rather than a real point in space) is located behind the retina (Fig 3-11B).

Astigmatism (*a* = without, *stigmos* = point) is an optical condition of the eye in which light rays from a point source on the eye's visual axis do not focus to a single point. Typically,

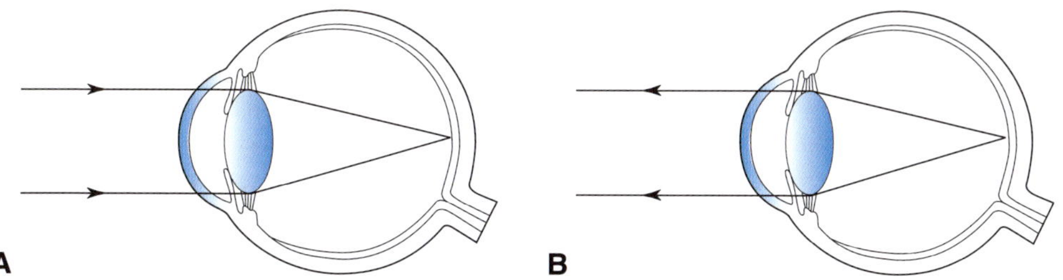

Figure 3-9 Emmetropia with accommodation relaxed. **A,** Parallel light rays from infinity focus to a point on the retina. **B,** Similarly, light rays emanating from a point on the retina focus at the far point of the eye at optical infinity. *(Illustration by C. H. Wooley.)*

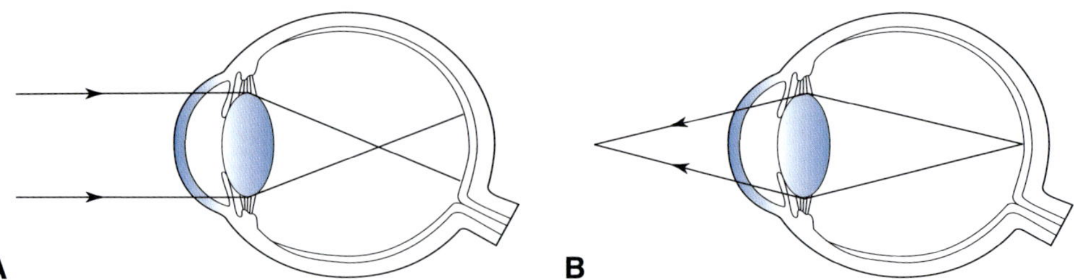

Figure 3-10 Myopia with accommodation relaxed. **A,** Parallel light rays from infinity focus to a point anterior to the retina, forming a blurred image on the retina. **B,** Light rays emanating from a point on the retina focus to a far point in front of the eye, between optical infinity and the cornea. *(Illustration by C. H. Wooley.)*

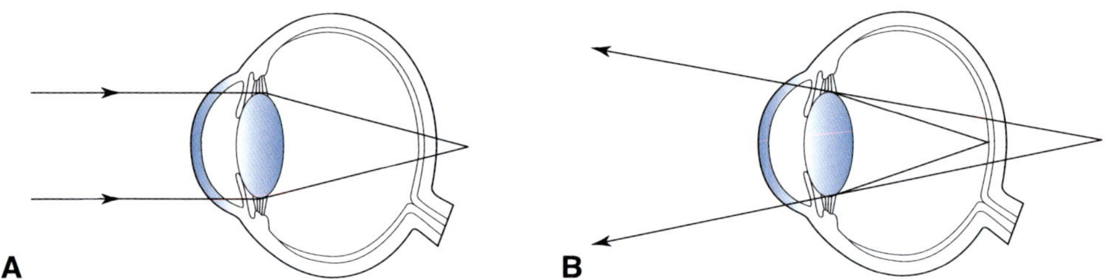

Figure 3-11 Hyperopia with accommodation relaxed. **A,** Parallel light rays from infinity focus to a point posterior to the retina, forming a blurred image on the retina. **B,** Light rays emanating from a point on the retina are divergent as they exit the eye, appearing to have come from a virtual far point behind the eye. *(Illustration by C. H. Wooley.)*

light rays from a single object point are refracted to form 2 *focal lines,* perpendicular to each other. Each astigmatic eye can be classified by the orientations and relative positions of these focal lines (Fig 3-12). If 1 focal line lies in front of the retina and the other is on the retina, the condition is classified as *simple myopic astigmatism.* If both focal lines lie in front of the retina, the condition is classified as *compound myopic astigmatism.* If, in a nonaccommodating eye, 1 focal line lies behind the retina and the other is on the retina, the astigmatism is classified as *simple hyperopic astigmatism.* If both focal lines lie behind the retina, the astigmatism is classified as *compound hyperopic astigmatism.* If, in a nonaccommodating eye, one focal line lies in front of the retina and the other behind it, the condition is classified as *mixed astigmatism.* The orientations of the focal lines reflect, in turn, the strongest and weakest meridians of the net refracting power of the anterior segment refracting surfaces (the cornea and lens). These are referred to as the *principal axes.*

If the principal axes of astigmatism have constant orientation at every point across the pupil, and if the amount of astigmatism is the same at every point, the refractive condition is known as *regular astigmatism.* Many cases of regular astigmatism may be classified as *with-the-rule* or *against-the-rule astigmatism.* In *with-the-rule* astigmatism (the more common type in children), the vertical corneal meridian is steepest (resembling an American football or a rugby ball lying on its side), and a correcting plus cylinder is placed with the cylinder axis near 90°. In *against-the-rule* astigmatism (the more common type in older

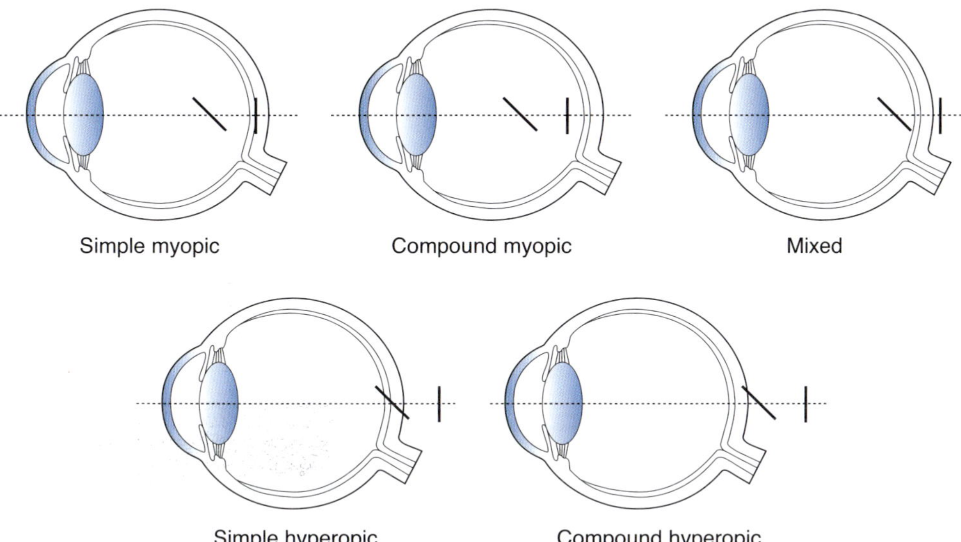

Figure 3-12 Types of astigmatism. The locations of the focal lines with respect to the retina define the type of astigmatism. The main difference between the types of astigmatism depicted in the illustration is the spherical equivalent refractive error. All of the astigmatisms depicted are with-the-rule astigmatisms—that is, they are corrected by using a plus cylinder with a vertical axis. If they were against-the-rule astigmatisms, the positions of the vertical and horizontal focal lines would be reversed.

adults), the horizontal meridian is steepest (resembling a football standing on its end), and a correcting plus cylinder should be placed with the axis near 180°. Alternatively, minus cylinders may be placed in the orthogonal directions. The term *oblique astigmatism* is used to describe regular astigmatism in which the principal meridians do not lie at, or close to, 90° or 180°, but instead lie nearer 45° or 135° (Fig 3-13).

In *irregular astigmatism*, the orientation of the principal meridians or the amount of astigmatism changes from point to point across the pupil. Although the principal meridians

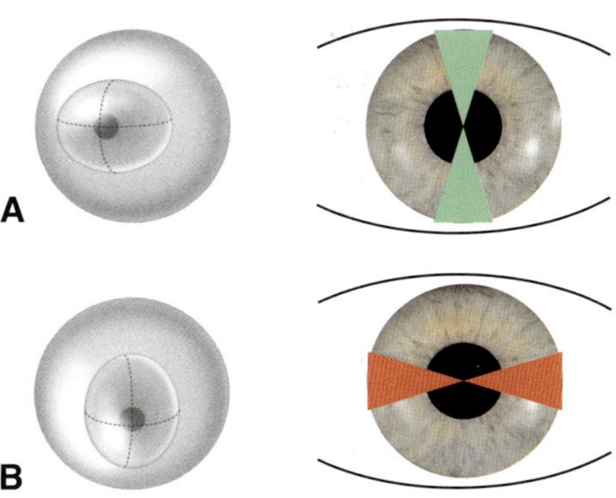

Figure 3-13 Regular astigmatism. Regular astigmatism may be classified as *with-the-rule* or *against-the-rule astigmatism*. **A,** In *with-the-rule* astigmatism the vertical corneal meridian is steepest and a correcting plus cylinder is placed with the cylinder axis near 90° *(green)*. **B,** In *against-the-rule* astigmatism the horizontal meridian is steepest and a correcting plus cylinder should be placed with the axis near 180° *(red)*. *(Black and white images developed by Scott E. Brodie, MD, PhD, and illustrated by Mark Miller. Color images courtesy of Uday Devgan, MD, and redrawn by C. H. Wooley.)*

are 90° apart at every point, it may sometimes appear with retinoscopy or keratometry that the principal meridians of the cornea, as a whole, are not perpendicular to one another. Most eyes have at least a small amount of irregular astigmatism, and instruments such as corneal topographers and wavefront aberrometers can be used to detect this condition clinically. These *higher-order* aberrations in the refractive properties of the cornea and lens may be characterized by Zernike polynomials, which are mathematical shapes that approximate various types of irregular astigmatism more closely than the simple "football" model. These aberrations include such shapes as spherical aberration, coma, and trefoil. See Chapters 1 and 7 of this book and BCSC Section 13, *Refractive Surgery,* for further discussion.

Binocular States of the Eyes

The spherical equivalent of a refractive state is defined as the algebraic sum of the spherical component and half of the astigmatic component. *Anisometropia* refers to any difference in the spherical equivalents between the 2 eyes. Uncorrected anisometropia in children may lead to amblyopia, especially if 1 eye is hyperopic. Although adults may be annoyed by uncorrected anisometropia, they may be intolerant of initial spectacle correction. Unequal image size, or *aniseikonia,* may occur, and the prismatic effect of the glasses will vary in different directions of gaze, inducing *anisophoria* (disparate ocular alignment in different directions of gaze). Anisophoria may be more bothersome than aniseikonia for patients with spectacle-corrected anisometropias. In most people, up to 7% of aniseikonia, which may result from approximately 3 diopters of anisometropia, is usually tolerated.

Even though aniseikonia is difficult to measure, anisometropic spectacle correction can be prescribed in such a manner as to reduce aniseikonia. Making the front surface power of a lens less positive can reduce magnification. Decreasing center thickness also reduces magnification. Decreasing vertex distance diminishes the magnifying effect of plus lenses as well as the minifying effect of minus lenses. These effects become increasingly noticeable as lens power increases. Contact lenses may provide a better solution than spectacles for some patients with anisometropia, particularly children, in whom fusion may be possible.

Unilateral aphakia is an extreme example of hyperopic anisometropia that arises from refractive ametropia. In the adult patient, spectacle correction produces an intolerable aniseikonia of about 25%; contact lens correction produces aniseikonia of about 7%. If necessary, the clinician may reduce aniseikonia further by adjusting the powers of contact lenses and simultaneously worn spectacle lenses to provide the appropriate minifying or magnifying effect via the Galilean telescope principle. With the near-universal adoption of intraocular lenses for the correction of aphakia, this problem is now rarely encountered. For further information on the correction of aphakia, see Chapter 6.

Accommodation and Presbyopia

Accommodation is the mechanism by which the eye changes refractive power by altering the shape and position of its crystalline lens. The changes in lens geometry that create this alteration were first described by Helmholtz. The posterior focal point is moved forward in the eye during accommodation (Fig 3-14A). Correspondingly, the far point moves closer to the eye (Fig 3-14B). *Accommodative effort* occurs when the ciliary muscle contracts in response to parasympathetic stimulation, thus allowing the zonular fibers to relax. The outward-directed tension on the lens capsule is decreased, and the lens becomes more convex, possibly in response to a pressure gradient pressing the lens forward against a "sling" formed by the zonular fibers and the anterior lens capsule ("catenary suspension"). *Accommodative response* results from the increase in lens convexity (primarily the anterior surface) and the net forward displacement of the lens. It may be expressed as the *amplitude of accommodation* (in diopters) or as the *range of accommodation,* the distance between the far point of the eye and the nearest point at which the eye can maintain focus *(near point).* It is evident that as the lens loses elasticity from the aging process, the accommodative response wanes, a condition called *presbyopia* (from Greek: "old eyes"), even though the amount of ciliary muscle contraction (or accommodative effort) is virtually unchanged. For an eye with presbyopia, the amplitude is a more useful measurement for calculating the power requirement of an eyeglass lens. For appraising an individual's ability to perform a specific visual task, the range is more informative.

Coleman DJ, Silverman RH, Lloyd H. Physiology of accommodation and role of the vitreous body. In: Sebag J, ed. *Vitreous: in Health and Disease.* Springer; 2014:495–507.

Eye Growth and Refractive Errors

An interplay among corneal power, lens power, anterior chamber depth, and axial length determines an individual's refractive status. All 4 elements change continuously as the eye grows. On average, babies are born with about 3.00 D of hyperopia. In the first few months of life, this hyperopia may increase slightly, but it then declines to an average of about 1.00 D of hyperopia by the end of the first year because of marked changes in corneal and

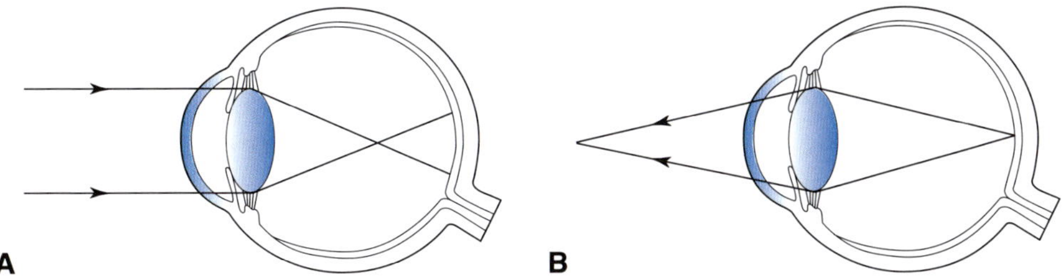

Figure 3-14 Emmetropia with accommodation stimulated. **A,** Parallel light rays now come to a point focus in front of the retina, forming a blurred image on the retina. **B,** Light rays emanating from a point on the retina focus to a near point in front of the eye, between optical infinity and the cornea. *(Illustration by C. H. Wooley.)*

lenticular powers as well as axial length growth. By the end of the second year, the anterior segment attains adult proportions; however, the curvatures of the refracting surfaces continue to change measurably. One study found that average corneal power decreased 0.10–0.20 D and lens power decreased about 1.80 D between ages 3 years and 14 years.

From birth to age 6 years, the axial length of the eye grows by approximately 5 mm; thus, one might expect a high prevalence of myopia in children. However, most children's eyes are actually emmetropic, with only a 2% incidence of myopia at 6 years. This phenomenon is due to a still-undetermined mechanism called *emmetropization.* During this period of eye growth, a compensatory loss of 4.00 D of corneal power and 2.00 D of lens power keeps most eyes close to emmetropia.

Prevent Blindness America; National Eye Institute. *Vision problems in the U.S.: prevalence of adult vision impairment and age-related eye disease in America.* Accessed November 22, 2021. https://preventblindness.org/wp-content/uploads/2013/04/VPUS_2008_update.pdf

Wolfram C, Höhn R, Kottler U, et al. Prevalence of refractive errors in the European adult population: the Gutenberg Health Study (GHS). *Br J Ophthalmol.* 2014;98(7):857–861.

Developmental Myopia

Myopia is defined as a spherical equivalent refractive error of −0.50 D or more when ocular accommodation is relaxed. High myopia is defined as a spherical equivalent refractive error of −6.00 D or greater when ocular accommodation is relaxed. These eyes are at increased risk of sight-threatening complications such as retinal detachment, myopic macular degeneration, and myopia-associated optic neuropathy.

In the United States, the prevalence of myopia has been estimated at 3% among children ages 5–7 years, 8% among those ages 8–10 years, 14% among those ages 11–12 years, and 25% among adolescents ages 13–17 years. In particular ethnic groups, a similar trend has been demonstrated, although the percentages in each age group may differ. Ethnic East Asian children have much higher rates of myopia at all ages. A study in Taiwan, China found that the prevalence was 12% among 6-year-olds and 84% among adolescents between the ages of 16 and 18 years. Similar rates have been found in Singapore and Japan. It has been estimated that the global number of myopic individuals (those with refractive errors of −0.50 D or more) could grow to 4758 million people (49.8% of the population; 95% CI, 3620–6056 million) by 2050 (Figure 3-15).

The development of myopia is a complex interaction of multiple genetic and environmental factors. Myopia is highly inheritable; genes account for up to 80% of the variance in refractive error from twin studies, and identical twins are more likely to have a similar degree of myopia than are fraternal twins, siblings, or a parent and their child. Recently, genome-wide association study approaches have confirmed that myopia is a complex trait, with many genetic variants influencing retinal signaling and eye growth. Environmental factors such as longer duration of education with near work and reduced outdoor activities have been associated with myopia progression. However, the exact mechanisms of how these factors contribute to myopia progression is still not completely understood.

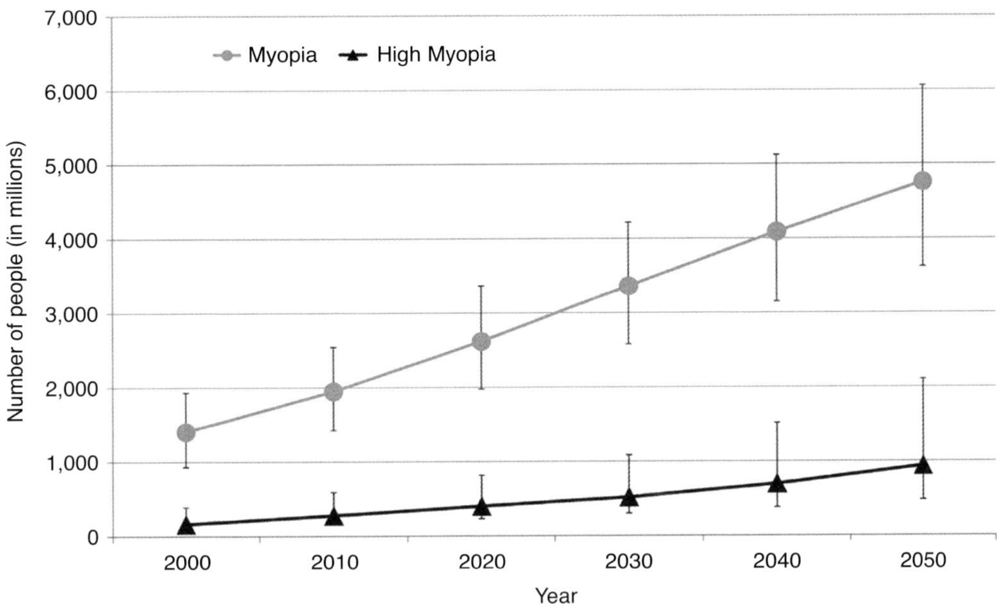

Figure 3-15 Line graph showing the historial and predicted prevalence of myopia and high myopia for each decade from 2000 through 2050. *(Reprinted from* Ophthalmology, *128(6), Bobeck S, et al,* Reducing the global burden of myopia by delaying the onset of myopia and reducing myopic progression in children: the Academy's task force on myopia, *pages 816–826, copyright 2021, with permission from Elsevier.)*

Ang M, Flanagan JL, Wong CW, et al. Review: Myopia control strategies recommendations from the 2018 WHO/IAPB/BHVI Meeting on Myopia. *Br J Ophthalmol.* 2020;104(11):1482–1487.

Modjtahedi BS, Abbott RL, Fong DS, Lum F, Tan D; Task Force on Myopia. Reducing the global burden of myopia by delaying the onset of myopia and reducing myopic progression in children: the Academy's task force on myopia. *Ophthalmology.* 2021;128(6):816–826.

Prevention of Myopia Progression

There is emerging evidence for various optical, pharmacological, and behavioral interventions that have been shown to be effective in reducing myopia progression. Because accommodation and/or the image falling behind the retina are postulated mechanisms for the progression of myopia, optical correction through the use of bifocal or multifocal spectacles or the removal of distance spectacles when one performs close work has been recommended to reduce the progression of myopia. Contact lens–based approaches, including orthokeratology and soft multifocal contact lens designs that provide myopic defocusing of light on the peripheral retina, have also been reported to be effective. Studies also suggest that low-dose atropine (eg, 0.01% eye drops) may slow myopia progression by 30%–60%, with less pupil dilatation and glare. From a public health perspective, encouraging more than 2 hours of outdoor activity per day and avoidance of excessive near work has also been shown to reduce myopia progression.

Developmental Hyperopia

Less is known about the epidemiology of hyperopia than that of myopia. There appears to be an increase in the prevalence of adult hyperopia with age that is separate from the development of nuclear sclerotic cataracts; nuclear sclerosis is usually associated with a myopic shift. A substantial increase in the prevalence of hyperopia from the fifth to the eighth decades of life has been observed across all races. In contrast to myopia, hyperopia has been associated with lower educational achievement.

Pan CW, Klein BE, Cotch MF, et al. Racial variations in the prevalence of refractive errors in the United States: the multi-ethnic study of atherosclerosis. *Am J Ophthalmol.* 2013;155(6): 1129–1138.

Appendix 3-1

Explanation of the ETDRS Visual Acuity Chart

Visual acuity eye charts with graduated lines of letters (or similar optotypes) have been routinely used since the work of Snellen and others in the nineteenth century. In the 1980s, the Early Treatment Diabetic Retinopathy Study introduced a modified Snellen chart based on the earlier work of Bailey and Lovie, which incorporated several refinements to the classic Snellen charts, and which has become the de facto standard for clinical research.

The ETDRS charts feature lines of 5 optotypes, with a uniform ratio between the size of the optotypes in successive lines of $10^{1/10} = 1.2589 \approx 2^{1/3}$. Any change of 3 lines in the acuity threshold represents a doubling or halving of the threshold angle of resolution. Since the base-10 logarithm of $2 = 0.301 \sim 0.3$, each line represents an increment or decrement of 0.1 logMAR ("logarithm of the minimum angle of resolution"). Note that since the logMAR notation is based on the *size* of the smallest features of the optotypes, *larger* logMAR values correspond to *poorer* visual acuity. The 20/20 optotypes, which are 5 minutes of arc in size, with key features (such as the gap in the letter "C") spaced 1 minute of arc apart, are assigned the MAR value of 1.0, and thus have a logMAR value of 0. Smaller optotypes yield negative logMAR values. Since each line contains 5 letters (or similar optotypes), each letter represents $0.1/5 = 0.02$ logMAR, and a gain or loss of 15 letters represents a change of 3 lines of vision, or a doubling or halving of the visual angle; thus, it is convenient to report *changes* in acuity by simply counting the increase or decrease in the number of letters read on the ETDRS chart.

The standard ETDRS chart is provided on a matte-finish plastic screen, which is displayed on an illuminated light box, which provides a standardized intensity of illumination. For informal measurements, a printed or projected chart may be used. (In the original ETDRS, 3 versions of the chart were provided: 1 for refraction, and 2 separate charts with different letters for testing the right eye and the left eye.) The standard chart is calibrated for viewing at a distance of 4.0 m (*not* 20 feet or 6 m). Equivalent Snellen fractions with the usual 20-ft denominators are provided for convenience. At this distance, the largest line reads 1.0 logMAR (20/200), and the smallest line reads –0.3 logMAR (20/10), for a total of 14 lines.

Because sizes of the optotypes on successive lines are in strict geometric progression, the chart can easily be used at other distances as well. For example, if patients are unable to read the largest line (calibrated for 20/200 at 4 m), it is recommended that they be tested using the same chart at a distance of 1 m (see Figure 10-1 in Chapter 10). At this distance, each line is effectively 4 times larger, corresponding to 0.6 logMAR greater than the value at 4 m, allowing measurement of acuities to a level of 20/800.

A table for converting visual acuity measurements between logMAR values and traditional Snellen fractions is provided on the inner front cover of this book. Note that if the acuity values are incremented in even logMAR steps, the corresponding Snellen fractions do not all have simple whole-number denominators, and, if one considers only the traditional Snellen fraction denominators, the logMAR values cannot appear in equal increments.

The original ETDRS charts featured Sloan letter optotypes. ETDRS-type charts are now available with many alternative optotype sets, including the Landolt C, HOTV, tumbling E, numerals, and picture optotypes such as the LEA symbols.

Chapter Exercises

Questions

3.1. Using the reduced schematic eye and the concept of the nodal point, what is the retinal image height of an 18-mm 20/40 Snellen letter at a distance of 20 ft (6 m)?

a. 0.5 mm
b. 0.05 mm
c. 1 mm
d. 0.1 mm

3.2. What is the approximate angle (in arcmin) subtended by the 20/40 Snellen letter at a distance of 20 ft (6 m)?

a. 1 arcmin
b. 2 arcmin
c. 5 arcmin
d. 10 arcmin
e. 40 arcmin

3.3. What is the relative size of target lights in a Goldmann perimeter (with a radius of 33 cm) relative to their corresponding retinal image?

a. same
b. 5 times larger
c. 10 times larger
d. 20 times larger

3.4. Describe the location of the far point of an emmetropic eye with relaxed accommodation. Do the same for a myopic eye and a hyperopic eye.

3.5. In an eye with mixed astigmatism, where are the focal lines located?
   a. Both are in front of the retina.
   b. One is in front of the retina; the other is on the retina.
   c. One is in front of the retina; the other is behind the retina.
   d. One is located on the retina; the other is behind the retina.

3.6. A patient with myopic vision is wearing eyeglasses that were prescribed incorrectly with an over-minus of 1.00 D. When he wears them, his near point of accommodation is 20 cm. What is his amplitude of accommodation?
   a. none
   b. 1.00 D
   c. 5.00 D
   d. 6.00 D

Answers

3.1. **b.** Utilizing the concepts of the nodal point and similar triangles, retinal image size is related to Snellen letter height (18 mm), the distance from the eye to the eye chart (6 m), and the distance from the nodal point to the retina (17 mm), as follows:

$$\frac{\text{Retinal Image Height}}{\text{Snellen Letter Height}} = \frac{\text{Nodal Point to Retina Distance}}{\text{Chart to Eye Distance}} = \frac{17\,\text{mm}}{6000\text{ mm}}$$

This implies

$$\text{Retinal Image Height} = \frac{18\text{ mm} \times 17\text{ mm}}{6000\text{ mm}} = 0.05\text{ mm}$$

The retinal image height of a 20/20 letter is half of this, about 0.025 mm.

3.2. **d.** Snellen letters are constructed such that they subtend an angle of 5 arcmin when located at the distance specified by the denominator (here, 40 ft). At a distance of 20 ft, the angle subtended by a 20/40 Snellen letter is twice that at 40 ft, or 10 arcmin.

3.3. **d.** The concept of the nodal point is applicable for the Goldmann perimeter, in which the target lights are located at 33 cm (330 mm) from the cornea. Because this distance is approximately 20 times greater than the 17-mm distance from the nodal point to the retina, the target lights in the perimeter are approximately 20 times larger than their corresponding retinal images.

3.4. The far point of an emmetropic eye is located at optical infinity. For a myopic eye, the far point is located at a finite distance in front of the cornea. For a hyperopic eye, the far point is located behind the retina.

3.5. **c.** One focal line is in front of the retina, the other is behind the retina. The circle of least confusion may be located very close to the retina (see Chapter 1), allowing such patients to see reasonably well even without optical correction if the magnitude of the astigmatism is not great.

3.6. **d.** The patient's amplitude of accommodation is 6.00 D, because it takes 1.00 D of accommodation to focus to infinity and an additional 5.00 D of accommodation to focus to the false near point at 20 cm.

CHAPTER 4

Clinical Refraction

Highlights

- Plus cylinder refracting equipment is preferable for retinoscopy and is frequently preferred for pediatric ophthalmology; minus cylinder equipment may be preferable for routine prescribing for adults. It is especially useful for contact lens practice.
- Cycloplegic refraction is recommended for children up to 10 years and for adults with inconsistent refractive findings, premature presbyopia, and unexplained or refractory asthenopic concerns. It may be necessary to recall the patient for a postcycloplegic refraction if the "wet" and "dry" refractive findings differ greatly or unexpectedly.
- The duochrome (red–green), alternate cover, and prism dissociation tests are useful to guard against inadvertent stimulation of accommodation and to ensure binocular balance.

Glossary

Amplitude of accommodation A measurement of the ability of an eye to change focus from a far point to a near point.

Autorefractor A computer-controlled instrument for determining the refractive error of the eye.

Jackson cross cylinder Combination of 2 cylinders of equal but opposite power, whose axes are perpendicular to each other; used in the determination of power and axis of refractive astigmatism.

Phoropter (refractor) An instrument containing a collection of spherical and cylindrical lenses for the performance of retinoscopy and manifest refraction. The instrument also commonly includes the Jackson cross cylinder, Risley prisms, and other accessories.

Presbyopia Functional loss of accommodation that occurs with aging.

Retinoscopy A manual, objective method of determining and evaluating the refractive status of an eye through the observation of the movement of a retinal reflex that is created by a beam of light seen through the pupil and the optical system of the eye.

Introduction

The process of clinical refraction represents one of the practical applications of geometric optics. Refraction is a critical component in ophthalmic examination. It allows the determination of the best-corrected vision of the eye. This determination is often necessary in determining the diagnosis and recommended treatment course. The refraction is necessary in determining visual correction with spectacles, contact lenses, lens implants, and refractive corneal surgery. Other techniques, such as the pinhole, corneal topography and tomography, and various forms of autorefraction, are valuable but, as yet, have not replaced manifest refraction in the ophthalmic examination.

Minus Cylinder and Plus Cylinder Terminology

The terms *minus cylinder* and *plus cylinder* are used in various ways in discussion of refraction and the prescription of eyeglasses. These include the measurement of refraction using the phoropter (refractor), the writing of the prescription for glasses, and the construction of spectacles with astigmatism correction.

The phoropter contains a full range of both plus and minus spherical lenses. For simplicity, the cylinder component contains lenses of only one type—either plus cylinder lenses or minus cylinder lenses. (Trial lens sets may be ordered with minus cylinder lenses, plus cylinder lenses, or both.) There is no consensus as to which type is preferable. In some communities, optometrists tend to prefer phoropters with minus cylinder lenses and ophthalmologists tend to prefer plus cylinder lenses. Minus cylinder phoropters may possess advantages for the fitting of contact lenses. In contrast, the axis of the plus cylinder may indicate the position of a tight suture in an eye after cataract surgery or penetrating keratoplasty. Plus cylinder equipment is also the better choice for retinoscopy and is often selected by pediatric ophthalmologists for that reason.

The prescription for a spectacle correction may be written in either minus cylinder or plus cylinder format. Normally this is transcribed directly from the phoropter or trial frame used to perform the refraction, so as to minimize the possibility of a transcription error; however, this is not mandatory. Either form may be easily converted to the other (Clinical Example 4-1).

CLINICAL EXAMPLE 4-1

This example demonstrates converting the specification of a spherocylindrical lens combination from plus cylinder notation to minus cylinder notation. The rules of thumb for this calculation are (1) add the cylinder power to the sphere power to find the new sphere power; (2) change the sign of the cylinder power (the magnitude of the power remains the same); and (3) change the axis of the cylinder by ±90° (making the adjustment so as to obtain a final axis greater than 0° and at most 180°). This procedure works when converting both from plus to minus notation and from minus to plus.

Take, for example, the following plus cylinder refraction:
−3.00 + 4.00 × 180°

Sphere power: −3.00 D
Cylinder power: +4.00 D
Axis of the cylinder: 180°

In the conversion to minus cylinder notation, the following transformations occur:

The cylinder power is added to the sphere power: +4.00 + (−3.00) = +1.00 D
The sign of the cylinder power is changed: +4.00 becomes −4.00 D
The axis of the cylinder is changed by 90°: 180° becomes 90°
Resultant minus cylinder notation: **+1.00 −4.00 × 090°**

In the fabrication of spherocylindrical spectacle lenses, the cylindrical component may be placed on the anterior surface (called plus cylinder grinding or front-cylinder grinding) or the posterior surface (called minus cylinder grinding or back-cylinder grinding) of the lens. Current preferred practice is for lenses to be fabricated in minus cylinder format regardless of which type of phoropter is used or how the prescription is written. This practice decreases the variation in the meridional magnification.

Examination Room Length

The room in which the refraction is carried out is important in achieving satisfactory results. For optical purposes, a 20-ft (approximately 6-m) distance from the patient to the vision chart approximates infinity (−0.17 diopters [D]). Many examination rooms are much shorter than this. If the vision chart is placed so that the distance to the patient is only 10 ft (3 m), the refraction will be overplussed by 0.33 D. Mirrors are often used to extend the viewing distance to the standard 20 ft in such rooms. Some patients (including many children) are not able to effectively fixate into a mirror and need to be examined in longer rooms or hallways. They may also tend to accommodate in a short room, even if it has a mirror to optically extend it. Simply correcting for the shorter working distance by decreasing the plus or increasing the minus in the measured refraction is not recommended because proper accommodative fogging techniques may not work as intended in such a situation.

Objective Refraction Technique: Retinoscopy

Although autorefractors are widely available, retinoscopy remains an important tool for the ophthalmologist to objectively determine the spherocylindrical refractive error of the eye. A *retinoscope* can also help the examiner detect optical aberrations, irregularities, and opacities, even through small pupils. Retinoscopy is especially useful for examination of infants, children, and adults who are unable to communicate.

If you have not already done so, please familiarize yourself with the basic concepts of retinoscopy as presented in Part 3 of the Quick-Start Guide in this volume.

Most retinoscopes in current use employ a streak projection system. The retinoscope provides illumination through a slit-shaped aperture; the slit-shaped beam of light is focused by adjusting the position of a convex lens with the sleeve of the retinoscope. The light then is directed toward the patient through a half-silvered or fully silvered mirror, depending on the type of retinoscope being used (Fig 4-1). If the light is slightly divergent, it appears to come from a point behind the retinoscope, as if the light were reflected off of a flat mirror (ie, a *plane mirror setting*) (Fig 4-2).

Alternatively, when the distance between the convex lens and the light source is increased by moving the sleeve on the handle, convergent light is emitted. In this situation, the image of the filament appears between the examiner and the patient, as if the light were reflected off of a concave mirror (Fig 4-3).

Note that when working with the concave mirror setting, with the apparent position of the light source between the retinoscope and the patient's eye, the apparent movement of the light source as seen by the patient is in the opposite direction from the apparent movement seen with the plane mirror setting. This causes the motion of the retinal reflexes to

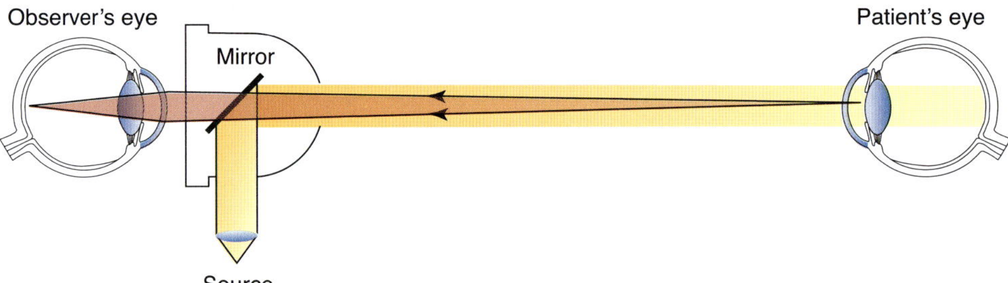

Figure 4-1 Illumination and observation systems of the retinoscope. Illumination system: Light path from the light source, through the patient's pupil, to the retina. Observation system: Light path from the patient's pupil, through the mirror, to the observer's retina. The observer views the patient's eye through a half-silvered mirror (with Welch-Allyn type retinoscopes) or a small central hole in a fully silvered mirror (Copeland retinoscopes). *(Illustration by C. H. Wooley.)*

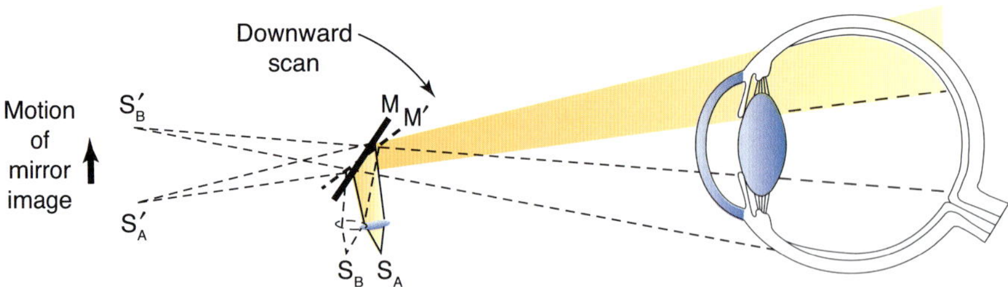

Figure 4-2 Illumination system: position of the source (S) with the plane mirror (M) effect. Note that in the plane mirror setting, the apparent light source (S_A') moves *upward* to S_B' when the retinoscope is tipped *downward.*

change direction when the retinoscope sleeve is moved to the extreme concave mirror setting (see Figures 4-2 and 4-3).

Retinoscopy may be performed with either a concave mirror setting or a plane mirror setting, determined by the sleeve of the scope. Retinoscopy is usually performed using the plane mirror setting so that light is slightly divergent as it enters the pupil of the patient's eye. We restrict most of our discussion to the plane mirror effect. With most modern retinoscopes, the plane mirror effect is produced with the sleeve in the maximally lowered position. (With Copeland retinoscopes, now rarely encountered, the plane mirror setting is produced with the sleeve maximally elevated, and the concave mirror setting with the sleeve maximally lowered.)

When viewing *with motion*, with the streak aligned with a principal axis of the eye, the streak image may be brought into somewhat sharper focus within the pupil by adjusting the height of the sleeve upward. This may facilitate accurate determination of the cylinder axis (Fig 4-4).

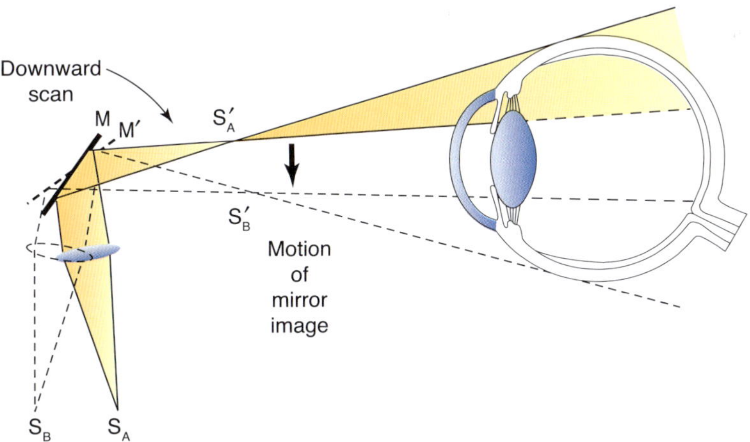

Figure 4-3 Illumination system: position of the source with the concave mirror effect. Note that in the concave mirror setting, the apparent light source (S'_A) moves *downward* to S'_B when the retinoscope is tipped *downward*.

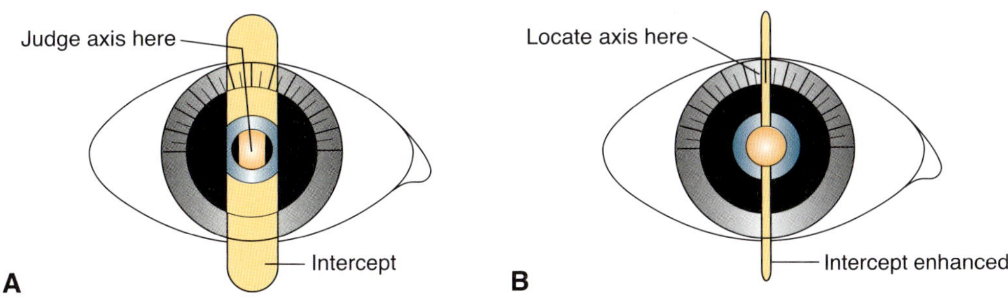

Figure 4-4 Locating axis on the protractor. **A,** First, determine the astigmatic axis. **B,** Second, adjust the sleeve to enhance the intercept until the filament is observed as a fine line that runs through the axis. *(Illustration by C. H. Wooley.)*

The axis can be confirmed through a technique known as straddling, which is performed with the estimated correcting cylinder in place (Fig 4-5). The retinoscope streak is turned 45° off-axis in both directions, and if the axis is correct, the width and intensity of the reflex should be equal in both off-axis positions. If the axis is not correct, the widths are unequal in these 2 positions. When plus cylinder correcting lenses are used, the axis of the correcting plus cylinder should be moved toward the brighter, narrower reflex (the "guideline") and the straddling repeated until the widths are equal. (When minus cylinder correcting lenses are used, which is not recommended, rotate the cylinder axis *away* from the narrower, brighter reflex.)

Fixation and Fogging

Retinoscopy should be performed with the patient's accommodation relaxed. The patient should fixate at a distance on a nonaccommodative target, for example, a dim light at the end of the room or a large Snellen letter (20/200 or 20/400 size). Plus lenses may be introduced in front of the eye not being examined to aid in the relaxation of accommodation. Accommodating after fogging is performed will only further blur the image. Children typically require pharmacologic cycloplegia (such as with cyclopentolate 1%).

Aberrations of the Retinoscopic Reflex

With irregular astigmatism, almost any type of aberration may appear in the reflex. *Spherical aberrations* tend to increase the brightness at the center or periphery of the pupil, depending on whether they are positive or negative.

As neutrality is approached, 1 part of the reflex may be myopic, whereas the other may be hyperopic relative to the position of the retinoscope. This situation produces a *scissors reflex.* Causes of the scissors reflex include keratoconus, irregular corneal astigmatism, corneal or lenticular opacities, and spherical aberration.

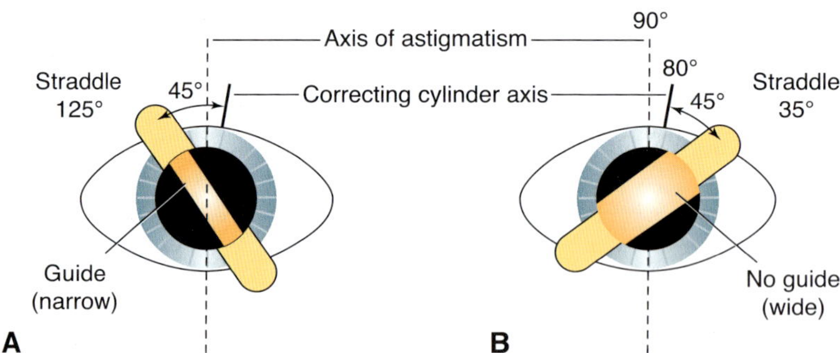

Figure 4-5 Straddling. The straddling meridians are 45° off the correcting cylinder axis, at roughly 35° and 125°. As the examiner moves back from the eye while comparing the meridians, the reflex at 125° remains narrow **(A)** at the same distance that the reflex at 35° has become wide **(B)**. This dissimilarity indicates an axis error; the narrow reflex (A) is the guide toward which the examiner must turn the correcting cylinder axis. (With minus cylinders [not recommended], rotate the correcting cylinder away from the guideline.) *(Illustration by C. H. Wooley.)*

All of these aberrant reflexes, in particular spherical aberration, are more noticeable in patients with large scotopic pupils. When a large pupil is observed during retinoscopy, the examiner should focus on neutralizing the central portion of the light reflex.

CLINICAL PEARL

Following placement of corneal sutures, as in penetrating keratoplasty or some cataract surgery procedures, the distortion of the cornea caused by a tight suture will distort the retinoscopic reflex so that the narrowest side of the retinoscopy beam points directly toward the tightest suture (Fig 4-6).

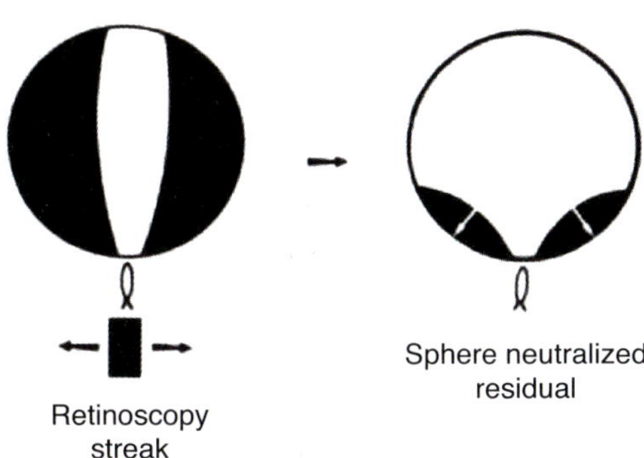

Figure 4-6 Distortion of the cornea caused by a tight suture. *Left:* Distortion of retinoscopic with reflex by a tight suture at the 6 o'clock position. *Right:* As the with reflex is neutralized with plus sphere power, the reflex broadens to fill the pupil, but residual distortion still causes the retinoscopic reflex to point toward the tight suture inferiorly. *(Rowsey JJ, Fowler WC, Terry MA, Scoper SV. Use of keratoscopy, slit-lamp biomicroscopy, and retinoscopy in the management of astigmatism after penetrating keratoplasty.* Refract Corneal Surg. *1991;7(1):33–41. Reprinted with permission from SLACK Incorporated.)*

Pseudoneutralization

As noted above, in general, *with reflexes* are brighter, sharper, and easier to perceive and interpret than *against reflexes.* In particular, the reflex in severely myopic eyes is seldom recognizable as an against reflex—rather, one sees only a dull, motionless illumination of the entire pupil. This is referred to as *pseudoneutralization.* This is best handled by reversing the sleeve of the retinoscope (to the maximal sleeve-up position). This will convert the dull pseudoneutral reflex to a readily recognizable with reflex, but in this case, the with reflex must be neutralized by adding *minus* sphere power. As true neutrality is approached, return the retinoscope sleeve to the usual position. The reflex will revert to an against reflex, as is usually seen in less myopic eyes. Continue to add minus sphere power until a with reflex is obtained, and then reduce the minus sphere so as to reach true neutrality from the with direction. Video Q-3 in the Quick-Start Guide demonstrates pseudoneutralization.

Cycloplegic Retinoscopy

Opinions differ as to when to perform retinoscopy with the aid of cycloplegia. While some recommend performing cycloplegic retinoscopy routinely, widely dilated pupils may paradoxically make retinoscopy more difficult, as the aberrations of the eye may result in different reflexes in the center and in the periphery of the pupil. Cycloplegic retinoscopy is recommended for all children younger than 10 years, as younger children can rarely maintain steady fixation on a distant target when distracted by the retinoscopist only 2 feet away. Older children and most adults can fixate steadily at distance, which allows accurate retinoscopy so long as the pupils are adequately large and the ocular media are clear. If the retinoscopic findings fluctuate rapidly, this suggests inconstant fixation, which may be remedied by repeating the retinoscopy under cycloplegia. Dilation may also be helpful for older patients with very small pupils or mild cataracts. As with subjective refraction under cycloplegia, it may be necessary to bring the patient back for a postcycloplegic manifest refraction to determine the patient's natural degree of accommodative tone, especially in patients with hyperopic refractive errors.

Subjective Refraction Techniques

In subjective refraction techniques, the examiner relies on the patient's responses to determine the refractive correction. If all refractive errors were spherical, subjective refraction would be easy. However, determining the astigmatic portion of the correction is more complex, and various subjective refraction techniques may be used. The Jackson cross cylinder is the most common instrument used in determining the astigmatic correction.

Stenopeic Slit Technique

The stenopeic slit is an opaque trial lens with an oblong slit whose width forms a pinhole with respect to vergence parallel to the slit (Fig 4-7). If an examiner is unable to decipher the astigmatism by performing standard retinoscopy because of the subject eye's irregular astigmatism or unclear media, they may neutralize the refractive error with spherical lenses and the slit at various meridians to find a spherocylindrical correction. This correction can then be refined subjectively. This process is especially useful for patients with small pupils, lenticular or corneal opacities, and/or irregular astigmatism. If the subject can accommodate, the examiner may fog and unfog with plus sphere to find the most plus power accepted. The slit can then be rotated in front of the eye until the subject says that the image is sharpest. If, for example, −3.00 D sphere is best when the slit is oriented vertically, this finding indicates −3.00 D at 90° in a power cross. If the best sphere with the slit oriented horizontally is −5.00 D (−5.00 × 180), the result is −3.00 − 2.00 × 090 when the power cross method is used. It is helpful to think of the "axis" of the stenopeic slit as a thin line *perpendicular* to the orientation of the slit.

Cross-Cylinder Technique

The cross-cylinder technique to measure astigmatism was described by Edward Jackson in 1887; he wrote that the cross-cylinder lens was probably "far more useful, and far more

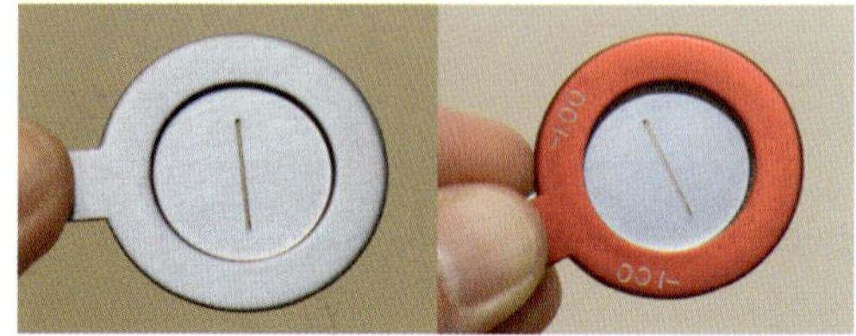

Figure 4-7 Stenopeic slit. The image on the right demonstrates the placement of a spherical lens in front of the stenopeic slit in order to determine the best visual acuity. *(Courtesy of Tommy Korn, MD.)*

used" than any other lens in clinical refraction. Every ophthalmologist should be familiar with the principles involved in its use. Although the cross cylinder is usually used to *refine* the cylinder axis and power of a refraction that has already been obtained, it can also be used for the entire astigmatic refraction.

A cross cylinder is a lens with a spherical equivalent power of 0 but with mixed astigmatism of equal amounts. Common cross cylinders are −0.50 +1.00 × 090 and −0.25 +0.50 × 090. They are mounted so they can readily be "flipped" about a line halfway between the axes (eg, 45° or 135°), which has the effect of interchanging the plus and minus cylinder axes.

The first step in cross-cylinder refraction is to adjust the sphere to yield the best visual acuity with accommodation relaxed. Begin by selecting a starting point: this may be based on the current prescription or the retinoscopy or autorefraction findings. Dial this into a trial frame or phoropter. Fog the eye to be examined with plus sphere while the patient views a visual acuity chart; then decrease the fog until the best visual acuity is obtained. If astigmatism is present, decreasing the fog places the circle of least confusion on the retina, creating a mixed astigmatism. Then use test figures that are 1 or 2 lines larger than the patient's best visual acuity. At this point, introduce the cross cylinder, first for refinement of cylinder axis and then for refinement of cylinder power.

Always refine cylinder axis before refining cylinder power. This sequence is necessary because the correct axis may be found without knowledge of the correct cylinder power, but the full cylinder power is found only in the presence of the correct axis. The axis may be rechecked after the power is determined and is more important with higher levels of astigmatism power. Use of the cross cylinder to detect the presence of astigmatism is discussed in the Quick-Start Guide.

Refinement of cylinder axis involves the combination of cylinders at oblique axes. When the axis of the correcting cylinder is not aligned with that of the astigmatic eye's cylinder, the combined cylinders produce residual astigmatism with a meridian roughly 45° away from the principal meridians of the 2 cylinders. To refine the axis, position the principal meridians of the cross cylinder 45° away from those of the correcting cylinder (if you are using a handheld Jackson cross cylinder, the stem of the lens handle will be parallel to the axis of the correcting cylinder). Present the patient with alternative flip choices, and select the choice that is the blackest and sharpest to the patient. Then rotate the axis of the correcting cylinder toward the corresponding plus or minus axis of the cross cylinder. (Plus cylinder axis is rotated toward the plus cylinder axis of the cross cylinder [indicated by the white dots], and minus cylinder axis is rotated toward the minus cylinder axis of the cross cylinder [indicated by the red dots].) Low-power cylinders are rotated in increments of 15°; high-power cylinders are rotated by smaller amounts, usually 5°, but can be as small as 1° for very high astigmatism. Repeat this procedure until the flip choices appear equal.

To refine cylinder power, align the cross-cylinder axes with the principal meridians of the correcting lens (Fig 4-8). Change cylinder power according to the patient's responses. The spherical equivalent of the refractive correction should remain constant to keep the circle of least confusion on the retina: this is done by changing the sphere half as much and in the opposite direction as the cylinder power is changed. In other words, for every 0.50 D of cylinder power change, change the sphere by 0.25 D in the opposite direction. Periodically, the sphere power should be adjusted for the best visual acuity.

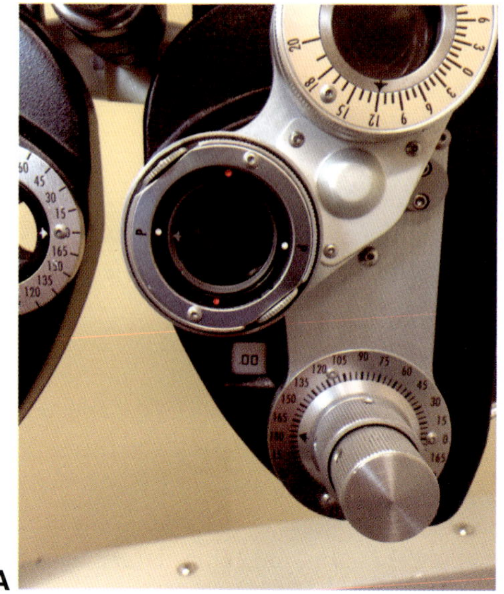

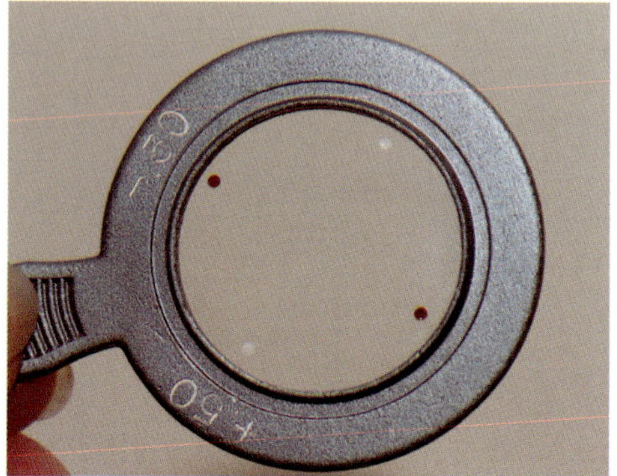

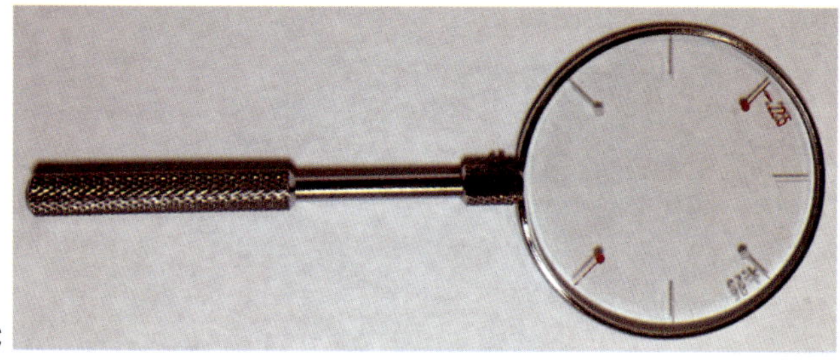

Figure 4-8 Jackson cross cylinder. **A,** In the phoropter. **B,** Manual trial lens. **C,** Rotating manual trial lens. *(Parts A and C courtesy of Thomas F. Mauger, MD. Part B courtesy of Tommy Korn, MD.)*

Continue to refine cylinder power until the patient reports that both flip choices appear equal. At that point, the 2 flip choices produce equal and opposite mixed astigmatism, blurring the visual acuity chart equally.

If the examiner is planning on prescribing for astigmatism at an axis *different* from that measured with the cross cylinder (eg, 90° or 180° instead of an oblique axis) the cross cylinder can be used to measure the cylinder power at the new axis.

If possible, use a cross cylinder with power similar to the patient's visual acuity level. For example, a ±0.25 D cross cylinder is commonly used with visual acuity levels of 20/30 and better. A high-power cross cylinder (±0.50 D or ±1.00 D) allows a patient with poorer vision to recognize differences in the flip choices.

The cross-cylinder refraction technique is summarized below. Also see Part 2 of the Quick-Start Guide.

1. Adjust sphere to the most plus or least minus that gives the best visual acuity.
2. Use test figures that are 1 or 2 lines larger than the patient's best visual acuity.
3. If cylindrical correction is not already present, look for astigmatism by testing with the cross cylinder at axes 90° and 180°. If none is found there, test at 45° and 135°.

4. Refine axis first. Position the cross-cylinder axes 45° from the principal meridians of the correcting cylinder. Determine the preferred flip choice and rotate the cylinder axis toward the corresponding axis of the cross cylinder. Repeat until the 2 flip choices appear equal.
5. Refine cylinder power. Align the cross-cylinder axes with the principal meridians of the correcting cylinder. Determine the preferred flip choice and add or subtract cylinder power according to the preferred position of the cross cylinder. Compensate for the change in position of the circle of least confusion by adding half as much sphere in the opposite direction each time the cylinder power is changed.
6. Refine sphere, cylinder axis, and cylinder power until no further change is necessary.

Jackson E. A trial set of small lenses and a modified trial size frame. *Trans Am Ophthalmol Soc.* 1887;4:595–598.

Refining the Sphere

After cylinder power and axis have been determined, the final step in determining monocular refraction is to refine the sphere. The endpoint in the refraction is the strongest plus sphere (or weakest minus sphere) that yields the best visual acuity. The following discussion briefly considers some of the methods used.

After the cross-cylinder technique has been used to determine the cylinder power and axis, add plus sphere in +0.25 D increments until the patient reports decreased vision. If no additional plus sphere is accepted, add minus sphere in –0.25 D increments until the patient achieves the optimal visual acuity.

Using accommodation, the patient can compensate for excess minus sphere. Therefore, it is important to use the least minus sphere necessary to reach the best visual acuity. In effect, accommodation creates a reverse Galilean telescope, whereby the eye generates more plus power as minus power is added to the trial lenses in front of the eye. As this minus power increases, the patient observes that the letters appear smaller and more distant (but also "darker," which the patient may misinterpret as "clearer").

The patient should be told what to look for. Before subtracting each 0.25 D increment, tell the patient that the letters may appear sharper and brighter or smaller and darker, and ask the patient to report any such change. Reduce the amount of plus sphere only if the patient can actually read additional letters.

To verify the spherical endpoint, the *duochrome test* (also known as the *red–green* or *bichrome test*) may be used (Fig 4-9). A split red and green filter makes the background of the visual acuity chart appear vertically divided into a red half and a green half. Because of the chromatic aberration of the eye, the shorter (green) wavelengths are focused in front of the longer (red) wavelengths. The eye typically focuses near the midpoint of the spectrum, between the red and green wavelengths. With optimal spherical correction, the letters on the red and green halves of the chart appear equally sharp. The commercial filters used in the duochrome test produce a chromatic interval of approximately 0.50 D between the red and green wavelengths; when the image is clearly focused in white light, the eye is 0.25 D myopic for the green letters and 0.25 D hyperopic for the red letters.

Each eye is tested separately for the duochrome test, which is begun with the eye slightly fogged (by 0.50 D) to relax accommodation. The letters on the red side should

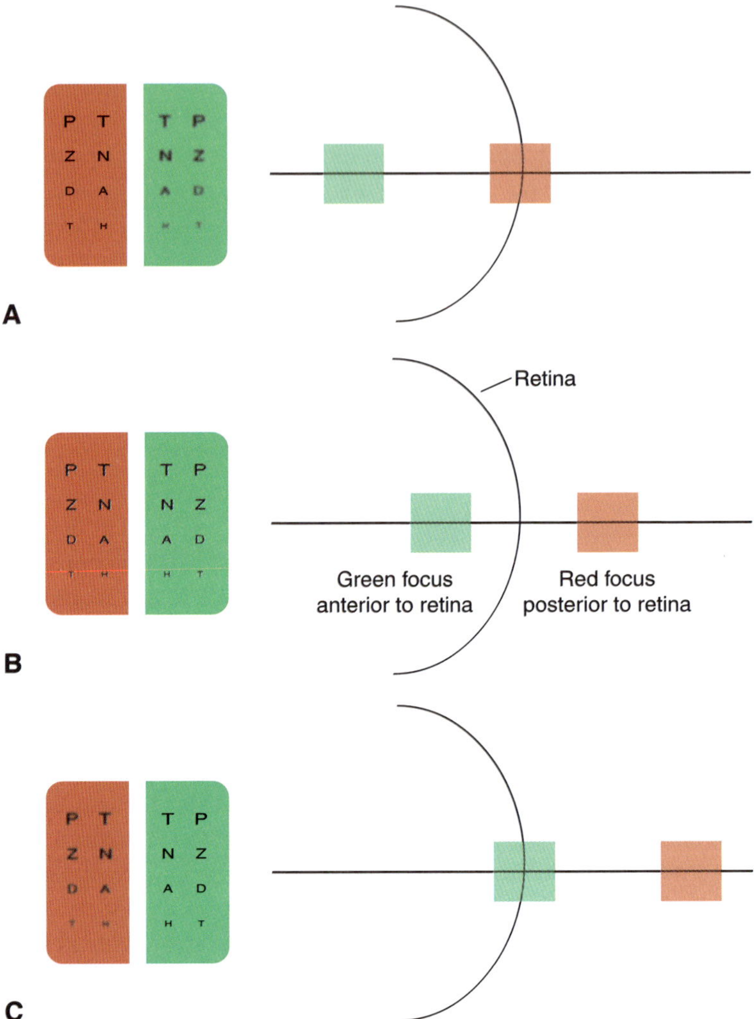

Figure 4-9 Diagram of duochrome test. **A,** Starting point; the eye is blurred with excess plus power—the red letters should be clearer. **B,** Plus power is decreased (or minus power is increased) until both sides of the chart have equal clarity. **C,** Plus power continues to be decreased (or minus power increased) until the green side of the chart is clearer. *(Illustration developed by Thomas F. Mauger, MD.)*

appear sharper; the clinician should add minus sphere until the 2 sides appear the same. If the patient responds that the letters on the green side are sharper, the patient is overminused, and more plus power should be added. When in doubt, it is preferable to err on the side of the more-plus or less-minus alternative ("leave 'em in the red"). Some clinicians use the RAM-GAP mnemonic—"*r*ed *a*dd *m*inus; *g*reen *a*dd *p*lus"—to recall how to use the duochrome test.

Because this test is based on chromatic aberration and not on color discrimination, it works equally well with color-blind patients (although it may be necessary to identify the sides of the chart as left and right rather than red and green). An eye with overactive accommodation may still require too much minus sphere in order to balance the red and green. Cycloplegia may be necessary. The duochrome test is not used with patients whose visual acuity is worse than 20/40 (6/12), because the 0.50 D difference between the 2 sides is too small to distinguish.

Binocular Balance

The final step of subjective refraction is to make certain that accommodation has been relaxed equally in both eyes. Several methods of binocular balance are commonly used. Most require that the corrected visual acuity be nearly equal in both eyes.

Alternate occlusion

When the endpoint refraction is fogged using a +0.75 D sphere before each eye, the visual acuity should be reduced to 20/40–20/50 (6/12–6/15). Alternately cover the eyes and ask the patient if the chart is equally blurred. If the eyes are not in balance, plus sphere should be added to the better-seeing eye until balance is achieved.

In addition to testing for binocular balance, the fogging method also provides information about appropriate sphere power. If either eye is overminused or underplussed, the patient should read smaller (better than 20/40) letters than expected. In this case, the refraction endpoints should be reconsidered.

Prism dissociation

The most sensitive test of binocular balance is prism dissociation (Fig 4-10). For this test, the refractive endpoints are fogged with +0.75 or +1.00 D spheres, and vertical prisms of 4 or 6 prism diopters (Δ) are placed before 1 eye (or divided equally between the 2 eyes) using the Risley prisms in the phoropter (or in a trial lens frame). Some phoropters have a built-in 6Δ setting for this test. Use of the prisms causes the patient to see 2 charts, 1 above the other. A single line, usually 20/40 (6/12), is isolated on the chart; the patient sees 2 separate lines simultaneously, 1 for each eye. The patient can readily identify differences between the fogged images in the 2 eyes of as little as 0.25 D sphere. In practice, +0.25 D sphere is placed before 1 eye and then before the other. In each instance, if the eyes are balanced, the patient reports that the image corresponding to the eye with the additional +0.25 D sphere

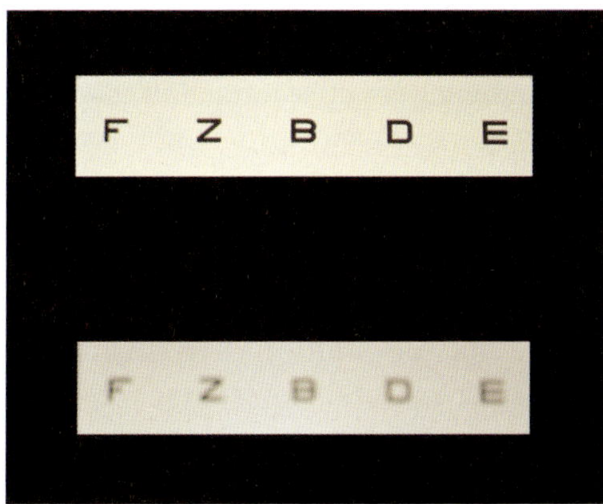

Figure 4-10 Binocular balancing by prism dissociation, from the patient's perspective. *(Courtesy of Tommy Korn, MD.)*

is blurrier. After a balance is established between the 2 eyes, remove the prism and reduce the fog binocularly until the best visual acuity is obtained.

Cycloplegic and Noncycloplegic Refraction

Ideally, refractive error is measured with accommodation relaxed. The amount of habitual accommodative tone varies from person to person, and even within an individual it varies at times and decreases with age. Because determining this variable may not always be possible, cycloplegic drugs are sometimes used. The indication and appropriate dosage for a specific cycloplegic drug depend on the patient's age, accommodative amplitude, and refractive error.

A practical approach to obtaining satisfactory refraction is to perform a careful noncycloplegic (or manifest) refraction, ensuring relaxed accommodation with fogging or other nonpharmacologic techniques. If the results are inconsistent or variable, a cycloplegic refraction should be performed. In some cases, comparison between the "dry" refraction and cycloplegic retinoscopy is all that is necessary. If the findings of these 2 refractions are similar, the prescription may be based on the manifest refraction. If there is a disparity, a postcycloplegic evaluation (performed at a time after the cycloplegic effects have abated, usually several days later) may be necessary. Most children require cycloplegic refraction because of their high amplitude of accommodation. For more details on the cycloplegic drugs used in adults and children, please refer to BCSC Section 2, *Fundamentals and Principles of Ophthalmology.*

Overrefraction

Phoropters may be used to refract the eyes of patients with highly ametropic vision. Variability in the vertex distance of the refraction (the distance from the back surface of the spectacle lens to the cornea) and other induced errors make prescribing directly from the phoropter findings unreliable.

Some of these problems can be avoided if highly ametropic eyes are refracted over the patients' current glasses (overrefraction). If the new lenses are prescribed with the same base curve and thickness (contributors to image size and aniseikonia) as the current lenses and are fitted in the same frames, many potential difficulties can be circumvented, including vertex distance error and pantoscopic tilt error (inducing effective refraction changes), as well as problems caused by oblique (marginal) astigmatism and chromatic aberration (if lens material remains the same). Overrefraction may be performed with loose lenses (using trial lens clips such as Halberg trial clips), with a standard phoropter in front of the patient's glasses, or with some automated refracting instruments.

If the patient is wearing spherical lenses, the new prescription is easy to calculate by combining the current spherical correction with the spherocylindrical overrefraction. If the current lenses are spherocylindrical and the cylinder axis of the overrefraction is not at 0° or 90° to the present correction, a *lensmeter* may be used to read the resultant lens power through the combination of the old glasses and the overrefraction correction. Care should be taken not to rotate cylindrical lenses on transfer to the lensmeter.

Overrefraction has other uses, too. For example, a patient wearing a soft toric contact lens may undergo overrefraction for the purpose of ordering new lenses. An overrefraction is especially useful for patients who wear rigid, gas-permeable, hard contact lenses for irregular corneal astigmatism or corneal transplants, as it can determine the amount of visual reduction that is caused by irregular astigmatism. Overrefraction can also be used in the retinoscopic examination of children.

Chapter Exercises

Questions

4.1. Which prescription represents a Jackson cross cylinder?
   a. −2.00 +4.00 × 180
   b. −1.00 +3.00 × 090
   c. +2.00 +3.00 × 180
   d. +1.00 −1.00 × 090

4.2. When performing cycloplegic retinoscopy on an anxious 7-year-old boy, you notice that the central reflex shows *with* movement while the peripheral reflex shows *against* movement. What is the most likely cause?
   a. keratoconus
   b. congenital cataract
   c. spherical aberration
   d. insufficient time for maximum cycloplegia

4.3. A wheelchair-bound aphakic patient has difficulty sitting at the phoropter, so refraction with the stenopeic slit is attempted. The apparent spherical equivalent correction is +10.00 sp. When the slit is rotated in front of the +10.00 sp lens, acuity is best with the slit oriented horizontally. With the slit in this position, the best acuity is obtained with a sphere of +10.50. With the slit oriented vertically, the best acuity is found with a sphere of +9.50. What is the estimated final correction in minus cylinder form?
   a. +10.00 sp
   b. +9.50 +1.00 × 090
   c. +10.50 −1.00 × 180
   d. +10.50 +1.00 × 180

Answers

4.1. **a.** The Jackson cross cylinder is a lens made of 2 cylinders of equal but opposite magnitude placed at 90°, relative to each other; the spherical equivalent of the resulting lens is zero (see Fig 4-8). High-power Jackson cross cylinders are especially useful for refining the refraction in patients with low vision.

4.2. **c.** Spherical aberration occurs in patients with large or dilated pupils. This aberration is caused when light rays are refracted as they travel through a widely dilated pupil and strike the peripheral crystalline lens. The periphery of the human lens is more curved than the center, so the incoming light rays show increased refraction compared with the light rays that strike the central lens. In retinoscopy, this can result in the appearance of different central and peripheral reflexes. Thus, it is always important to concentrate on the central light reflex when retinoscopy is performed.

4.3. **c.** The stenopeic slit findings directly translate to +9.50 +1.00 × 090. Remember, one can think of the slit together with the lens behind it as equivalent to a cylinder with axis *perpendicular* to the slit. But in this case, the answer is requested in minus cylinder form.

CHAPTER 5

Eyeglasses

Highlights

- Vertex distance should be taken into account when glasses with corrections stronger than ±5.00 D are prescribed.
- If a strong astigmatic correction is contemplated, place the proposed correction in trial frames and ask the patient to walk around the office with the correction in place. If distortion or tilted images are noted, adjust the prescription accordingly. (The experience of wearing the correction in motion is important—merely experiencing the new correction while seated is not an adequate trial.)
- Prescribe the minimal bifocal add that meets the patient's needs. Stronger adds unnecessarily narrow the range of near vision.
- Progressive-add lenses are a good choice for patients with recent-onset presbyopia, as the adaptation to these lenses is easiest with low-power adds. Subsequent adjustment as stronger adds are needed is usually effortless.

Glossary

Image displacement Change in the apparent position of an object, as seen through the periphery of a spectacle lens.

Image jump Sudden movement of an image when gaze is shifted across the border between the distance and the near portions of a multifocal spectacle lens.

Meridional aniseikonia Unequal magnification of retinal images in different meridians that is induced by astigmatic lenses.

Oblique (marginal) astigmatism Astigmatism induced by the tilting of a spherical lens or by viewing through the periphery of a spherical lens.

Prentice's rule Each centimeter of lens decentration induces 1 prism diopter (Δ) of prism for each diopter of power of the lens.

Presbyopia Functional loss of accommodation that accompanies aging.

Slab-off prism (bicentric grinding) Creation of base-up prism in the area of a bifocal to correct induced prismatic effect in downgaze through the bifocal reading segment.

Vertex distance Distance from the back surface of a spectacle or contact lens to the anterior surface of the cornea.

Spectacle Correction of Ametropias

Ametropia is a refractive error; it is the absence of emmetropia. The most common method of correcting refractive error is through prescription of spectacle lenses.

Spherical Correcting Lenses and the Far Point Concept

In the Quick-Start Guide, the action of a correcting lens is envisioned as moving the focal point of the eye's natural optics forward or backward so as to coincide with the fovea. In many contexts, it is more useful to envision the role of the correcting lens as relocating the source image so as to coincide with the "far point" of the eye. The far point of the non-accommodated eye is the location in space conjugate with the fovea. Source objects at the far point will automatically be focused on the retina. Recall that for a simple lens (plus or minus sphere), distant objects (those at optical infinity) come into sharp focus at the *secondary focal point* (F_2) of the lens. To correct the refractive error of an eye, a correcting lens should place the image it forms (or its F_2) at the eye's far point. The image at the far point plane becomes the object that is focused onto the retina. For example, in a myopic eye, the far point lies somewhere in front of the eye, between the cornea and optical infinity. In this case, the correct *diverging lens* forms a virtual image of distant objects at its F_2, coincident with the far point of the eye (Fig 5-1).

The same principle holds for the correction of hyperopia (Fig 5-2). However, because the far-point plane of a hyperopic eye is behind the retina, a *converging lens* with appropriate power to focus parallel rays of light to the far point plane must be chosen.

The Importance of Vertex Distance

For any spherical correcting lens, the distance from the lens to its focal point is constant. Changing the position of the correcting lens relative to the eye also changes the

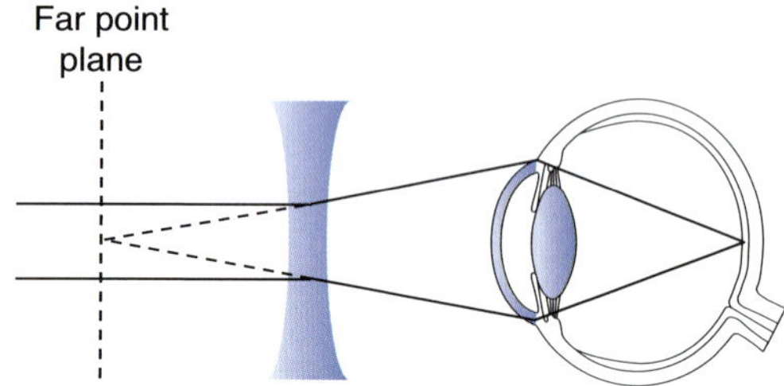

Figure 5-1 A diverging lens is used to correct myopia.

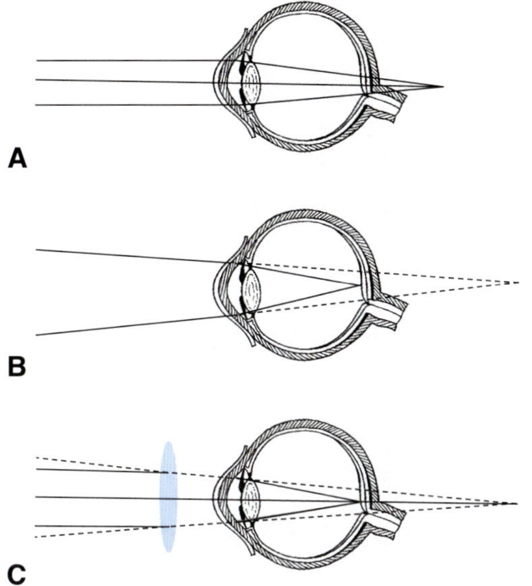

Figure 5-2 Correction of hyperopia. **A,** A hyperopic eye focuses parallel incoming light rays behind the retina. **B,** The far point of the hyperopic eye is a point behind the retina that is conjugate to the fovea. **C,** A convex lens that images parallel rays from optical infinity at the far point thus corrects the refractive error. *(Courtesy of Scott E. Brodie, MD, PhD.)*

relationship between the F_2 of the correcting lens and the far point plane of the eye. With high-power lenses, as are used in the spectacle correction of aphakia or high myopia, a small change in the placement of the lens produces considerable blurring of vision unless the lens power is altered to compensate for the new lens position, so that the secondary focal point of the lens again coincides with the far point of the eye.

With refractive errors greater than ±5.00 D, the vertex distance must be accounted for in prescribing the power of the spectacle lens. A *distometer* (also called a *vertexometer*) is used to measure the distance from the back surface of the spectacle lens to the cornea with the eyelid closed (Fig 5-3A). Moving a correcting lens closer to the eye—whether the lens has plus or minus power—reduces its effective focusing power (the image moves posteriorly away from the fovea), whereas moving it farther from the eye increases its focusing power (the image moves anteriorly away from the fovea).

For example, in Figure 5-4 the +10.00 D lens placed 10 mm in front of the cornea provides sharp retinal imagery. Because the focal point of the correcting lens is identical to the far point plane of the eye and because this lens is placed 10 mm in front of the eye, the far point plane of the eye must be 90 mm behind the cornea. If the correcting lens is moved to a new position 20 mm in front of the eye, the far point plane of the eye remains 90 mm behind the cornea, so the focal length of the new lens must be 110 mm, requiring a +9.10 D lens for correction. The equivalent contact lens will need to have a power of 11.10 D. This example demonstrates the significance of vertex distance in spectacle correction of large refractive errors. Thus, the prescription must indicate not only the lens power but also the vertex distance at which the refraction was performed. The optician must recalculate the lens power as necessary for the actual vertex distance of the chosen spectacle–frame combination. Clinical Example 5-1 demonstrates examples of vertex distance. See also Chapter 1, Example 1-6.

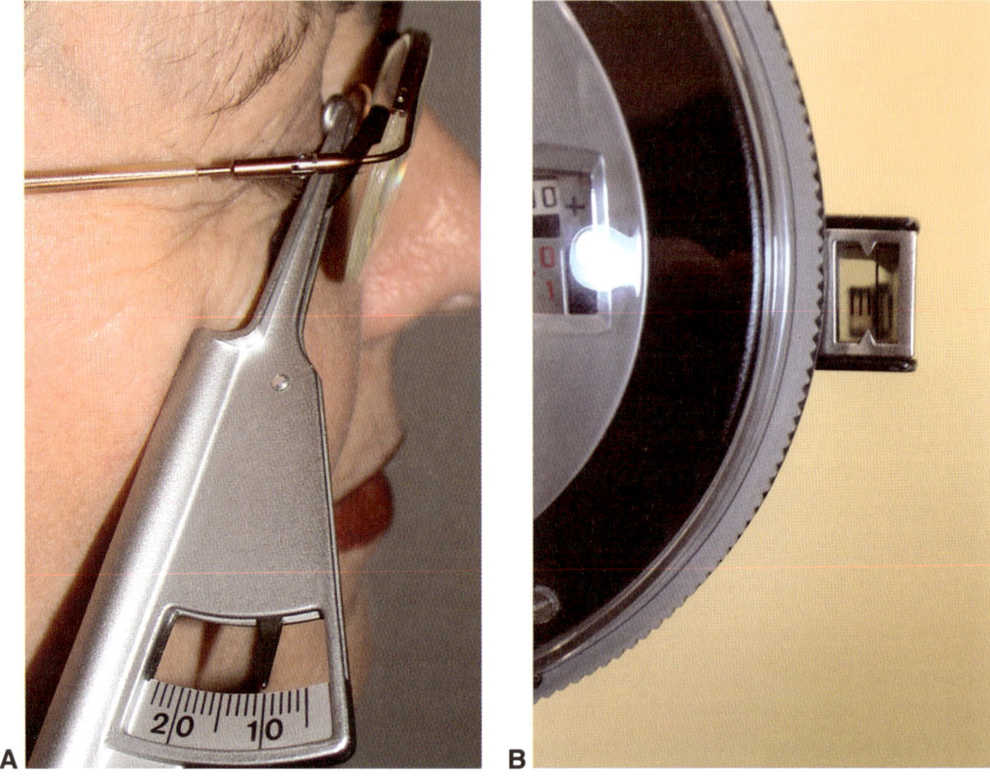

Figure 5-3 Measuring vertex distance. **A,** Vertexometer (distometer). **B,** Corneal alignment tool. *(Part A courtesy of Tommy Korn, MD; part B courtesy of Thomas F. Mauger, MD.)*

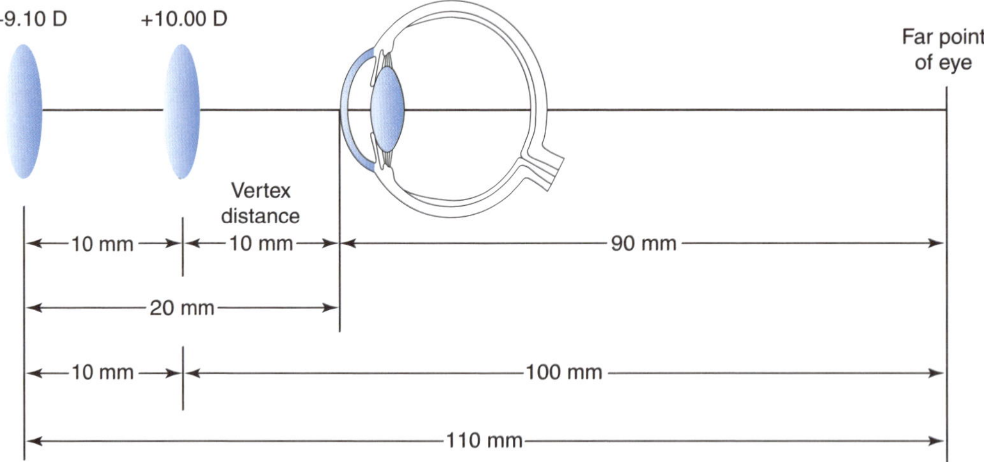

Figure 5-4 The importance of vertex distance in the correction of high refractive errors.

CLINICAL PEARL

The effect of changing the vertex distance can also be used by patients to their advantage. For example, a myopic patient with presbyopia can facilitate viewing of a near target by sliding their glasses down their nose, increasing the vertex distance. This will move the image of near objects forward (farther away from the eye), lessening the accommodative demand. The same is true, to a lesser degree, for hyperopes.

CLINICAL EXAMPLE 5-1

A +10.00 D lens at a vertex distance of 10 mm corrects an eye for distance. A new frame is used and the vertex distance is now 15 mm. What should the power of the lens be to correct the eye for distance?

The far point is 1/10 = 0.1 m (100 mm) behind the original lens. At the new vertex distance (15 mm), the lens needs to correct for a far point that is now 105 mm behind the lens. Therefore, the correcting lens power is 1/0.105 = +9.50 D.

A −10.00 D lens that corrects an eye for distance with an original vertex distance of 10 mm that is changed to 15 mm will need to be changed to −10.50 D.

Note: If the glasses are simply moved out 5 mm without changing the lens power, the eye will be 0.50 D myopic. This is one reason that people with high spectacle corrections move their glasses down their noses to read.

Allowing for vertex distance with the phoropter is made easier by 2 commonly found features. The first feature is that the lenses within the phoropter, even though found in different planes, have their power referenced to the back surface of the most posterior lens in the system. The second feature is that if the cornea of the eye is aligned at the zero mark on the corneal alignment tool (Fig 5-3B), the vertex distance equals that assumed for the phoropter (13.75 mm for the Reichert Phoroptor). A table is provided by the manufacturer to allow for adjustment of lens power for eyes refracted closer to or farther from the instrument. The patient should be refracted in a trial frame or overrefracted in their current spectacles if the vertex distance varies significantly (>6 mm) from that assumed in the phoropter.

Cylindrical Correcting Lenses and the Far Point Concept

The far point principles used in the correction of hyperopia and myopia are also employed in the correction of astigmatism with spectacle lenses. However, in astigmatism, the required lens power must be determined separately for each of the 2 principal meridians.

Cylinders in spectacle lenses produce both monocular and binocular distortion. The primary cause is *meridional aniseikonia*—that is, unequal magnification of retinal images in the various meridians. Although aniseikonia may be decreased by special iseikonic spectacles, such corrections may be complicated and expensive, and most practitioners prefer to prescribe cylinders according to their clinical judgment. Clinical experience also suggests that adult patients vary in their ability to tolerate distortion, whereas young children nearly always adapt to their cylindrical corrections.

The following guidelines may prove helpful in prescribing astigmatic spectacle corrections:

- For *children,* astigmatic errors of 1.50 D or greater are generally corrected. Prescribe the full astigmatic correction at the correct axis.
- For *adults,* try the full correction initially. Give the patient the chance to experience the proposed correction by walking around the clinic with the correction in trial frames before writing the prescription, if appropriate. (The experience of seeing the effects of motion is an important part of this process—the patient's sitting in a chair with the proposed prescription in trial frames is not an adequate test.) Inform the patient of the need for adaptation. To reduce distortion, use minus cylinder lenses (now standard) and minimize vertex distance.
- Because spatial distortion from astigmatic spectacles is often a binocular phenomenon, occlude 1 eye to verify that spatial distortion is the cause of the patient's difficulty.
- If necessary, reduce distortion by rotating the axis of the cylinder toward 180° or 90° (or toward the old axis) and/or reduce the cylinder power. Adjust the sphere to maintain spherical equivalent, but rely on a final subjective check to obtain the most satisfactory visual result.
- If distortion cannot be reduced sufficiently, consider contact lenses or iseikonic corrections.

For a more detailed discussion of the problem of, and solutions for, spectacle correction of astigmatism, see the reference.

Guyton DL. Prescribing cylinders: the problem of distortion. *Surv Ophthalmol.* 1977;22(3): 177–188.

Pantoscopic Tilt

A spectacle lens works best when the line of sight passes through the optical center of the lens, and when the lens is oriented perpendicularly to the line of sight. This alignment prevents unwanted prismatic effects and minimizes aberrations such as astigmatism of oblique incidence. However, when lenses are mounted in eyeglass frames, such an alignment cannot be maintained in all directions of gaze, as the eyes rotate behind the spectacle frames. In practice, it is helpful to rotate the lenses slightly downward, so as to compromise between the line of sight during straight-ahead distance viewing and the depressed line of sight often used for reading, especially with bifocal or progressive-add lenses. This downward rotation is referred to as pantoscopic tilt. This adjustment is particularly important for multifocal lenses, which are used for both distance and near. Typical values for the pantoscopic tilt are approximately 7° (Fig 5-5).

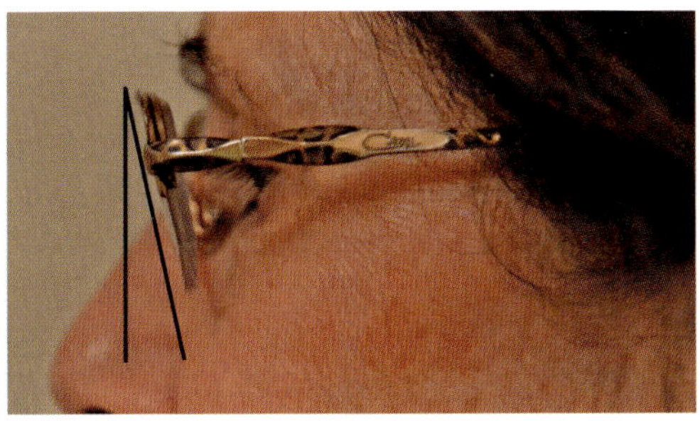

Figure 5-5 In order to optimize image quality for both straight-ahead viewing and downgaze (as for reading), eyeglass frames typically rotate the plane of the lenses downward, a correction known as pantoscopic tilt. Values of about 7° are typical. *(Courtesy of Scott E. Brodie, MD, PhD.)*

Prescribing for Children

The correction of ametropia in children presents several special and challenging problems. In adults, the correction of refractive errors has 1 measurable endpoint: the best-corrected visual acuity. Prescribing visual correction for children often has 2 goals: providing a focused retinal image and achieving the optimal balance between accommodation and convergence.

In some young patients, *subjective refraction* may be impossible or inappropriate, often because of the child's inability to cooperate with subjective refraction techniques. In addition, the optimal refraction in infants or small children (particularly those with esotropia) requires the *paralysis of accommodation* with complete cycloplegia. In such cases, objective techniques such as retinoscopy are the best way to determine the refractive correction. Moreover, the presence of *strabismus* may require modification of the normal prescribing guidelines.

Myopia

There are 2 types of childhood myopia: *congenital* (usually high) myopia and *developmental* myopia, which usually manifests itself between the ages of 7 and 10 years. Developmental myopia is less severe and easier to manage because the patients are older and refraction is less difficult. However, both forms of myopia are progressive; frequent refractions (every 6–12 months) and periodic prescription changes are necessary. The following are general guidelines for correction of significant childhood myopia.

- Cycloplegic refractions are mandatory (until age 10 years, or so). In infants, children with esotropia, and children with very high myopia (>10.00 D), atropine refraction may be necessary if tropicamide or cyclopentolate fails to paralyze accommodation in the office.
- In general, the full refractive error, including cylinder, should be corrected. Young children tolerate cylinder well.
- Some ophthalmologists intentionally undercorrect myopia, and others use bifocal lenses with or without atropine, based on the theory that accommodation hastens or increases the development of myopia. This topic remains controversial among ophthalmologists. (See the discussion in Chapter 3 of this volume.)

- Intentional undercorrection of a child's myopic esotropia to decrease the angle of deviation is rarely tolerated.
- Intentional overcorrection of a myopic error (or undercorrection of a hyperopic error) may help control intermittent exodeviations. However, such overcorrection can cause additional accommodative stress.
- Parents should be educated about the natural progression of myopia and the need for frequent refractions and possible prescription changes.
- In older children, contact lenses may be desirable to avoid the problem of image minification that arises with high-minus lenses.

Hyperopia

The appropriate correction of childhood hyperopia is more complex than that of myopia for 2 reasons. First, children who are significantly hyperopic (>5.00 D) are more visually impaired than are their myopic counterparts, who can at least see clearly at near. Second, childhood hyperopia is more frequently associated with strabismus and abnormalities of the *accommodative convergence/accommodation (AC/A)* ratio (see BCSC Section 6, *Pediatric Ophthalmology and Strabismus*). The following are general guidelines for correcting childhood hyperopia:

- Unless there is esodeviation or evidence of reduced vision, it is not necessary to correct low hyperopia. Most children have very high amplitude of accommodation. As with myopia, significant astigmatic errors should be fully corrected.
- When hyperopia and esotropia coexist, initial management includes full correction of the cycloplegic refractive error. Reductions in the amount of correction may be appropriate later, depending on the amount of esotropia and level of stereopsis with the full cycloplegic correction in place.
- In a school-aged child, the full refractive correction may cause blurring of distance vision because of the inability to relax accommodation fully. Reducing the amount of correction is sometimes necessary for the child to accept the glasses. A short course of cycloplegia may help a child accept the hyperopic correction.

Anisometropia

A child or infant with anisometropia is typically prescribed the full refractive difference between the 2 eyes, regardless of age, presence or amount of strabismus, or degree of anisometropia. Anisometropic amblyopia is frequently present and may require occlusion therapy, but many children recover equal or near equal acuity simply by wearing the anisometropic refractive correction full-time, without patching. *Bilateral amblyopia* occasionally occurs when there is significant hyperopia, myopia, and/or astigmatism in both eyes. Refractive amblyopia is less common with bilateral myopia because these patients have clear near vision.

Clinical Accommodative Problems

See Chapter 3 for a discussion of the terminology and mechanisms of accommodation.

Presbyopia

Presbyopia is the gradual loss of accommodative response resulting from reduced elasticity of the crystalline lens. Accommodative amplitude diminishes with age. It becomes a clinical problem when the remaining accommodative amplitude is insufficient for the patient to read and carry out near-vision tasks comfortably. Fortunately, appropriate convex lenses can compensate for the waning of accommodative power.

Symptoms of presbyopia usually begin to appear in patients older than 40 years. The age at onset depends on preexisting refractive error, depth of focus (pupil size), the patient's visual tasks, and other variables. Table 5-1 presents a simplified overview of age norms.

Accommodative Insufficiency

Accommodative insufficiency is the premature loss of accommodative amplitude. This problem may manifest itself by the blurring of near visual objects (as in presbyopia) or by the inability to sustain accommodative effort. The onset may be heralded by the appearance of asthenopic symptoms; the ultimate development is blurred near vision. Such "premature presbyopia" may signify concurrent or past debilitating illness, or it may be induced by medications such as tranquilizing drugs or the parasympatholytics used in treating some gastrointestinal disorders. In both cases, the condition may be reversible; however, permanent accommodative insufficiency may be associated with neurogenic disorders such as encephalitis or closed head trauma. In some cases, the etiology may never be determined. These patients require additional plus power for near vision. The most common causes of premature presbyopia, however, are unrecognized (latent) hyperopia and overcorrected myopia.

Accommodative Excess

Ciliary muscle spasm, often incorrectly termed spasm of accommodation, causes accommodative excess. A ciliary spasm has characteristic symptoms: headache, brow ache, variable

Table 5-1 Average Accommodative Amplitudes for Different Ages

Age	Average Accommodative Amplitude [a]
8	14.0 (±2.00 D)
12	13.0 (±2.00 D)
16	12.0 (±2.00 D)
20	11.0 (±2.00 D)
24	10.0 (±2.00 D)
28	9.0 (±2.00 D)
32	8.0 (±2.00 D)
36	7.0 (±2.00 D)
40	**6.0 (±2.00 D)**
44	4.5 (±1.50 D)
48	3.0 (±1.50 D)
52	2.5 (±1.50 D)
56	2.0 (±1.00 D)
60	1.5 (±1.00 D)
64	1.0 (±0.50 D)
68	0.5 (±0.50 D)

[a] Until age 40, accommodation decreases by 1.00 D for each 4 years. After age 40, accommodation decreases more rapidly. From age 48 on, 0.50 D is lost every 4 years. Thus, one can recall the entire table by remembering the amplitudes at age 40 and age 48.

blurring of distance vision, and an abnormally close near point. Ciliary spasm may be a manifestation of local disease such as iridocyclitis, it may be caused by medications such as the anticholinergics used in the treatment of glaucoma, or it may be associated with uncorrected refractive errors—usually hyperopia but also astigmatism. In some patients, ciliary spasm exacerbates preexisting myopia. Cycloplegic refraction often helps determine the patient's true refractive error in such cases.

Ciliary spasm may also occur after prolonged and intense periods of near work. *Spasm of the near reflex* is a characteristic clinical syndrome often observed in tense or anxious persons who present with (1) excess accommodation, (2) excess convergence, and (3) miosis.

Accommodative Convergence/Accommodation Ratio

Normally, accommodative effort (A) is accompanied by a corresponding convergence (AC) effort. For practical purposes, the AC/A ratio is ordinarily expressed in terms of prism diopters (Δ) of deviation per diopter of accommodation. Using this type of expression, the normal AC/A ratio is 3:1–5:1.

The AC/A ratio is relatively constant in a particular patient, but it should be noted that there is some variability among individuals. For example, a patient with an uncorrected 1.00 D of hyperopia may accommodate 1.00 D for clear distance vision without exercising a convergence effort. Conversely, a patient with uncorrected myopia must converge without accommodative effort to fuse at the far point.

The AC/A ratio can be measured by varying the stimulus to accommodation in several ways. These methods are described in the following subsections.

Heterophoria method

The heterophoria method involves moving the fixation target. The heterophoria is measured at 6 m and again at 0.33 m.

$$\frac{\mathrm{AC}}{\mathrm{A}} = PD + \frac{\Delta n - \Delta d}{D}$$

Where

PD = interpupillary distance in centimeters
Δn = near deviation in prism diopters
Δd = distance deviation in prism diopters
D = amount of accommodation in diopters

Sign convention:

Esodeviations: +
Exodeviations: –

Gradient methods

The AC/A ratio can be measured in 1 of 2 ways with the gradient method. The first way is by *stimulating accommodation.* Measure the heterophoria with the target distance fixed at 6 m. Then remeasure the induced phoria after interposing a –1.00 D sphere in front of both eyes. The AC/A ratio is the difference between the 2 measurements.

The second way is by *relaxing accommodation.* With the target distance fixed at 0.33 m, measure the phoria before and after interposing +3.00 D spheres. The phoria difference divided by 3 is the AC/A ratio.

An abnormal AC/A ratio can place stress on the patient's fusional mechanisms at one distance or another, causing asthenopia or manifest strabismus. Abnormal AC/A ratios should be accounted for when corrective lenses are prescribed.

Effect of Spectacle and Contact Lens Correction on Accommodation and Convergence

Both accommodation and convergence requirements differ between contact lenses and spectacle lenses. The effects become more noticeable as the power of the correction increases.

Let us first consider accommodative requirements (see also Chapter 6). Recall that because of vertex distance considerations, particularly with high-power corrections, the dioptric power of the distance correction in the spectacle plane is different from that in the contact lens plane: for a near object held at a constant distance, the amount that an eye needs to accommodate depends on the location of the refractive correction relative to the cornea. Patients with myopia must accommodate more for a given near object when they wear contact lenses than when they wear glasses. For example, patients in their early 40s with myopia who switch from single-vision glasses to contact lenses may suddenly experience presbyopic symptoms. The reverse is true with patients with hyperopia; spectacle correction requires more accommodation for a given near object than does contact lens correction. Patients with spectacle-corrected high myopia, when presbyopic, need only weak bifocal add power (or none at all). For example, a patient with high myopia who wears –20.00 D glasses needs to accommodate only approximately 1.00 D to see an object at 33 cm.

Now let us consider convergence requirements and refractive correction. Because contact lenses move with the eyes and spectacles do not, different amounts of convergence are required for viewing near objects. Spectacle correction gives a myopic patient a base-in prism effect when converging and thus reduces the patient's requirement for convergence. (Fortunately, this reduction parallels the lessened requirement for accommodation.) In contrast, a patient with spectacle-corrected hyperopia encounters a base-out prism effect that increases the requirement for convergence. This effect is beneficial in the correction of residual esotropia at near in patients with hyperopia and accommodative esotropia. These effects may be the source of a patient's symptoms on switching between glasses and contact lenses.

Prescribing Multifocal Lenses

A multifocal lens has 2 or more refractive elements. The power of each segment is prescribed separately, relative to the power of the main lens. A prescription additional to that for the main lens is called an *add.*

Determining the Add Power of a Bifocal Lens

The information necessary to prescribe bifocal lenses includes (1) an accurate baseline refraction, (2) the accommodative amplitude, and (3) the patient's social or occupational activities that require near-vision correction (eg, reading, sewing, or computer use).

Measuring accommodative amplitude

Any of the following tests can provide useful information for determining the accommodative amplitude: (1) the near point of accommodation with accurate distance refractive correction in place, (2) the accommodative rule (eg, with a Prince rule [Royal Air Force Rule]), and (3) the use of plus and minus spheres at near distance until the fixation target blurs. *Binocular amplitude of accommodation* is normally greater than the measurement for either eye alone by 0.50–1.00 D.

Near point of accommodation A practical method for measuring the near point of accommodation is to have the patient fixate on a near target (usually small print such as a 5-point typeface or Jaeger 2–print) and move the test card toward the eye until the print blurs. If the eye is emmetropic (or rendered emmetropic by proper refractive correction), the far point of the eye is effectively at infinity, and the near point can be converted into diopters of amplitude.

This method is subject to certain errors, including the apparent increased amplitude resulting from angular magnification of the letters as they approach the eye. In addition, if the eye is ametropic and not corrected for distance, the near point of accommodation cannot be converted into diopters of amplitude. In the following examples, each eye has 3.00 D of accommodative amplitude:

- A person with emmetropia would have a near point of 33 cm and a far point at optical infinity.
- A patient with an uncorrected 3.00 D of myopia would have a near point at 16.7 cm because at the far point of 33 cm, no accommodation is needed.
- A patient with an uncorrected 3.00 D of hyperopia would have a near point at infinity because all of the available accommodation is needed to overcome the hyperopia.

Accommodative rule Amplitude of accommodation can be measured with a device such as a Prince rule (Fig 5-6), which combines a reading card with a ruler calibrated in centimeters and diopters. Placing a +3.00 D lens before the emmetropic (or accurately corrected ametropic) eye places the far point of accommodation at 33 cm, and the near point is also brought closer by a corresponding 3.00 D. The amplitude is then determined by subtraction of the far point (in diopters) from the near point (in diopters).

Method of spheres Amplitude of accommodation may also be measured by having the patient fixate on a reading target at 40 cm. Accommodation is stimulated by the placement

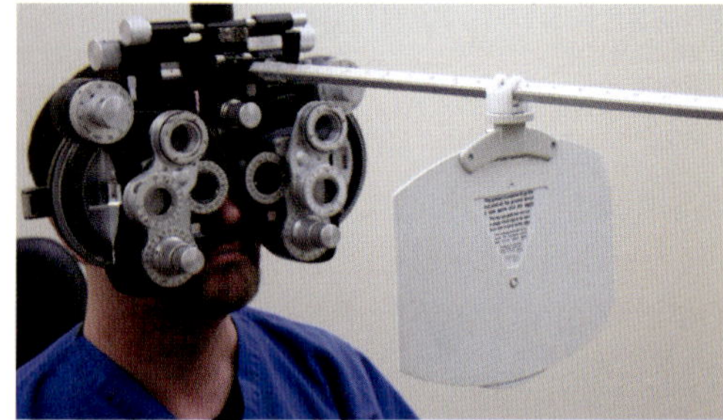

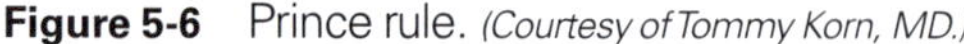

Figure 5-6 Prince rule. *(Courtesy of Tommy Korn, MD.)*

of successively stronger minus spheres before the eye until the print blurs; accommodation is then relaxed by the use of successively stronger plus lenses until blurring begins. The difference between the 2 lenses is a measure of accommodative amplitude. For example, if the patient accepts −3.00 D to blur (stimulus to accommodation) and +2.50 D to blur (relaxation of accommodation), the amplitude is 5.50 D.

Range of accommodation

Determining the range of accommodation, like measuring the amplitude of accommodation, is valuable in ensuring that the prescribed bifocal add power meets the patient's visual needs. The range of accommodation measures the useful range of clear vision when a given lens is employed. For this purpose, a measuring tape, meter stick, or accommodation rule may be used.

Selecting an add power

Determination of the amount of accommodation required for the patient's near-vision tasks is a clinical assessment. For example, reading at 40 cm requires a total of 2.50 D of plus lens power, taking into account a contribution from the patient's own accommodation together with a plus lens correction beyond any correction needed for distance. From the patient's measured accommodative amplitude, the ophthalmologist generally allows one-half to be held in reserve. This reserve allows for some comfortable movement, should the patient move the reading material either closer or farther away than the nominal reading distance. For instance, if the patient has 2.00 D of accommodation, 1.00 D may be comfortably contributed by the patient. (Some patients may use more than one-half of their available accommodation with comfort.) Subtract the patient's available accommodation (1.00 D) from the total amount of near focusing power required (2.50 D); the difference (1.50 D) is the approximate additional plus lens power (add) needed.

Place a lens with this add power in front of the distance refractive correction and measure the range of accommodation (near point to far point of accommodation, in centimeters). Does this range adequately meet the requirements of the patient's near-vision activities? If the accommodative range is too close, reduce the add power in increments of 0.25 D until the range is appropriate for the patient's requirement. Because binocular accommodative amplitude is usually 0.50–1.00 D greater than the monocular measurement, using the binocular measurement generally guards against prescribing an add power that is too high.

CLINICAL PEARL

Initial estimates of the appropriate bifocal add are frequently based simply on patient age: 40–50 years, about +1.00 D; 50–60 years, about +2.00 D; 65 years and older, about 2.50–3.00 D. It is of course advisable to check this estimate by placing the proposed correction in a trial frame or dialing it into the phoropter on top of the distance correction and using a near card to verify the near point and far point of accommodation and adjust the add as indicated.

Types of Bifocal Lenses

Most bifocal lenses currently dispensed are 1-piece lenses that are made by generating the different refracting surfaces on a single lens blank (Fig 5-7). One-piece *round segment bifocal lenses* have their segment on the concave surface. One-piece *molded plastic bifocal lenses* are available in various shapes, including (1) round top with button on convex surface, (2) flat top with button on convex surface, and (3) Franklin (executive) style with split bifocal.

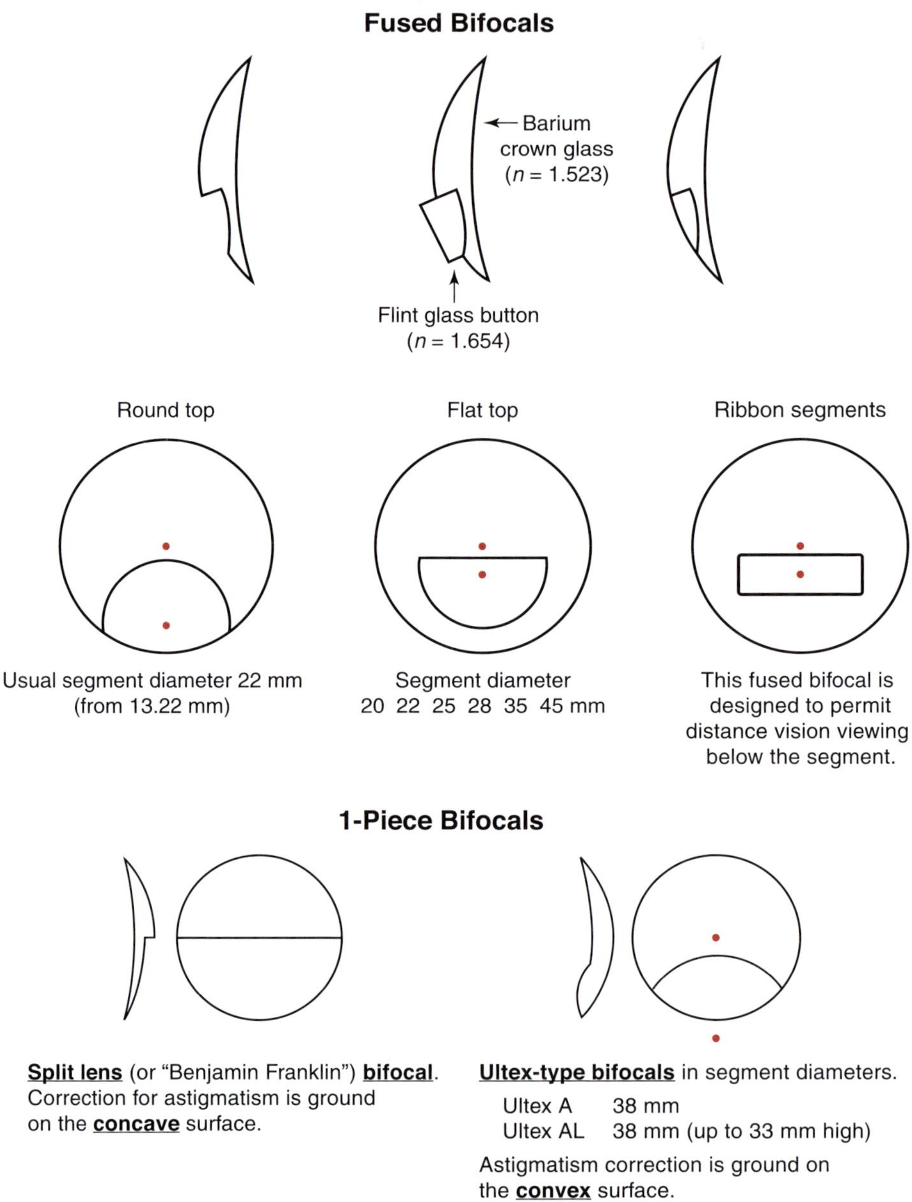

Figure 5-7 Bifocal lens styles. The red dots indicate the optical centers of carrier lenses and bifocal segments. *n* = index of refraction.

With *fused bifocal lenses*, the increased refracting power of the bifocal segment is produced by fusing a button of glass that has a higher refractive index than the basic crown glass lens into a countersink in the crown glass lens blank. With all such bifocal lenses, the add segment is fused into the convex surface of the lens; astigmatic corrections, when necessary, are ground on the concave surface.

Trifocal Lenses

A bifocal lens may not fully satisfy all the visual needs of an older patient with limited accommodation. Even when near and distant ranges are corrected appropriately, vision is not clear in the intermediate range, approximately at arm's length. The loss of intermediate-range vision may be exacerbated by a stronger bifocal add than is really needed. This problem can be solved with trifocal spectacles, which incorporate a third segment of intermediate strength (typically one-half the power of the reading add) between the distance correction and the reading segment. The intermediate segment allows the patient to focus on objects beyond the reading distance but closer than 1 m (Clinical Example 5-2). In contemporary practice, progressive addition lenses have supplanted trifocals in most instances.

CLINICAL EXAMPLE 5-2

This example demonstrates the advantage of trifocal lenses. Consider a patient with 1.00 D of available accommodation. He wears a bifocal lens with a +2.00 add. His accommodative range for each part of the spectacle lens is:

Distance segment: Infinity to 100 cm
Bifocal segment: 50–33 cm

He now has a blurred zone between 50 and 100 cm. An intermediate segment, in this case +1.00 D (half the power of the reading segment), would provide sharp vision from 50 cm (using all of his available accommodation plus the +1.00 D add) to 100 cm (using the add only). This trifocal lens combination therefore provides the following ranges of clear vision:

Distance segment: Infinity to 100 cm
Intermediate segment: 100–50 cm
Near segment: 50–33 cm

Progressive Addition Lenses

Both bifocal and trifocal lenses have an abrupt change in power as the line of sight passes across the boundary between 1 portion of the lens and the next; image jump and diplopia can occur at the segment lines. Progressive addition lenses (PALs) avoid these difficulties by supplying power gradually as the line of sight is depressed toward the reading level. Unlike bifocal and trifocal lenses, PALs offer clear vision at all focal distances. Other advantages of PALs include lack of intermediate blur and absence of any visible segment lines.

The PAL layout has 4 types of optical zones on the convex surface: a spherical distance zone, a reading zone, a transition zone (or "corridor"), and zones of peripheral distortion.

The progressive change in lens power is generated on the convex surface of the lens by progressive aspheric changes in curvature from the top to the bottom of the lens. The concave surface is reserved for the cylinder of the patient's distance lens prescription, as in traditional minus cylinder lens designs.

However, there are certain drawbacks to PALs. Most notably, some degree of peripheral distortion is inherent in the design of all PALs. This peripheral aberration is caused by astigmatism resulting from the changing aspheric curves; these curves are most pronounced in the lower inner and outer quadrants of the lens. These distortions may produce a "swimming" sensation with head movement.

The vertical meridian joining the distance and reading optical centers is free of surface astigmatism and provides the optimal visual acuity. To either side of this distortion-free vertical meridian, induced astigmatism and a concomitant degradation of visual acuity occur. If the lens is designed such that the peripheral distortions are spread out over a relatively wide portion of the lens, there is a concomitant decrease in the distortion-free principal zones. This effect is the basis of *soft-design PALs* (Fig 5-8). Conversely, a wider distortion-free zone for distance and reading means a more intense lateral deformity. This effect is the basis of *hard-design PALs*. If the transition corridor is lengthened, the distortions are less pronounced, but problems arise because of the greater vertical separation between the distance optical center and the reading zone. Therefore, each PAL design represents a series of compromises. Some manufacturers prefer less distortion at the expense of less useful aberration-free distance and near visual acuity; others opt for maximum acuity over a wider usable area, with smaller but more pronounced lateral distortion zones.

Good candidates for progressive lenses may be patients with new presbyopia who have not experienced traditional lined bifocals or trifocals, those who only occasionally need intermediate vision, and those with strong aversions to lined lenses. Less successful candidates are those who are currently happy with other alternatives (lined bifocals/trifocals or single-vision correction); patients with anisometropia; and those requiring prism or high

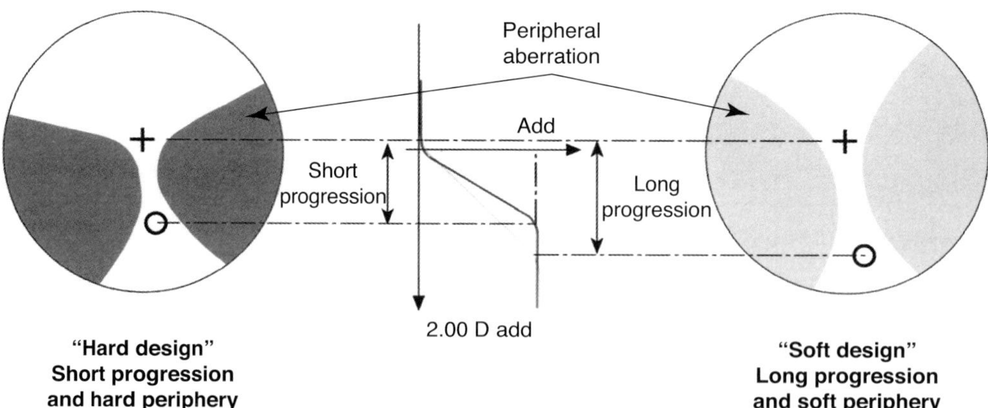

Figure 5-8 Comparison of hard-design and soft-design progressive addition lenses (PALs). These illustrations compare the power progression and peripheral aberration of these 2 PAL designs. *(From Wisnicki HJ. Bifocals, trifocals, and progressive-addition lenses.* Focal Points: Clinical Modules for Ophthalmologists. *American Academy of Ophthalmology; 1999, module 6.)*

adds, a large field of view, or multiple near-fixation lines of sight, or those whose eye movements are extreme/dynamic (often involved in the playing of sports). These factors should be taken into consideration, as should personality, which may play a role in acceptance of progressive lenses.

Fitting of these lenses is a critical process. Measurement of pupillary distance should be performed monocularly, as any asymmetry must be accounted for. Frame selection is important; the frame must have adequate vertical depth to allow the full progressive add and reasonable zones for distance and near vision to be present. The distance and near reference areas should be marked with the frame in place. Frames with adjustable nose pads allow future adjustment of the PAL position. A shorter back vertex distance will give greater binocular field of vision. Greater pantoscopic tilt gives increased near visual field but must be accounted for in the effective lens power.

PALs are readily available from −12.00 to +8.00 D spheres and up to 4.00 D cylinders; the available add powers are from +1.50 to +3.50 D. Some vendors also make custom lenses with parameters outside these limits. Prism can be incorporated into PALs.

Patients who change from conventional multifocal lenses to PALs should be advised that distortion will be present and that adaptation will be necessary. Small-frame PALs can reduce the usable reading zone to a small area at the bottom edge of the lens. Also, the differential magnification through the progressive zone can make computer screens appear trapezoidal (wider at the bottom than the top, though in sharp focus throughout). Progressive designs are also available for indoor use, with large zones devoted to computer monitor use and reading distances (eg, 23 inches and 16 inches from the eye).

Prentice's Rule and Bifocal Lens Design

There are special considerations when prescribing lenses for patients with significant anisometropias.

Prismatic effects of lenses

All lenses act as prisms when one looks through the lens at any point other than the optical center. The amount of the induced prismatic effect depends on the power of the lens and the distance from the optical center. Specifically, the amount of prismatic effect (measured in prism diopters) is equal to the distance (in centimeters) from the optical center multiplied by the lens power (in diopters). This equation is known as *Prentice's rule:*

$$\Delta = hD$$

Where

Δ = prismatic effect (in prism diopters)
h = distance from the optical center (in centimeters)
D = lens power (in diopters)

Note that the distance from the optical center in Prentice's rule is measured in *centimeters,* unlike all other distances in optical calculations, which are expressed in *meters.* This reflects the use of centimeters, rather than meters, in the measurement of deflection of light by a prism in the definition of *prism diopter.*

Image displacement

When reading at near through a point below the optical center, a patient wearing spectacle lenses of unequal power may notice vertical double vision. With a bifocal segment, the gaze is usually directed 8–10 mm below and 1.5–3.0 mm nasal to the distance optical center of the distance lens (in the following examples, we assume the usual 8 mm down and 2 mm nasal). As long as the bifocal segments are of the same power and type, the induced vertical prismatic displacement is determined by the power in the vertical meridian of the distance lens alone.

If the lens powers are the same for the 2 eyes, the displacement of each is the same (Figs 5-9, 5-10). However, if the patient's correction is anisometropic, a phoria is induced by the unequal prismatic displacement of the 2 lenses (Figs 5-11, 5-12). The amount of *vertical phoria* is determined by subtracting the smaller prismatic displacement from the larger if both lenses are myopic or hyperopic (see Fig 5-10) or by adding the 2 lenses if the patient is hyperopic in 1 eye and myopic in the other (see Fig 5-11).

For determination of the induced *horizontal phoria,* the induced prisms are added if both eyes are hyperopic or if both eyes are myopic. If 1 eye is hyperopic and the other is myopic, the smaller amount of prismatic displacement is subtracted from the larger (see Fig 5-11).

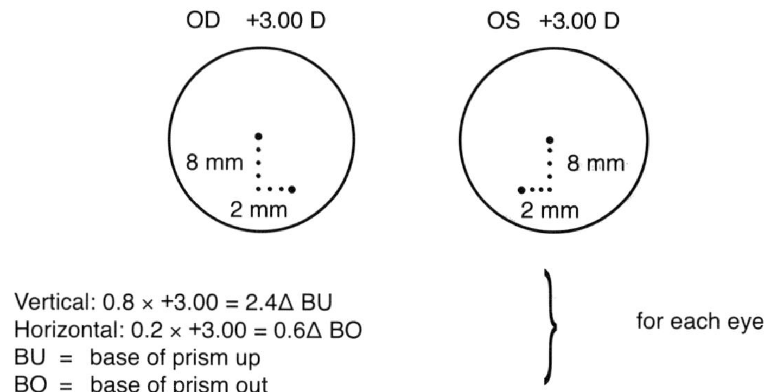

Figure 5-9 Prismatic effect of bifocal lenses in isometropic hyperopia.

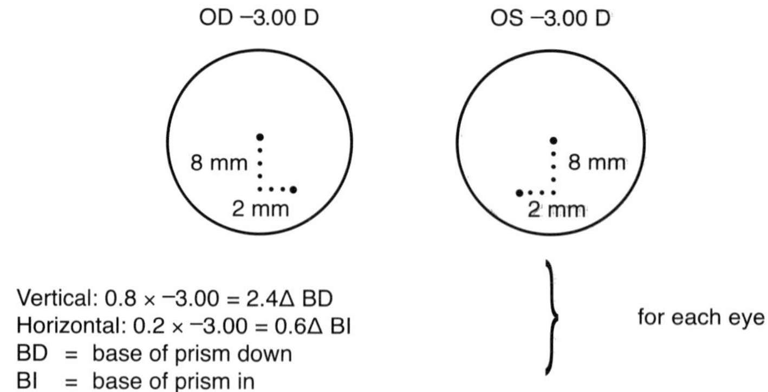

Figure 5-10 Prismatic effect of bifocal lenses in isometropic myopia.

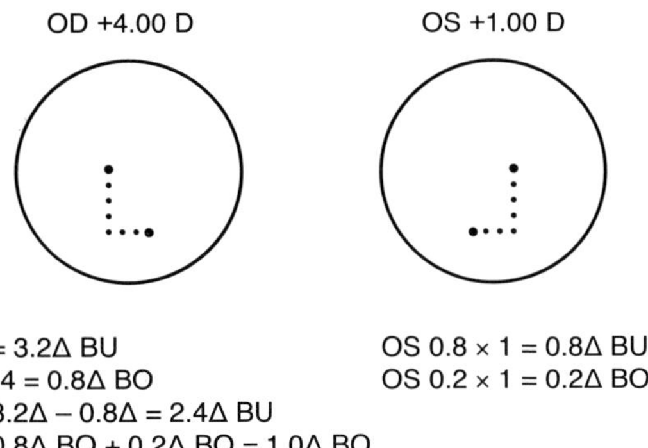

Vertical: OD 0.8 × 4 = 3.2Δ BU — OS 0.8 × 1 = 0.8Δ BU
Horizontal: OD 0.2 × 4 = 0.8Δ BO — OS 0.2 × 1 = 0.2Δ BO
Induced phoria: OD 3.2Δ − 0.8Δ = 2.4Δ BU
OD 0.8Δ BO + 0.2Δ BO = 1.0Δ BO

Figure 5-11 Prismatic effect of bifocal lenses in anisometropic hyperopia.

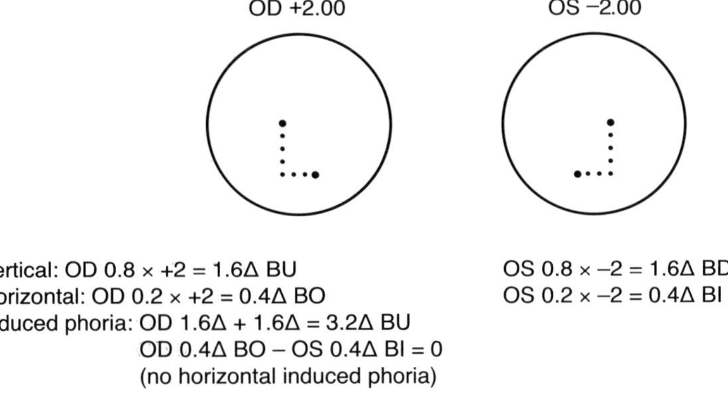

Figure 5-12 Prismatic effect of bifocal lenses in antimetropia.

Image displacement is minimized when round-top segment bifocal lenses are used with plus lenses and flat-top segment bifocal lenses are used with minus lenses (Fig 5-13).

Image jump

The usual position of the top of a bifocal segment is 5 mm below the optical center of the distance lens. As the eyes are directed downward through a lens, the prismatic displacement of the image increases (downward in plus lenses, upward in minus lenses). When the eyes encounter the top of a bifocal segment, they meet a new plus lens with a different optical center, and the object appears to jump upward unless the optical center of the add is at the very top of the segment (Fig 5-14). (Executive-style segments have their optical centers at the top of the segment.) The optical center of a typical flat-top segment is located 3 mm below the top of the segment. The closer the optical center of the segment approaches the top edge of the segment, the less the image jump. Thus, flat-top segments produce less image jump than do round-top segments because the latter have much lower optical centers. Patients with myopia who wear round-top bifocal lenses would be more bothered by image jump than would patients with hyperopia because the jump occurs in the direction of image displacement.

With plus lenses:

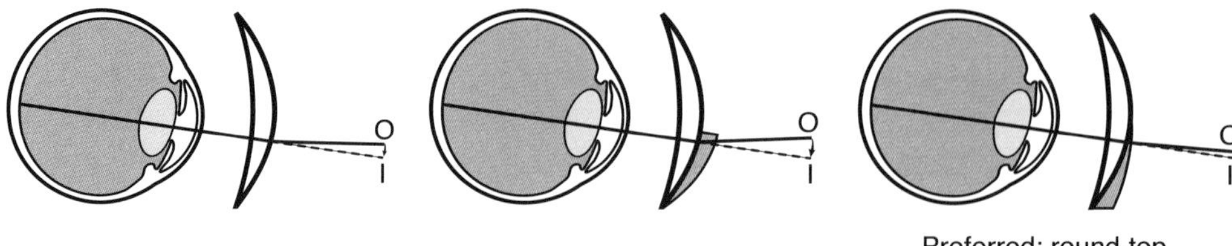

With minus lenses:

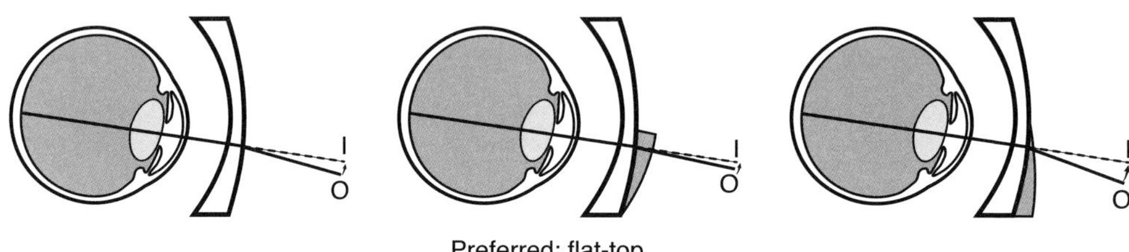

Figure 5-13 Image displacement through bifocal segments. *(From Wisnicki HJ. Bifocals, trifocals, and progressive-addition lenses.* Focal Points: Clinical Modules for Ophthalmologists. *American Academy of Ophthalmology; 1999, module 6. Reprinted with permission from Guyton DL.* Ophthalmic Optics and Clinical Refraction. *Prism Press; 1998. Redrawn by C. H. Wooley.)*

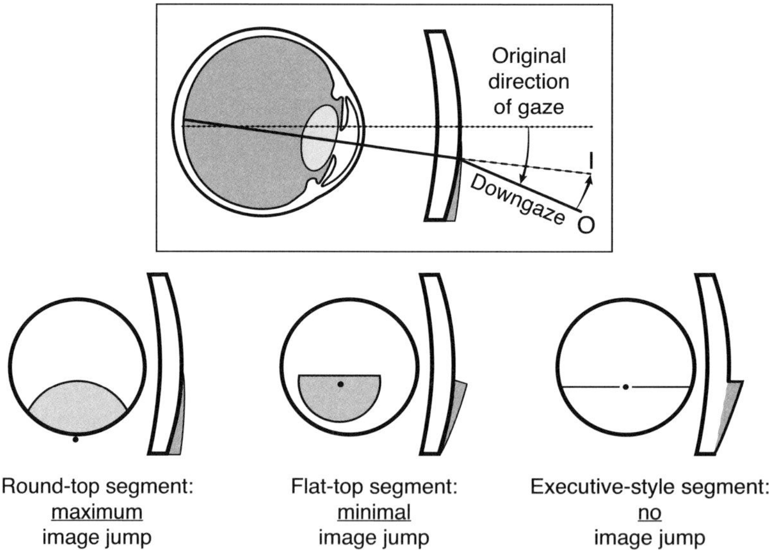

Figure 5-14 Image jump through bifocal segments. If the optical center of a segment is at its top, no image jump occurs. *(From Wisnicki HJ. Bifocals, trifocals, and progressive-addition lenses.* Focal Points: Clinical Modules for Ophthalmologists. *American Academy of Ophthalmology; 1999, module 6. Reprinted with permission from Guyton DL.* Ophthalmic Optics and Clinical Refraction. *Prism Press; 1998. Redrawn by C. H. Wooley.)*

Compensating for induced anisophoria

When anisometropia is corrected with spectacle lenses, unequal prism is often introduced in all secondary positions of gaze. This prism may be the source of symptoms, even diplopia. *Symptomatic anisophoria* occurs especially when a patient with early presbyopia uses his or her first pair of bifocal lenses or when the anisometropia is of recent and/or sudden origin, as occurs after retinal detachment surgery, with gradual asymmetric progression of cataracts, or after unilateral intraocular lens implantation. The patient usually adapts to horizontal imbalance by increasing head rotation but may have symptoms when looking down, in the reading position. Recall that horizontal vergence amplitudes are large compared with vertical fusional amplitudes, which are typically less than 2Δ. We can calculate the amount of induced phoria by using Prentice's rule (Fig 5-15; Clinical Example 5-3).

Rx: OD +4.00 sphere
OS +1.00 sphere
Add +2.50 OU

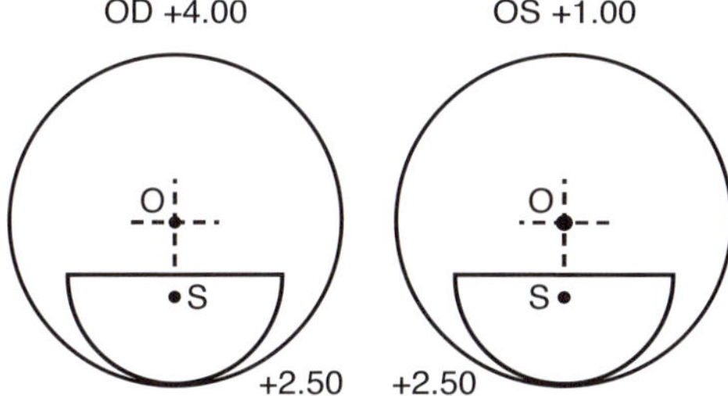

O = optical center, distance
S = optical center of segment
R (= S): Reading position 8 mm below distance optical center

Figure 5-15 Calculation of induced anisophoria.

CLINICAL EXAMPLE 5-3

This example demonstrates Prentice's rule. Consider a patient with the following reading point, 8 mm below distance optical center:

OD 4.00 D × 0.80 cm	=	3.20Δ base up (BU)
OS 1.00 D × 0.80 cm	=	0.80Δ BU
Net difference		2.40Δ BU

In this example, there is an induced right hyperdeviation of 2.40Δ. Conforming to the usual practice in the management of heterophorias, approximately two-thirds to three-fourths of the vertical phoria should be corrected—in this case, 1.75 D.

The correction of induced vertical prism may be accomplished in several ways:

Press-on (Fresnel) prisms With press-on prisms, 2Δ of base-down (BD) prism may be added to the right segment in the preceding example or 2Δ of base-up (BU) prism to the left segment.

Slab-off The most satisfactory method of compensating for the induced vertical phoria in anisometropia is the technique of bicentric grinding, known as *slab-off* (Fig 5-16). In this method, 2 optical centers are created in the lens that has the greater minus (or less plus) power, thereby counteracting the base-down effect of the greater minus lens in the reading position. It is convenient to think of the slab-off process as creating *base-up prism* (or removing base-down prism) over the reading area of the lens.

Bicentric grinding is used for single-vision lenses as well as for multifocal lenses. By increasing the distance between the 2 optical centers, this method achieves as much as 4Δ of prism compensation at the reading position.

Reverse slab-off Prism correction in the reading position is achieved not only by removing *base-down prism* from the lower part of the more minus lens (slabbing off) but also by adding base-down prism to the lower half of the more plus lens. This technique is known as *reverse slab-off.*

Historically, it was easy to remove material from a standard lens. Currently, because plastic lenses are fabricated by molding, it is more convenient to add material to create a base-down prism in the lower half of what will be the more plus lens. Because plastic lenses account for most lenses dispensed, reverse slab-off is the most common method of correcting anisometropically induced anisophoria. In theory, a minus-powered spectacle lens will have less edge thickness with slab-off than with reverse slab-off.

When the clinician orders a lens that requires prism correction for an anisophoria in downgaze, it is often appropriate to leave the choice of slab-off versus reverse slab-off to the optician by including a statement in the prescription, such as, "Slab-off right lens 3Δ (or reverse slab-off left lens)." In either case, the prescribed prism should be measured in the reading position, not calculated, because the patient may have partially adapted to the anisophoria.

Dissimilar segments In anisometropic bifocal lens prescriptions, vertical prism compensation can also be achieved by using dissimilar bifocal segments with their optical centers at 2 different heights. The segment with the lower optical center should be placed in front of the more hyperopic (or less myopic) eye to provide base-down prism. (This method contrasts with the bicentric grinding method, which produces base-up prism and is therefore employed on the lesser plus or greater minus lens.)

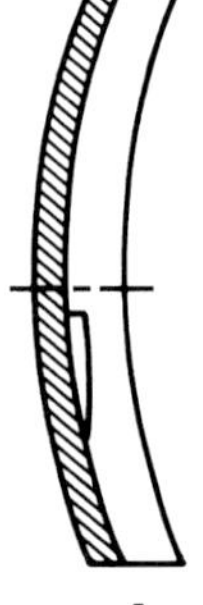

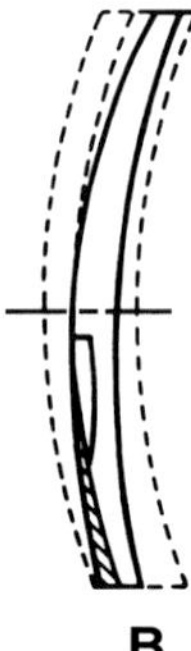

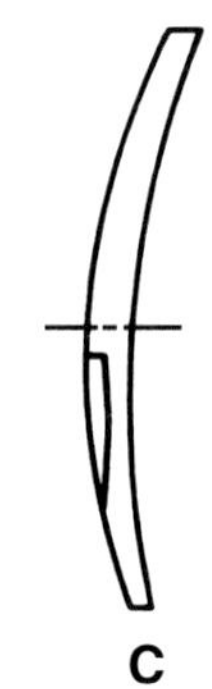

Figure 5-16 Bicentric grinding (slab-off). **A,** Lens form with a dummy lens cemented to the front surface. **B,** Both surfaces of the lens are reground with the same curvatures, but base-up prism is removed from the top segment of the front surface and base-down prism is removed from the entire rear surface. **C,** The effect is a lens from which base-down prism has been removed from the lower segment only.

In the example in Figure 5-17, a 22-mm round segment is used for the right eye, and the top of its segment is at the usual 5 mm below the distance optical center. For the left eye, a 22-mm flat-top segment is used, again with the top of the segment 5 mm below the optical center.

Because the optical center of the flat-top segment is 3 mm below the top of the segment, it is at the patient's reading position; that segment will introduce no prismatic effect. However, for the right eye, the optical center of the round segment is 8 mm below the patient's reading position; according to Prentice's rule, this 2.50 D segment will produce $2.50 \times 0.8 = 2\Delta$ base-down prism.

Single-vision reading glasses with lowered optical centers Partial compensation for the induced vertical phoria at the reading position can be obtained with single-vision reading glasses when the optical centers are placed 3–4 mm below the pupillary centers in primary gaze. The patient's gaze will be directed much closer to the optical centers of the lenses when they read.

Contact lenses Contact lenses can be prescribed for patients with significant anisometropia that causes a symptomatic anisophoria in downgaze with spectacles. Reading glasses can be worn over the contacts if the patient's vision is presbyopic.

Refractive surgery Corneal refractive surgery may be an option for some patients with symptomatic anisometropia or anisophoria.

Occupation and Bifocal Segment

The *dioptric power* of a segment depends on the patient's accommodative reserve and the working distance required for a specific job. Such focal length determinations are a characteristic not of the job but of the individual patient's adaptation to that job. If the patient is allowed to use half of their available accommodation (which should be measured), the remainder of the dioptric requirement will be met by the bifocal add. For example,

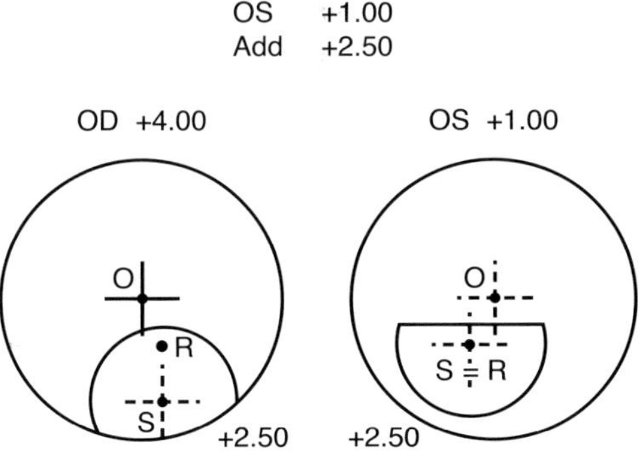

Figure 5-17 Dissimilar segments used to compensate for anisophoria in anisometropic bifocal prescriptions.

O = optical center, distance
S = optical center of segment
R (= S): Reading position 8 mm below distance optical center

if the job entails proofreading at 40 cm, the dioptric requirement for that focal length is 2.50 D. If the patient's accommodative amplitude is 2.00 D, and half of that (1.00 D) is used for the job, the balance of 1.50 D becomes the necessary bifocal add. It is essential that the accommodative range (near point to far point) be measured and that it be adequate for the tasks required by the patient's job.

Lens design

The most important characteristic of the bifocal segment is the *segment height* in relation to the patient's pupillary center. The lenses will be unsuitable if the segment is placed too high or too low for the specific occupational need.

Segment width is substantially less important. The popular impression that very large bifocal lenses mean better reading capability is not supported by projection measurements. At a 40-cm reading distance, a 25-mm flat-top segment provides a horizontal reading field of 50–55 cm.

At a 40-cm distance, an individual habitually uses face rotation to increase their fixation field when it exceeds 45 cm (30° of arc); therefore, a 25-mm-wide segment is more than adequate for all but a few special occupations, such as a graphic artist or an architectural drafter who uses a drawing board. Furthermore, with a 35-mm segment producing a horizontal field 75 cm wide, the focal length at the extremes of the fixation field would be 55 cm, not 40 cm; therefore, the split bifocal is useful not because it is a wider bifocal lens but because of its monocentric construction.

The *shape* of the segment must also be considered. For example, round-top segments require the user to look far enough down in the segment to employ their maximum horizontal dimension. In addition, these segments exaggerate image jump, especially in myopic corrections.

Segment decentration To avoid inducing a base-out prism effect when the bifocal lens–wearing patient converges for near-vision tasks, the reading segment is generally decentered inward. This design is especially important in aphakic spectacles. Consider the following points for determination of proper decentration:

- *Working distance.* Because the convergence requirement increases as the focal length decreases, additional inward decentration of the bifocal segment is required.
- *Interpupillary distance.* The wider the interpupillary distance, the greater the convergence requirement and, correspondingly, the need for inward decentration of the segments.
- *Lens power.* If the distance lens is a high-plus lens, it will create a greater base-out prism effect (ie, induced exophoria) as the viewer converges. Additional inward decentration of the segments may be helpful. The reverse is true for high-minus lenses.
- *Existing heterophoria.* As with lens-induced phorias, the presence of an existing exophoria suggests that increasing the inward decentration would be effective. An esophoria calls for the opposite approach.

Prescribing Special Lenses

Aphakic Lenses

The problems of correcting aphakia with high-plus spectacle lenses include:

- magnification of approximately 20%–35%
- altered depth perception resulting from the magnification
- pincushion distortion; for example, doors appear to bow inward
- difficulty with hand–eye coordination
- ring scotoma generated by prismatic effects at the edge of the lens (causing a "jack-in-the-box" phenomenon)
- extreme sensitivity of the lenses to minor misadjustment in vertex distance, pantoscopic tilt, and height
- in monocular aphakia, loss of useful binocular vision because of differential magnification

In addition, aphakic spectacles create cosmetic problems. The patient's eyes appear magnified and, if viewed obliquely, may seem displaced because of prismatic effects. The high-power lenticular lens is itself unattractive, given its "fried-egg" appearance (Fig 5-18).

For these reasons, intraocular lenses and aphakic contact lenses now account for nearly all aphakic corrections. Nevertheless, spectacle correction of aphakia is sometimes appropriate, as in bilateral infantile pediatric aphakia.

Refracting technique

Because of the sensitivity of aphakic glasses to vertex distance and pantoscopic tilt, it is difficult to refract an aphakic eye reliably with a phoropter. The vertex distance and the pantoscopic tilt are not well controlled, nor are they necessarily close to the values for the final spectacles. Rather than a phoropter, trial frames or lens clips are preferred.

The trial frame allows the refractionist to control vertex distance and pantoscopic tilt. It should be adjusted for minimal vertex distance and for the same pantoscopic tilt planned for the actual spectacles (approximately 5°–7°, not the larger values that are appropriate for conventional glasses). Pantoscopic tilt is desirable in spectacle lenses to maintain the vertex distance in downgaze. Excess tilt will induce oblique (marginal) astigmatism in the axis of rotation.

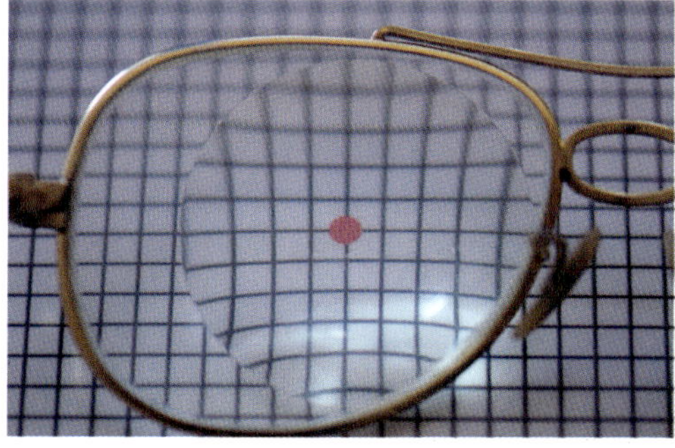

Figure 5-18 Aphakic lens with magnification and pincushion distortion. *(Courtesy of Tommy Korn, MD.)*

Refracting with clip-on trial lens holders placed over the patient's existing aphakic glasses (overrefraction) keeps vertex distance and lens tilt constant. Take care that the center of the clip coincides with the optical center of the existing lens. Even if the present lens contains a cylinder at an axis different from what is needed, it is possible to calculate the resultant spherocylindrical correction with an electronic calculator, by hand, or with measurement of the combination in a lensmeter.

Absorptive Lenses

In certain high-illumination situations, sunglasses allow for better visual function in a number of ways.

Improvement of contrast sensitivity

On a bright, sunny day, irradiance from the sun ranges from 10,000–30,000 foot-lamberts. These high light levels tend to saturate the retina and therefore decrease finer levels of contrast sensitivity. The major function of dark (often gray, green, or brown) sunglasses is to allow the retina to remain at its normal level of contrast sensitivity. Most dark sunglasses absorb 70%–80% of the incident light of all wavelengths.

Improvement of dark adaptation

A full day at the beach or on the ski slopes on a sunny day (without dark sunglasses) can impair dark adaptation for more than 2 days. Thus, dark sunglasses are recommended for prolonged periods in bright sun.

Reduction of glare sensitivity

Various types of sunglasses can reduce glare sensitivity. Because light reflected off a horizontal surface is polarized in the horizontal plane, properly oriented *polarized lenses* reduce the intensity of glare from road surfaces, glass windows, metal surfaces, and lake and river surfaces. *Graded-density sunglasses* are deeply tinted at the top and gradually become lighter toward the lens center. They are effective in removing glare from sources above the line of sight, such as the sun. Wide-temple sunglasses work by reducing glare from temporal light sources.

Use of photochromic lenses

When short-wavelength light (300–400+ nm) interacts with photochromic lenses, the lenses darken by means of a chemical reaction that converts silver ions to elemental silver. This process is similar to the reaction that occurs when photographic film is exposed to light. Unlike that in photographic film, however, the chemical reaction in photochromic lenses is reversible. Current photochromic lenses incorporate complex organic compounds in which ultraviolet light changes the molecules into different configuration states (ie, *cis* to *trans*); this process darkens the lenses (Fig 5-19). Photochromic lenses can darken enough to absorb approximately 80% of the incident light; when the amount of illumination falls, they can lighten to absorb only a small amount of the incident light. Note that these lenses take some time to darken and, in particular, take longer to lighten than to darken. This discrepancy can be problematic in patients who move frequently between outdoor and indoor environments. Because automobile glass and the window glass in many residences

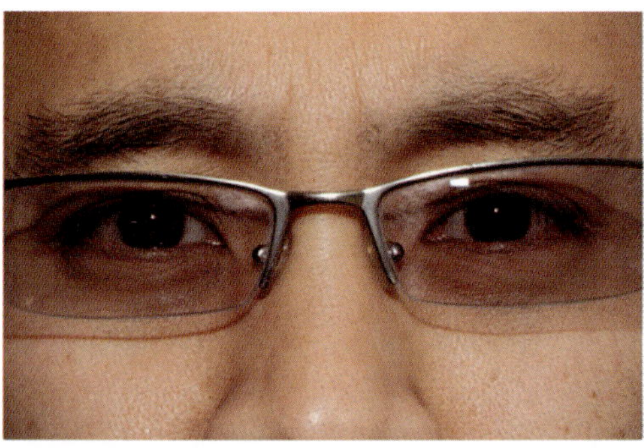

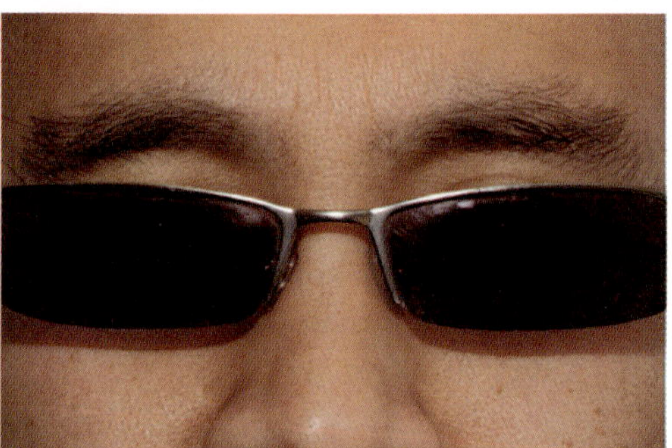

Figure 5-19 Photochromic lenses. *(Courtesy of Tommy Korn, MD.)*

and commercial buildings absorb light in the UV spectrum, most photochromics do not darken inside cars or buildings. Patients should also be warned that in colder weather, these lenses darken more than usual, especially on cloudy days. Nevertheless, photochromic lenses are excellent UV absorbers.

Ultraviolet-absorbing lenses

The spectrum of ultraviolet (UV) light is divided into 3 types: UVA contains wavelengths of 400–320 nm, UVB contains wavelengths of 320–290 nm, and UVC contains wavelengths below 290 nm. The ozone layer of the atmosphere absorbs almost all UVC that comes from the sun. Most exposure to UVC is from manufactured sources, including welding arcs, germicidal lamps, and excimer lasers. Of the total solar radiation falling on the earth, approximately 5% is UV light, of which 90% is UVA and 10% is UVB.

The amount of UV light striking the earth varies with season (greatest in the summer), latitude (greatest near the equator), time of day (greatest at noon), and elevation (greatest at high elevation). UV light can also strike the eye by reflection. Fresh snow reflects between 60% and 80% of incident light; sand (beach, desert) reflects approximately 15% of incident light; and water reflects approximately 5% of incident light.

Laboratory experiments have shown that UV light damages living tissue in 2 ways. First, chemicals such as proteins, enzymes, nucleic acids, and cell-membrane components absorb UV light. When they do so, their molecular bonds (primarily the double bonds) may become disrupted. Second, these essential biochemicals may become disrupted by the action of free radicals (such as the superoxide radical). Free radicals can often be produced by UV light in the presence of oxygen and a photosensitizing pigment. For a fuller discussion of free radicals, see BCSC Section 2, *Fundamentals and Principles of Ophthalmology.*

Because it may take many years for UV light to damage eye tissue, a tight linkage between cause and effect is difficult to prove. Therefore, proof that UV light damages the eye comes primarily from acute animal experiments and epidemiologic studies covering large numbers of patients.

Some surgeons routinely prescribe UV-absorbing glasses after surgery. Intraocular lenses incorporating UV-absorbing chromophores are now the norm. For further information regarding the effects of UV radiation on various ocular structures, see BCSC Section 8, *External Disease and Cornea,* and Section 12, *Retina and Vitreous.*

Almost all dark sunglasses absorb most incident UV light. The same is true for certain coated clear-glass lenses and clear plastic lenses made of CR-39 or polycarbonate. One suggestion has been that certain sunglasses (primarily light-blue ones) may cause light damage to the eye. Proponents of this theory contended that the pupil dilates behind dark glasses and that if the sunglasses do not then absorb significant amounts of UV light, they will actually allow more UV light to enter the eye than if no sunglasses were worn. In fact, dark sunglasses reduce light levels striking the eye on a bright, sunny day to the range of 2000–6000 foot-lamberts. Such levels are approximately 10 times higher than those of an average lighted room. At such light levels, the pupil is significantly constricted. Thus, contrary to the preceding argument, dark sunglasses used on a bright day allow pupillary dilation of only a fraction of a millimeter and do not lead to light injury to the eye.

There is no convincing evidence in the literature of any health or vision benefits of "blue-blocking" glasses.

Special Lens Materials

It is important for the ophthalmologist to be aware of the variety of spectacle lens materials available. Four major properties are commonly discussed in relation to lens materials. Lens materials are compared in Table 5-2.

1. *Index of refraction.* As the refractive index increases, the thickness of the lens can be decreased to obtain the same optical power.
2. *Specific gravity.* As the specific gravity of a material decreases, the lens weight can be reduced.

Table 5-2 Properties of Common Materials for Eyeglass Lenses

Material	Refractive Index	Specific Gravity	Abbe Number	Impact Resistance? FDA 21CFR801.410	ANSI Z87.1	Remarks
Standard glass	1.52	2.54	59	✓		High-index versions available
Standard plastic	1.49	1.32	58	✓		
Polycarbonate	1.58	1.2	30	✓	✓	Scratches easily
Trivex	1.53	1.11	45	✓	✓	Scratches easily

3. *Abbe number (value).* This value indicates the variation in refractive index with wavelength, which governs the degree of dispersion of light. The degree of dispersion of light is responsible for chromatic aberration; materials with a higher Abbe number exhibit less chromatic aberration and allow higher optical quality.
4. *Impact resistance.* All lenses dispensed in the United States must meet impact-resistance requirements defined by the U.S. Food and Drug Administration (FDA) (in 21CFR801.410), except in special cases wherein the physician or optometrist communicates in writing that such lenses would not fulfill the visual requirements of the particular patient. Lenses used for occupational and educational personal eye protection must also meet the impact-resistance requirements defined in the American National Standards Institute (ANSI) high-velocity impact standard (Z87.1). Lenses prescribed for children and active adults should also meet the ANSI Z87.1 standard, unless the patient is duly warned that they are not getting the most impact-resistant lenses available.

Standard glass

Glass lenses provide superior optics and are scratch resistant but also have several limitations, including low impact resistance, increased thickness, and heavy weight. Once the standard in the industry, glass lenses are less frequently used in current practice; many patients select plastic lenses. Without special treatment, glass lenses may be easily shattered. Chemical or thermal *tempering* increases the shatter resistance of glass, but if it is scratched or worked on with any tool after tempering, the shatter resistance is lost. Farmers appreciate photoreactive glass for its scratch resistance and easy care. Welders and grinders are better off with plastic, as small hot particles can become embedded in glass. Persons with myopia who desire thin glasses may choose high-index glass. The highest-index versions cannot be tempered and require that waivers be signed by patients who accept the danger of their breakage. Glass does not block UV light unless a coating is applied.

Standard plastic

Due to its high optical quality and light weight, standard plastic (also known as hard resin or CR-39) is the most commonly used lens material and is inexpensive. Standard plastic lenses are almost 50% lighter than glass lenses owing to the lower specific gravity of their material. They block 80% of UV light without treatment, can be tinted easily if desired, and can be coated to resist scratching and to provide further UV-light blocking. The index of refraction is not high, so the lenses are not thin. CR-39 lenses do not have the shatter resistance of polycarbonate or Trivex.

Polycarbonate

Introduced in the 1970s for ophthalmic lens use, the high-index plastic material polycarbonate has a low specific gravity and a higher refractive index, which allow for a light, thin lens. Polycarbonate is also durable and meets the high-velocity impact standard. One disadvantage of this material is the high degree of chromatic aberration, as indicated by its low Abbe number (30). Thus, color fringing can be an annoyance, particularly in strong prescriptions. Another disadvantage is that polycarbonate is the most easily scratched plastic, so a scratch-resistant coating is required. Also, if polycarbonate is cut too thin, it can flex on impact and pop out of the frame.

Trivex

Introduced in 2001, Trivex is a highly impact-resistant, low-density material that delivers strong optical performance and provides clear vision because of its high Abbe number. Its impact resistance is close to that of polycarbonate, and it blocks all UV light. Its index of refraction is not high, however, so the lenses are not thin. Trivex is the lightest lens material currently available and meets the high-velocity impact standard. A scratch-resistant coating is required.

High-index materials

A lens with a refractive index of 1.60 or higher is referred to as a *high-index lens*. High-index materials can be either glass or plastic and are most often used for higher-power prescriptions to create thin, cosmetically attractive lenses. The weight, optical clarity, and impact resistance of high-index lenses vary depending on the specific material used and the refractive index; in general, as the index of refraction increases, the weight of the material increases and the Abbe number decreases. None of the high-index materials passes the ANSI Z87.1 standard for impact resistance. Plastic high-index materials require a scratch-resistant coating.

Therapeutic Use of Prisms

Small horizontal and vertical deviations can be corrected conveniently in spectacle lenses by the addition of prisms.

Horizontal heterophorias

Asthenopic symptoms may develop in patients (usually adults) if fusion is disrupted by inadequate vergence amplitudes; if fusion cannot be maintained, diplopia results. Thus, in patients with an exophoria at near, symptoms develop when the convergence reserve is inadequate for the task at hand. Some patients can compensate for this fusional inadequacy through the improvement of fusional amplitudes. Younger patients may be able to do so through orthoptic exercises, which are sometimes used in conjunction with prisms that further stimulate patients' fusional capability (base-out prisms to enhance convergence reserve).

Symptoms may arise in some patients because of abnormally high accommodative convergence. Thus, an esophoria at near may be improved by full hyperopic correction for distance and/or by the use of bifocal lenses to decrease accommodative demand. In adult patients, orthoptic training and maximum refractive correction may be inadequate, and prisms or surgery may be necessary to restore binocularity.

Prisms are especially useful if a patient experiences an abrupt onset of symptoms secondary to a basic heterophoria or heterotropia. The prisms may be needed only temporarily, and the minimum amount of prism correction necessary to reestablish and maintain binocularity should be used.

Vertical heterophorias

Vertical fusional amplitudes are small ($<2\Delta$). Thus, if a vertical muscle imbalance is sufficient to cause asthenopic symptoms or diplopia, it should be compensated for by the incorporation of prisms into the refractive correction. Once again, the minimum amount of prism needed to eliminate symptoms should be prescribed. In a noncomitant vertical heterophoria, the prism used should be sufficient to correct the imbalance in primary gaze. With combined vertical and horizontal muscle imbalance, correcting only the vertical deviation may help improve control of the horizontal deviation as well. If the horizontal deviation is not adequately corrected, an oblique Fresnel prism may be helpful. A brief period of clinical heterophoria testing may be insufficient to unmask a latent muscle imbalance. Often, after prisms have been worn for a time, the phoria appears to increase, and the prism correction must be correspondingly increased.

Methods of prism correction

The potential effect of prisms should be evaluated by having the patient test the indicated prism in trial frames or trial lens clips over the current refractive correction. Temporary prisms in the form of clip-on lenses or Fresnel press-on prisms can be used to evaluate and alter the final prism requirement. The Fresnel prisms have several advantages: (1) they are light in weight, thin (1 mm thick), and more acceptable cosmetically because they are affixed to the concave surface of the spectacle lens, and (2) they allow much larger prism corrections (up to 40Δ). With higher prism powers, however, it is not uncommon to observe a decrease in the visual acuity of the corrected eye. Patients may also observe chromatic fringes.

Prisms can be incorporated into spectacle lenses within the limits of cost, appearance, weight, and the technical skill of the optician. Prisms should be incorporated into the spectacle lens prescription only after an adequate trial of temporary prisms has established that the correction is appropriate and the deviation is stable. It may be helpful to suggest frames with relatively small lens openings, as the edges of large-diameter prismatic lenses will be very thick.

Prism correction may also be achieved by decentering the optical center of the lens relative to the visual axis, although a substantial prism effect by means of this method is possible only with higher-power lenses. Aspheric lens designs are not suitable for decentration. (See earlier discussion of lens decentration and Prentice's rule.) Bifocal segments may be decentered *in* more than the customary amount to give a modest additional base-in effect to help patients with convergence insufficiency.

Management of Anisometropia

The bulleted list below highlights approaches to the management of anisometropia. These include full correction with adaptation, undercorrection of 1 eye to reduce anisometropia, contact lens wear (1 or both eyes), refractive surgery, reducing aniseikonia, and reducing induced vertical prismatic effect.

- Full correction with adaptation: If the full correction of the more hyperopic eye is not tolerated, correct as much of the hyperopia as the patient can tolerate, and preserve the accurate difference between the 2 eyes. In children with refractive amblyopia, full correction of both eyes is frequently well tolerated, and may be sufficient to correct the amblyopia even without patching or atropine penalization.

- Undercorrection of one eye to reduce anisometropia: In children under treatment for amblyopia, fully correct the amblyopic eye; in adults, fully correct the better-seeing (or dominant) eye.
- Contact lens wear (one or both eyes).
- Refractive surgery.
- Reducing aniseikonia: Adjust the lens base curve and center thickness of the lenses to minimize the effect on image size. Consider high–refractive index lenses. Maintain the base curve and center thickness of current spectacles if they are well tolerated.
- Reducing induced vertical prismatic effects: Separate single-vision distance and near glasses; slab-off prism or dissimilar segment styles for bifocal corrections.

Troubleshooting for Dissatisfied Spectacle Wearers

The management of dissatisfied spectacle wearers is both an art and a science. As in many areas of medicine, the management of expectations is critical. Demonstrations with trial frames and overrefracting with the patient's existing spectacles may be helpful tools. Major changes (such as cylinder axis changes) should be carefully evaluated and discussed with the patient prior to prescribing.

Many potential problems can be prevented with appropriate attention during the prescribing and fitting process. A good working relationship with the optometrist and dispensing optician is critical, and the written prescription is helpful in preventing problems. The interpupillary distance (monocular for PALs) should be included in it, and the vertex distance should be specified for high-strength prescriptions. The exact type of bifocal, trifocal, or PAL should be specified or noted if it should remain the same as in the current glasses. Any prismatic correction should be carefully noted, as should whether it is the same as in the current glasses, so that the dispensing optician can verify this. The dispensing optician has extensive latitude in the actual materials and coatings of the lenses as well as the type and style of the bifocal and the vertex distance unless these are written on the prescription. For instance, if the prescriber wishes to keep the same base curve as the current spectacles (to decrease changes in image size, in the case of anisometropia) this should be specified on the prescription. The lens material should be indicated, especially if it is a high-index or impact-resistant material. Any photochromic or lens tint or other coatings that the prescriber wants the spectacles to have should be specified.

A "balance lens" may be specified for a completely blind eye; this indicates that the dispensing optician should place in the glasses frames for the blind eye a lens that is cosmetically similar to that being prepared for the fellow eye. In some cases, this may lessen the cost of the patient's lenses. Care must be taken in prescribing a lens for an eye with limited but usable vision (eg, with amblyopia or macular degeneration).

Once the patient presents with dissatisfaction with a new spectacle correction, a detailed history of the problem should be obtained. The nature of the concern should be isolated, if possible, to its source: does it involve distance or near vision, static or dynamic objects/images, blurring, distortion, and/or diplopia? The spectacle power and optic center should be measured and compared with those of the prescription. The refraction should be rechecked, especially in the case of a significant difference from the previous spectacle correction.

When the previous spectacle correction is not different from the new one, a comparison of the spectacles' other properties is helpful. The optical centers (induced prism), prismatic correction, or slab-off in the previous correction should match those in the new prescription. Changes in base curve and center thickness (from old to new) may cause aniseikonia symptoms. If the previous prescription is very old, it should be checked with a Geneva lens clock for plus (front) cylinder design. Differences in bifocal type and position should be noted. Positioning and alignment of PALs should be noted, as a change in model of PAL may cause significant problems. A change from traditional bifocals or trifocals to PALs may also be a source of problems. Changes in vertex distance and pantoscopic tilt may lead to effective lens power differences. Finally, lens material changes may cause chromatic aberrations.

Milder B, Rubin M. *The Fine Art of Prescribing Glasses: Without Making a Spectacle of Yourself.* 3rd ed. Triad Publishing Company; 2004.

Pharmacologic Treatment of Presbyopia

In 2021, the FDA approved the sale of pilocarpine 1.25% eyedrops, marketed as Vuity (AbbVie, Inc.), for the management of presbyopia. The eyedrops are to be administered once daily. In clinical trials, acuity at near was improved by 3 lines in 26%–31% of patients between the ages of 40 and 55 years, presumably due to a combination of increased accommodative tone and depth of field that result from pupillary constriction. The benefit decreased by 50% after 6 hours. Dimming of vision is to be expected, and patients are advised to avoid night driving and similar activities in poor illumination. Adverse reactions of headache and conjunctival hyperemia were reported in more than 5% of patients. Other adverse reactions included blurred vision (possibly due to myopic shift), eye pain, visual impairment, eye irritation, and increased lacrimation. (A small risk of retinal detachment has been reported with the use of other miotic eyedrops; this may apply to Vuity, as well.)

Chapter Exercises

Questions

5.1. What type of distortion is shown in Figure 5-20?
   a. pincushion distortion
   b. barrel distortion
   c. image jump
   d. image displacement

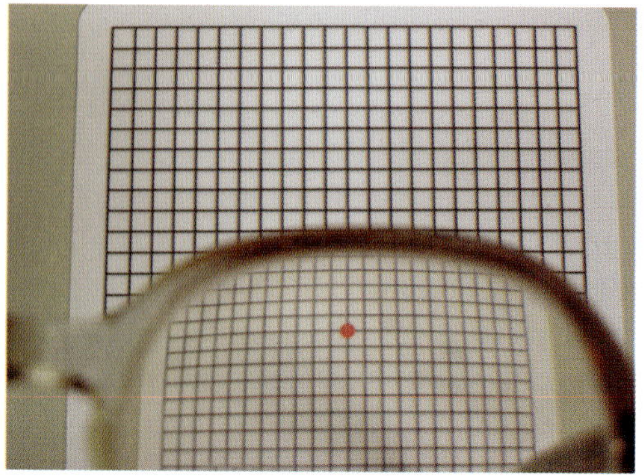

Figure 5-20 Example of lens distortion; see Question 5.1. *(Courtesy of Tommy Korn, MD.)*

5.2. A patient with +9.00 D spectacle lenses (vertex distance is 12 mm) requires a new spectacle frame because of recent nasal surgery. The vertex distance of the new frame is required to be 22 mm to avoid any nasal discomfort. What power is required for the new spectacles?
   a. +7.25 D
   b. +8.25 D
   c. +9.25 D
   d. +10.25 D

5.3. Based on the type of spectacle lenses shown in Figure 5-21, what is a likely occupation of the owner of these spectacles?
   a. retired investment banker or stockbroker
   b. professional senior golfer
   c. airline pilot
   d. jewelry or watch-repair technician

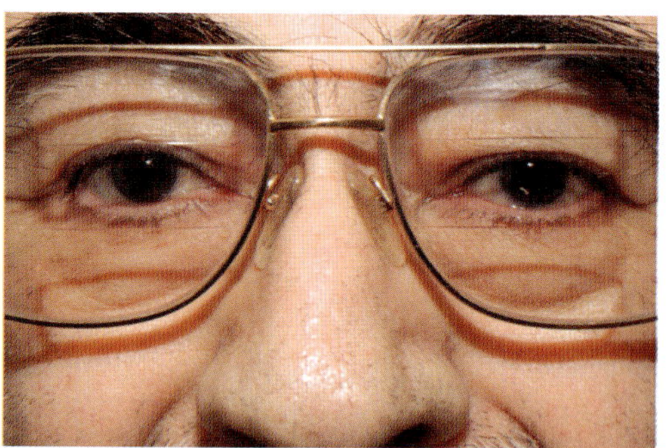

Figure 5-21 Example of occupational spectacle design; see Question 5.3. *(Courtesy of Tommy Korn, MD.)*

5.4. The Abbe number is a measure of what characteristic?
   a. spherical aberration
   b. chromatic aberration
   c. image displacement in plus lenses
   d. curvature of spectacle lenses

5.5. Your refraction determines that a −8.00 D lens in a trial frame with a vertex distance of 10 mm from the patient's cornea provides 20/15 visual acuity. What is the minus power lens needed if the patient requires a vertex distance of 14 mm to use their favorite existing spectacle frame?

a. −7.25 D
b. −8.25 D
c. −9.25 D
d. −10.25 D

5.6. What is the primary reason that patients with presbyopia cannot tolerate significant anisometropia in bifocal lenses?

a. asthenopia
b. inability of the lens to accommodate and correct any hyperopic error
c. reduced vertical fusion amplitude
d. spherical aberration

5.7. In bifocal lens design, image jump may be minimized by which step?

a. placing the optical center of the segment as close as possible to the top of the segment
b. placing the top of the segment as close as possible to the distance optical center
c. using a smaller bifocal segment
d. using a blended bifocal segment that has no visible line of separation
e. lowering the bifocal segment by 3 mm

5.8. An angle of 45° corresponds to how many prism diopters (Δ)?

a. 45Δ
b. 22Δ
c. 90Δ
d. 100Δ

5.9. Which statement applies to bifocal lenses that are prescribed for a patient with myopia?

a. The practitioner should leave the choice of the segment type to the optician.
b. A round-top segment is preferred because of its thin upper edge, which causes less prismatic effect.
c. A flat-top segment is preferred because it lessens image jump.
d. The 1-piece shape is indicated for adds greater than +2.00 D.
e. A split bifocal should be used because patients with myopia do not accept bifocal lenses easily.

5.10. An aphakic contact lens wearer (+13.00 soft contact lens in each eye) needs to switch to spectacles but finds that they experience diplopia at near. What prismatic correction would you expect to correct their diplopia?

a. base-up prism
b. base-in prism
c. oblique prism
d. base-out prism

5.11. A patient who has just been prescribed new progressive addition lenses returns with the concern that they need to tilt their chin up in order to see clearly at distance. What is the most likely source of the problem?
   a. add power that is too strong
   b. add power that is positioned too high
   c. undercorrected hyperopia or overcorrected myopia
   d. incorrect optical centers

5.12. Following cataract surgery in the left eye, the patient has a refraction of right, –3.50 D; left, –0.50 D. You prescribe this with a +2.50 flat-top bifocal set 3 mm below the optical center of the lens. How much induced prism will there be when the patient is looking 4 mm below the top of the bifocal?
   a. no induced prism
   b. 0.9Δ base down in the right eye
   c. 1.2Δ base down in the right eye
   d. 2.1Δ base down in the right eye

Answers

5.1. **b.** Figure 5-20 depicts a high-minus spectacle lens that effects minification of the image. Note the barrel-shaped distortion of the Amsler grid as viewed through the lens.

5.2. **b.** The far point of a +9.00 D lens is 111 mm (1/9 m) behind the lens. However, for the old lens to focus the image on the retina, it must be held by the frame 12 mm in front of the cornea. Thus, the far point of the patient's hyperopia is located 99 mm (111 mm – 12 mm) behind the cornea. If the new frame is to be located 22 mm in front of the cornea, it should be placed 121 mm (99 mm + 22 mm) in front of the far point of the patient's hyperopia. The power required for this new lens, therefore, is 1/0.121 m = +8.26 D. Because spectacle lenses come in 0.25 D steps, the answer is +8.25 D.

5.3. **c.** Figure 5-21 depicts an occupational multifocal lens known as a *double D.* This type of lens has the additive near power at the top and bottom of the spectacle lens; the distance power is in the middle. This design is especially useful for airline pilots, who must frequently look up at cockpit instrument panels that are in close proximity to one another and look down at printed flight material.

5.4. **b.** The Abbe number is a measure of chromatic aberration. The lower the Abbe number, the higher the amount of chromatic aberration present in the lens material. Spectacle lenses with a low Abbe number often require antireflective coating to minimize chromatic aberration that arises particularly when bright indoor light reflects off the lenses.

5.5. **b.** The far point of a –8.00 D lens is 125 mm (1/8 m) and is located in front of the lens. A patient's myopic refractive error is corrected with a –8.00 D trial lens when the lens is placed 10 mm in front of the cornea (Fig 5-22). If the lens is moved to 14 mm in front of the cornea with their existing frame, the far point remains the same distance from the original –8.00 D lens. The location of the

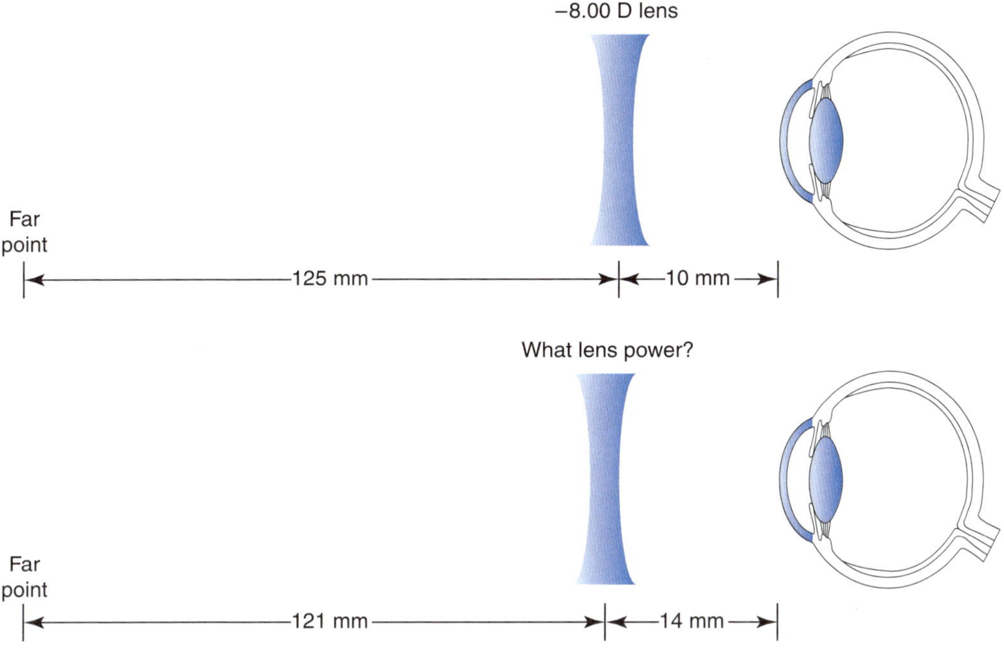

Figure 5-22 *(Illustration developed by Tommy Korn, MD.)*

existing frame from the far point is 135 mm – 14 mm = 121 mm. The power of the lens must then be 1/0.121 m = –8.26 D. Because spectacle lenses come in 0.25 D increments, the answer is –8.25 D.

5.6. **c.** When a patient has anisometropia, which may arise after cataract surgery, for example, a large vertical prismatic effect is induced in the bifocal add. When the patient suddenly looks through the top of the bifocal segment, image jump occurs because of vertical prismatic effects through the spectacle lenses. Image jump is a problem because the human brain has a very limited capacity to fuse 2 images that are separated vertically, as in the case of a bifocal lens with anisometropia.

5.7. **a.** As the eyes look down to read through the add segment, there is an abrupt upward image jump at the top edge of the segment. This jump is due to the prismatic effect of the plus lens (the add segment). On the basis of Prentice's rule, the amount of jump depends on the power of the segment and on the distance from the top of the segment to the optical center of the segment.

5.8. **d.** As a general rule, the number of prism diopters is approximately twice the angle in degrees. However, this equation works only for small angles (<20°). An angle of 45° means that at 1 m, a beam is deviated by 1 m (100 cm). Thus, 45° corresponds to 100Δ. An angle of 90° corresponds to infinity in prism diopters.

5.9. **c.** In general, patients perceive image jump as a greater problem than image displacement. Flat-top segments minimize image jump because the optical center is near the top. In patients with myopia, flat-top segments also reduce prism displacement because the base-down effect of the distance portion is reduced by the base-up effect of the segment.

5.10. **b**. Aphakic spectacles will generate base-out prism with convergence when compared to contact lens correction. Adjustment of the optical centers, addition of base-in prism, or single-vision reading glasses may improve this problem.

5.11 **c**. In the chin-up position, the patient is effectively adding plus power to the distance prescription by viewing through the upper portion of the add. The patient has either undercorrected hyperopia or overcorrected myopia.

5.12 **d**. The induced prism is a result of the anisometropia of the distance correction. The bifocal add is equal, and there should be no induced prism contribution from that. If the top of the bifocal is 3 mm below the optical center of the lens and the patient is looking 4 mm below that, then the distance for Prentice's rule is 7 mm and the power difference is 3.00 D—therefore, 2.1Δ with the induced prism base in the more myopic correction (right side).

CHAPTER 6

Contact Lenses

Highlights

- Contact lenses induce fewer aberrations and less magnification/minification than spectacles. This can be helpful for treating significant anisometropia.
- Compared with spectacle correction, contact lenses increase accommodative and convergence demands in myopes and decrease both demands in hyperopes.
- Rigid gas-permeable, hybrid, and scleral contact lenses are especially useful for treating irregular corneal astigmatism; however, spherical contact lenses do not correct lenticular astigmatism.
- In contact lens fitting, the SAM *(steeper add minus)* and FAP *(flatter add plus)* rules help determine the power for rigid gas-permeable lenses, and the LARS (*left add; right subtract)* rule is useful for adjusting the rotation of soft toric lenses.
- Contact lens–related problems can include infections, hypoxia, lens solution toxicity, mechanical issues, inflammation, and dry eye.

Glossary

Apical zone of the cornea, corneal apex The steepest part of the cornea, normally including its geometric center, usually 3–4 mm in diameter.

Base curve The curvature of the central posterior surface of the lens, which is adjacent to the cornea, described by its radius of curvature (mm). Base curves and peripheral curvatures of contact lenses are chosen to achieve a good fit of the lens to the cornea.

Diameter (chord diameter) The width of the contact lens, from edge to edge. The diameter of soft contact lenses, for example, ranges from 13 mm to 15 mm, whereas that of corneal rigid gas-permeable (RGP) lenses ranges from 9 mm to 10 mm and that of scleral RGP lenses, from 15 mm to 24 mm.

Optical zone The central area of the contact lens. The curvature of its anterior surface is designed to yield the desired refractive power of the lens.

Oxygen permeability The ability of a contact lens material to transmit oxygen by diffusion. It is an inherent property of the material.

Peripheral curves Secondary curves of the posterior lens surface away from the center, nearer the lens edge. These curves are flatter than the central posterior "base" curve to approximate the normal flattening of the peripheral cornea and achieve a desired fit. Junctions between central and more peripheral curvatures are smoothed (or "blended") or may be continuously graduated.

Sagittal depth or vault The distance between the center of the posterior surface to the plane of the edges of the lens. If the diameter of the lens is held constant, the sagittal depth decreases as the base curve radius increases.

Tear lens The lens formed by the tears that fill in the space between the posterior surface of the contact lens and the anterior surface of the cornea.

Wetting angle The wettability of a lens surface. A low wetting angle means that water will spread over the surface, increasing surface wettability, whereas a high wetting angle means that water will bead up, decreasing surface wettability. A lower wetting angle (greater wettability) generally translates into better lens comfort and vision.

Introduction

About 50% of adults in the United States use glasses or contact lenses. A quarter of those use contact lenses: 90% wear soft lenses, and 10% wear corneal rigid gas-permeable (RGP) lenses. There is increasing use of scleral RGP lenses. These preferences vary around the world; for example, about a third of the lenses fit in France and the Netherlands are RGP material.

Morgan PB, Woods CA, Tranoudis IG, et al. International contact lens prescribing in 2020. *Contact Lens Spectrum.* 2021;36(1):32–38.
Nichols JJ, Fisher D. Contact lenses 2020. *Contact Lens Spectrum.* 2021;36(1):24–29, 51.

Contact Lens Optics

When a contact lens is in place on the cornea, most of the refraction occurs at the interface between air and the tear film on the anterior surface of the contact lens. A corneal contact lens is located only 3 mm or so in front of the eye's first principal plane, where refraction may be considered to occur. The lens turns with the eye, so that compared to a spectacle lens 12 mm in front of a rotating eye, there is less aberrational blur, distortion, and magnification/minification. Spectacle lenses have different optical advantages: they offer stable vision and the possibility of adding more useful bifocals or applying prism when needed. Table 6-1 summarizes optical considerations of various types of contact lenses.

Anisometropia and Image Size

When one eye is much more myopic or hyperopic than the other, spectacle correction creates retinal images of unequal size, unless the difference is caused primarily by unequal axial lengths (Clinical Example 6-1). Also, as the eyes look off-axis, through parts of

Table 6-1 Optical Considerations of Contact Lenses

Type of Lens	Indications	Optical Characteristics
Soft spherical	Mild myopia or hyperopia with mild to moderate amount of regular astigmatism	May mask mild astigmatism.
Soft toric	Myopia, hyperopia, mild to moderate amount of regular astigmatism	Lens must maintain toric axis position through ballast, thin areas, or edge shape. May be used to correct corneal and lenticular astigmatism.
Soft bifocal alternating vision	Presbyopia, regular refractive errors	The lens is transposed upward on the cornea during downgaze by the action of the lower eyelid. The inferior periphery of the lens contains the near prescription.
Soft bifocal simultaneous vision	Presbyopia, regular refractive errors	Concentric rings or aspheric design give simultaneous focus of distant and near objects.
Corneal RGP spherical	Myopia, hyperopia, regular and irregular astigmatism	Corrects corneal but not lenticular astigmatism.
Corneal RGP posterior toric	Has a posterior toric surface to match the cornea; especially effective to treat against-the-rule astigmatism	The toric surface, which matches that of the cornea, helps position the lens.
Corneal RGP bitoric	Useful for higher amounts of astigmatism, has toric shape on both sides	The anterior toric shape can be used to correct whatever residual refractive error is not corrected by the posterior surface.
Corneal RGP bifocal alternating or simultaneous	May be used with regular and irregular corneas	Similar to soft bifocal lenses.
Hybrid	Keratoconus, postkeratoplasty; other irregular corneas	Combines the comfort and fitting properties of soft contact lenses with the ability of rigid lenses to correct irregular corneas.
Scleral RGP	Keratoconus, postkeratoplasty; other irregular corneas. Also useful in creating a therapeutic environment in ocular surface disease such as Stevens-Johnson syndrome and graft-vs-host disease	Can correct significant irregular corneal astigmatism.

RGP = rigid gas-permeable

the spectacle lenses farther from their optical centers, the eyes encounter unequal prism (Prentice's rule; see Chapter 5). This is particularly disturbing when one looks down through bifocal segments, as even a small amount of unequal vertical prism can cause discomfort or diplopia. To manage this, it may be necessary to "slab-off" prism on one of the bifocal segments (see Chapter 5).

Conversely, contact lenses of unequal powers yield retinal images that are of almost equal size, if the eyes are of similar axial length. The lenses move with the eyes, so there is little induced prismatic effect. Unilateral aphakia is an extreme example of anisometropia, with the aphakic eye usually much more hyperopic than its fellow eye. Typically, the aphakic spectacle lens creates a retinal image about 25% larger than it would be in an emmetropic eye of the same axial length, whereas a contact lens creates an image only about 7% larger. To understand this "relative spectacle magnification," imagine starting with emmetropic eyes: instead of removing the natural lens of one eye, neutralize the lens's power with a minus lens just in front of the natural lens, and place a correcting plus-powered spectacle lens 12 mm in front of the eye. These 2 lenses create a magnifying Galilean telescope effect, which enlarges the retinal image.

CLINICAL EXAMPLE 6-1

Fitting a unilateral aphakic eye causes diplopia that persists in the presence of prisms that superimpose the 2 images. The refractive error of the fellow eye is −5.00 D, and the image produced by the aphakic eye is described as larger than that produced by the fellow myopic eye. How can the diplopia be resolved?

The goal is to reduce the aniseikonia of the 2 eyes by magnifying the image size in the phakic eye and/or reducing the image size in the contact lens–corrected aphakic eye. To achieve the former, correct the myopic phakic eye with a contact lens to increase the size of the image on the retina. If this is inadequate, overcorrect the contact lens for the aphakic eye by +5.00 D and prescribe a spectacle lens of −5.25 D for that eye, in effect introducing a reverse Galilean telescope. If, however, the phakic eye were hyperopic, its retinal image would be increased in size by correcting the eye's refractive error with a spectacle lens rather than a contact lens.

Accommodation

When an eye is corrected for distance, how much accommodation is required to focus the image of a near object? Compared with spectacles, contact lenses increase the accommodative demand for myopic eyes and decrease it for hyperopic eyes in proportion to the size of the refractive error.

Clinical Example 6-2 and Figure 6-1 illustrate accommodative demand. For an emmetropic eye to read print that is one-third meter away, it needs to accommodate by 3 diopters. Suppose that the eye is myopic, instead of emmetropic, and has a −7.00 D spectacle lens 15 mm in front of it, which exactly corrects its myopia for distance viewing. Parallel rays passing through the lens have divergence of −6.30 D when they reach the cornea, and the eye effortlessly focuses those rays on the retina. A pencil of rays coming from an object one-third meter in front of that eye has about −3.00 D divergence when it reaches the −7.00 D lens, and therefore −10.00 D leaving the lens. After traversing the 15 mm from the lens to the cornea, it has −8.70 D divergence. In order to focus the pencil on the retina, which requires the pencil to have −6.30 D divergence at the cornea, the required accommodation is the difference, which is 2.40 D. This is the "near effectivity" of the myopic spectacles, which reduces accommodative demand, in this case, from 3.00 D to 2.40 D. If we correct the same eye with a contact lens, a –6.30 D contact lens is required to replace the –7.00 D spectacle lens for distance viewing, and the full 3.00 D of accommodation is required to read the print at one-third meter. Thus, contact lenses eliminate the *accommodative advantage* enjoyed by those with spectacle-corrected myopia and the *disadvantage* experienced by those with spectacle-corrected hyperopia. A 42-year-old person with myopia who is getting along well enough with –5.00 D glasses may find reading with contact lenses difficult, even though both the glasses and contacts are correct for distance. Conversely, a 38-year-old person with hyperopia, beginning to have symptoms of presbyopia with glasses, will have easier near vision with contact lenses fitted to correct distance vision than they will with the glasses.

CLINICAL EXAMPLE 6-2

What is the accommodative demand of a –7.00 D myopic eye corrected with a spectacle lens compared with a contact lens? What is it for a +7.00 D hyperopic eye? Assume a vertex distance of 15 mm and a near-object distance of 33.3 cm.

The myopic refractive error of the first eye is –7.00 D at a vertex distance of 15 mm, and the object distance is 33.3 cm. The vergence of rays originating at infinity and exiting the spectacle lens is –7.00 D. Due to the vertex distance, the vergence of these rays at the front surface of the cornea (which is approximately the location of the first principal point) is –6.30 D. Use the focal point of the –7.00 D spectacle lens, 1/7 = 0.143 m, plus the vertex distance of 0.015 m (0.158 m) to find the vergence at the corneal surface: 1/0.158 m = –6.33 D (rounded to 6.30 in Fig 6-1A).

The vergence of rays originating at 33.3 cm after exiting the spectacle lens is –10.00 D (see Fig 6-1B). The vergence is calculated by using the vergence of the light after it leaves the spectacle lens: –3 + (–7) = –10. Due to the vertex distance, the vergence of these rays at the front surface of the cornea (which is approximately the location of the first principal point) is –8.70 D. Use the focal point of the rays after the light travels through the lens, –10.00 D, 1/10 = 0.1 m, plus the vertex distance of 0.015 m (0.115 m) to find the vergence at the corneal surface: 1/0.115 m = –8.70 D).

Accommodative demand is the difference between the vergence at the first principal point between rays originating at infinity and the vergence of rays originating at 33.3 cm. In this case, the accommodation is 2.40 D: –6.3 – (–8.7) = 2.4. In contrast, the accommodation required with contact lens correction is approximately 3.00 D (see Fig 6-1C, D). Therefore, this myopic eye would need 0.60 D more accommodation to focus an object at 33.3 cm with a contact lens than with a spectacle lens. Similarly, the accommodative demand of an eye corrected with a +7.00 D spectacle lens would be 3.50 D, compared with approximately 3.00 D for a contact lens (Table 6-2).

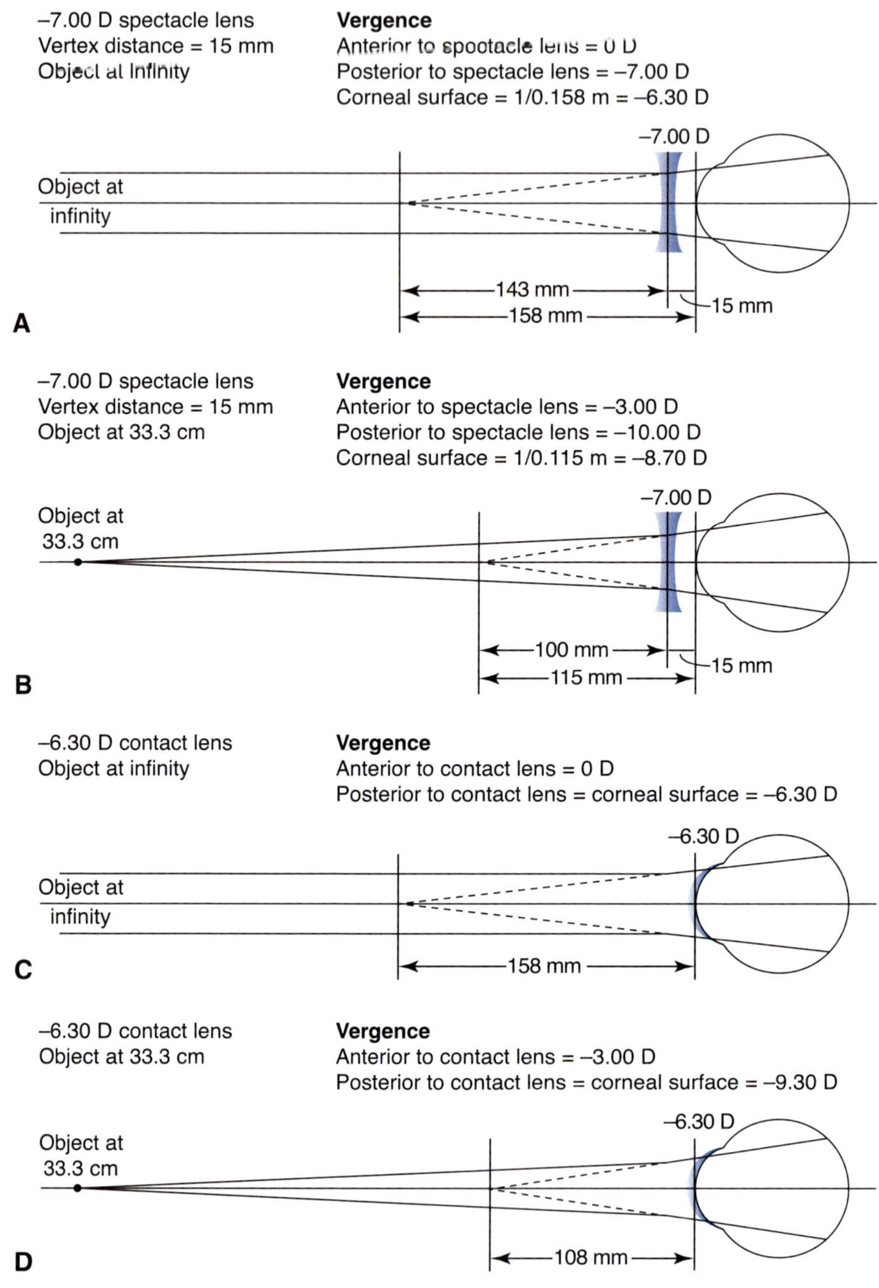

Figure 6-1 Accommodative demand. (Diopter measurements have been rounded to the nearest tenth.) **A,** Effective spectacle lens power at the corneal surface. **B,** Accommodative demand with a –7.00 D spectacle lens. **C,** Correction with a –6.30 D contact lens. **D,** Accommodative demand with a –6.30 D contact lens. *(Illustrations developed by Thomas F. Mauger, MD.)*

Table 6-2 Accommodative Demand Through Spectacles and Contact Lenses

	−7.00 D Spectacle Lens		−6.30 D Contact Lens[a]	
Object at:	Infinity	33.3 cm	Infinity	33.3 cm
Vergence (D) at anterior spectacle lens surface	0	−3.00		
Power of lens	−7.00	−7.00	−6.30	−6.30
Vergence at posterior spectacle lens surface	−7.00	−10.00		
Vergence at corneal surface with 15 mm vertex distance	−6.30	−8.70	−6.30	−9.30
Accommodative demand	−6.30 − (−8.70) = **2.40 D**		−6.30 − (−9.30) = **3.00 D**	
	+7.00 D Spectacle Lens		**+7.80 D Contact Lens[b]**	
Vergence (D) at anterior spectacle lens surface	0	−3.00		
Power of lens	+7.00	+7.00	+7.80	+7.80
Vergence at posterior spectacle lens surface	+7.00	+4.00		
Vergence at corneal surface with 15-mm vertex distance	+7.80	+4.30	+7.80	+4.80
Accommodative demand	+7.80 − (+4.30) = **3.50 D**		+7.80 − (+4.80) = **3.00 D**	

D = diopter; diopter measurements are rounded to the nearest tenth.
[a] The equivalent power at the cornea of a −7.00 D spectacle lens with a vertex distance of 15 mm is −6.30 D.
[b] The equivalent power at the cornea of a +7.00 D spectacle lens with a vertex distance of 15 mm is +7.80 D.

Depending on their power, spectacle lenses (whose optical centers are positioned for distance viewing) and contact lenses require different amounts of convergence to achieve fusion when one looks at a near object. Contact lenses turn with the eyes; therefore, no prism is encountered when one looks through the contact lenses when the eyes converge. Myopic spectacle lenses induce *base-in prisms* for near objects, following Prentice's rule, so that the eyes do not have to turn in as much to look at the near object. Hyperopic spectacles increase the convergence needed for fusion by inducing *base-out prisms.*

In summary, correction of myopia with contact lenses, as opposed to spectacle lenses, increases both accommodative and convergence demands of focusing and fusion for near objects, proportional to the size of the refractive error, and decreases both demands in hyperopia (Fig 6-2). These effects may be welcome, unwelcome, or of no consequence, depending on the patient's muscle balance and ability to accommodate.

Correcting Astigmatism

Rigid lenses with a spherical rear surface form a *tear lens* in the space between the lens and the cornea (see the discussion of corneal rigid gas-permeable contact lenses in the section Contact Lens Fitting later in this chapter). When rigid (and toric soft) contact

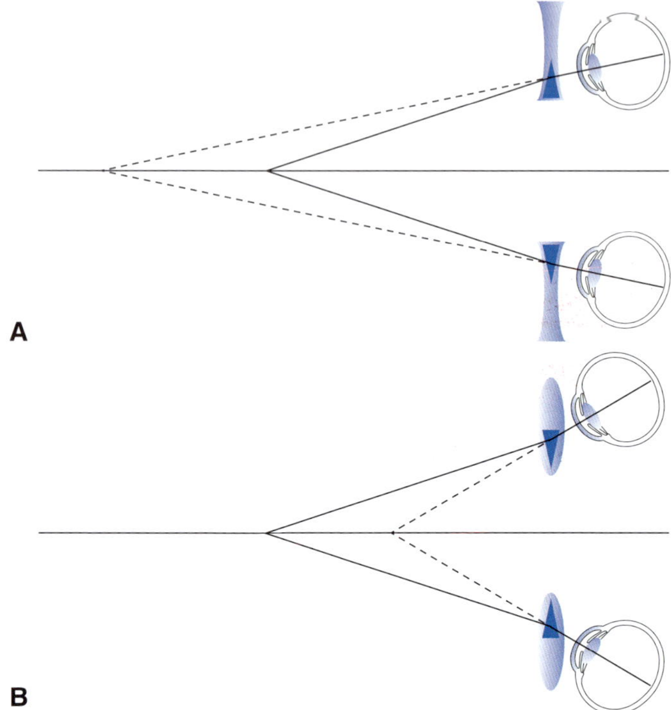

Figure 6-2 Effect of spectacle lenses on convergence demands. **A,** Lenses for correction of myopia create induced base-in prism, which decreases the convergence demand. **B,** Lenses for correction of hyperopia create induced base-out prism, which increases the convergence demand. *(Illustrations developed by Thomas F. Mauger, MD.)*

lenses neutralize astigmatism at the corneal surface, the meridional aniseikonia created with toric-surface spectacle lenses is avoided. For this reason, people whose astigmatism has been corrected with contact lenses often experience an annoying change in spatial orientation when they switch to spectacles. However, refractive astigmatism is the sum of *corneal* and *lenticular astigmatism.* Lenticular astigmatism, if present, is not corrected by spherical contact lenses, so it persists as "residual" astigmatism when the corneal astigmatism component is neutralized by spherical rigid contact lenses. This finding is more common among older patients and often explains why their hard contact lenses fail to provide full correction. These cases can be identified by refracting the patient while their contact lenses are in place. If it happens that the eye has lenticular astigmatism against the rule and a similar amount of corneal astigmatism with the rule, a soft contact lens may be used so that the astigmatism of the cornea and of the lens continue to compensate for each other.

For example, consider a patient whose refraction is –3.50 –0.50 × 180 and whose keratometry measurements of the affected eye are 42.50 D (7.94 mm) horizontal and 44.00 D (7.67 mm) vertical. Would a soft or rigid contact lens provide better vision (ie, less residual astigmatism)? The disparity between the corneal astigmatism of 1.50 D and the refractive astigmatism of 0.50 D reveals 1.00 D of against-the-rule lenticular astigmatism that neutralizes a similar amount of with-the-rule corneal astigmatism. Neutralizing the corneal component of the refractive astigmatism with a rigid contact lens exposes the 1.00 D of lenticular residual astigmatism. Therefore, a spherical soft contact lens would, in this case, provide better vision than a spherical RGP lens.

Contact Lens Materials

What would we ask of a material used to make a contact lens? The material would fit a variety of corneal shapes, be durable, easy to handle, comfortable, and transparent. Its surface would be "wettable" and stay wet between blinks, but we would not want deposits to stick to it, or for *Pseudomonas* to find it a congenial home. We would want the lens to transmit oxygen and carbon dioxide and flush new tears under it with each blink to maintain corneal metabolism. We would not want the lens to contribute to dry eye problems by soaking up water from the cornea.

Dk, Dk/t, and *wetting angle* are some terms used to describe oxygen permeability and wettability: *Dk* refers to the oxygen permeability of a *lens material,* where *D* is the diffusion coefficient for oxygen movement in the material, and *k* is the solubility constant of oxygen in the material. *Dk/t* refers to the oxygen transmissibility of a *lens,* depending on its material and central thickness *(t). Wetting angle* refers to the wettability of a lens surface (Fig 6-3). With a low wetting angle, water will spread over the surface, increasing surface wettability. Both a high Dk/t and a low wetting angle are desirable.

"Hard" contact lenses were introduced in the 1940s and were originally made of *polymethylmethacrylate (PMMA),* the same plastic used subsequently for the first intraocular lenses. These lenses were very durable, but oxygen passed only around them (via tear exchange), not through them.

Soft contact lenses are made of a hydrogel polymer, *hydroxyethylmethacrylate,* or, more often now, a silicone hydrogel. Hydrogels have more oxygen permeability when they have higher water content, but the lenses with higher water content tend to cause dryness of the cornea if they are particularly thin, and they may form deposits and require frequent

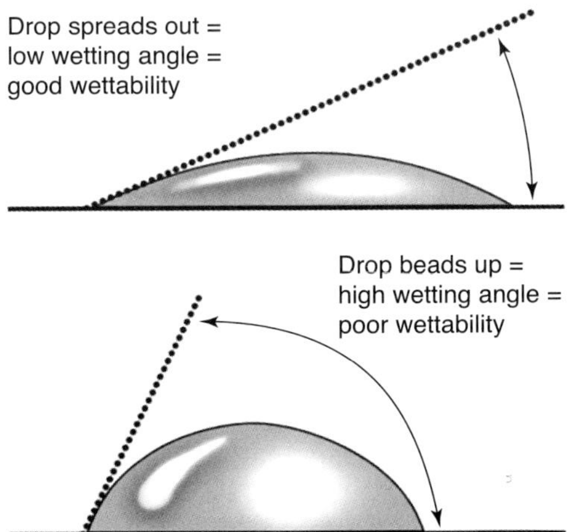

Figure 6-3 The wettability of a lens surface determines whether a wetting angle will be low (greater wettability, greater comfort) or high (less wettability, less comfort). *(Modified with permission from Stein HA, Freeman MI, Stein RM.* CLAO Residents Contact Lens Curriculum Manual. *Contact Lens Association of Ophthalmologists; 1996. Redrawn by Christine Gralapp.)*

replacement. Modifying the hydrogels yielded "silicone hydrogels," which are used for daily and extended wear. These lenses achieve their oxygen permeability with less water content; they use pores induced by the presence of silicon atoms, rather than high water content. Some patients are more comfortable with the hydrogels than the silicone hydrogels. Available lenses differ in chemistry throughout the lens or at its surfaces with differing wettability, flexibility, clarity, resistance to deposit retention, and suitability for those with dry eye. They also differ in their longevity and should be replaced at recommended intervals.

Corneal RGP lenses were developed in the latter 20th century; these use the architecture of large-polymer plastics to allow passage of oxygen. RGP lenses allow oxygen to pass through and allow more tear exchange around the lens with each blink than soft lenses allow, so that oxygen-depleted tears are not trapped between the lens and the cornea. The addition of fluorine to the silicone/acrylate material increases oxygen permeability and encourages the coating of the lens with mucin, which improves wettability. Corneal RGP lenses can employ various other chemical makeups for different advantages.

Table 6-3 summarizes the comparative advantages of soft and corneal RGP contact lenses.

Table 6-3 Comparative Advantages of Soft and Corneal Rigid Gas-Permeable Contact Lenses

Soft Contact Lenses	Corneal RGP Contact Lenses
Shorter adaptation period	Clear vision
More comfortable for occasional wear than RGP lenses	Correction of regular and irregular corneal astigmatism
Variety of lens types (eg, disposable lenses, lenses replaced frequently)	Ease of handling
Ability to change eye color	Stability and durability
Easier to fit, inexpensive to replace	Ease of care

Patient History and Examination

Factors that increase the risk of complications with contact lens use include diabetes mellitus, especially if it is poorly controlled; immunosuppression; long-term use of topical ocular medications, such as corticosteroids; and occupational chemical or foreign-body exposure. Other relative contraindications to contact lens use include an inability or history of failure to care for contact lenses, monocularity, abnormal eyelid function such as Bell palsy, severe dry eye, and corneal neovascularization.

The eyes and adnexa are examined for abnormalities of eyelid and eyelash position, the tear film, and the ocular surface. Eyelid movement should be observed. The cornea and conjunctiva should be evaluated carefully for signs of allergy, scarring, symblepharon, or other indications of conjunctival scarring diseases, such as ocular cicatricial pemphigoid and giant papillary conjunctivitis or abnormal vascularization resulting from previous lens wear. Through refraction and keratometry, the ophthalmologist can determine whether there is significant corneal, lenticular, or irregular astigmatism. The identification of irregular astigmatism may suggest other pathologies, such as keratoconus.

Contact Lens Selection

The main advantages of soft contact lenses are their comfort and shorter period of adaptation (see Table 6-3). They are available in a wide range of shapes and materials and are usually easier to fit than rigid lenses. A lost or damaged lens is readily replaced without much cost.

Soft lenses are generally designed for daily replacement or replacement every 1, 2, or 4 weeks. Very few soft lenses dispensed now are intended for replacement cycles longer than 1 month.

Daily wear lenses have been favored in the United States ever since reports in the 1980s showed increased incidence of keratitis with extended-wear lenses. Improved materials that have greater oxygen permeability ($Dk = 60–140$) have been approved for extended wear but should be used with caution. Use of these materials may decrease the risk of infection compared with the risk associated with earlier materials, but patients who want extended-wear lenses should understand the increased risk of bacterial keratitis and the signs and symptoms that require the attention of a physician. Additional risk factors for complications with extended-wear lenses include previous eye infections, lens use while swimming, exposure to smoke, dry eye, eyelid margin disease, and allergy. Daily wear users are exposed to the same risks, only less so.

About 10% of contact lenses fitted in the United States are corneal RGP lenses. Some with high oxygen permeability are approved for extended wear. They are typically replaced yearly. The main advantages of RGP lenses are the high quality of vision they offer, including the correction of corneal astigmatism, durability, and simplicity of lens care (See Table 6-3). The main disadvantages of RGP contact lenses are initial discomfort, longer periods of adaptation, greater knowledge and effort required for fitting, and the greater cost of replacing lost or damaged lenses. People who use contact lenses only sporadically are generally more comfortable with a soft lens.

Contact Lens Fitting

The goals of lens fitting are good vision that does not fluctuate with blinking or eye movement, comfort for the entire day, and low risk of complications. Terms used to describe lens geometry, illustrated in Figure 6-4, include the following: The *base curve* is the curvature of the central posterior surface of the lens, which is adjacent to the cornea, described by its radius of curvature. The *diameter (chord diameter)* is the width of the contact lens from edge to edge. The *optical zone* is the central area of the lens; curvature of its front surface is chosen to achieve the desired power of the lens. *Peripheral* or *secondary curves* of the posterior lens surface farther from its center are designed to follow the shape of the cornea, which is normally flatter toward its periphery. *Sagittal depth,* or *vault,* is the distance between the center of the posterior surface to the plane of the edges of the lens.

Contact lenses are described by their rear vertex power, which can be checked for rigid lenses by placing the back of the lens on the nose cone of a lensmeter (this is done less frequently for soft lenses and typically requires placing the lens in a liquid chamber and correcting for the index of refraction). The contact lens power differs from the corresponding spectacle power due to the difference in the position of the correcting lens. This disparity is known as the correction for the effectivity of lenses and is discussed in Chapter 1. The magnitude of the correction depends on the strength of the lenses and can be readily obtained from standard tables (Table 6-4).

Soft Contact Lenses

Soft contact lenses are comfortable, thanks to the thin edges encountered by the eyelids. The lenses extend beyond the cornea to the conjunctiva overlying the sclera. A good soft contact lens fit is often described as having a "light 3-point touch": the lens touching the

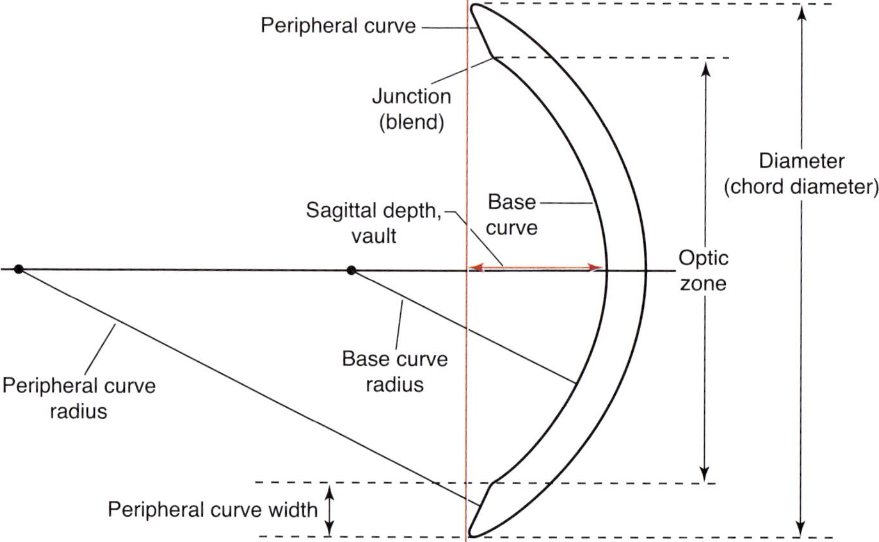

Figure 6-4 Contact lens. Note the relationship among the parts. *(Modified with permission from Stein HA, Freeman MI, Stein RM.* CLAO Residents Contact Lens Curriculum Manual. *Contact Lens Association of Ophthalmologists; 1996. Redrawn by Christine Gralapp.)*

Table 6-4 "Vertexing" Chart for Converting From Spectacle Prescription to Expected Contact Lens Prescription

Spectacle Lens Power[a]	Contact Lens Power
−5.00 D	−4.75 D
−6.00 D	−5.50 D
−8.00 D	−7.25 D
−10.00 D	−9.00 D
−14.00 D	−12.00 D
+5.00 D	+5.25 D
+6.00 D	+6.50 D
+8.00 D	+9.00 D
+10.00 D	+11.25 D
+14.00 D	+17.00 D

[a] Rear vertex at 12 mm

surface of the eye at the corneal apex and at the limbus on either side of the cornea. A soft or rigid lens can be made to fit tighter either by choosing a smaller radius to steepen the base curve or by increasing the lens chord diameter without changing the radius. Either way, the sagittal depth, the height of the lens's rear surface, is increased (Table 6-5 and Fig 6-5).

When evaluating the soft lens fit, the clinician should observe the lens movement and centration after the lens has been in the eye for a while, until the fit has stabilized. In a good fit, the lens will move about 1 mm with upward gaze or blink, or with gentle pressure on the lower eyelid. A tight lens resists movement, and a loose lens will move too much. By evaluating a patient's vision and comfort, slit-lamp findings (eg, lens movement, lens edge, limbal injection), and keratometry mires, the clinician can determine whether the lens fits well (see Table 6-5). Once a fit is deemed adequate, an overrefraction is performed to check whether the power needs to be adjusted.

When the initial fitting process is complete, the final lens parameters should be clearly identified (Table 6-6). The clinician should teach the patient how to insert and remove the contact lenses, how to care for them, and how to recognize the signs and symptoms of eye emergencies. Follow-up appointments are scheduled depending on the lens and patient.

Table 6-5 Basic Soft Contact Lens Fitting

Initial Lens Selection	
Parameter	**Description**
Diameter	Approximately 2 mm larger than the horizontal corneal diameter
Base curve	0.2–0.6 mm greater (flatter) than the radius of the flattest *K* reading
Power	Close to the patient's refraction corrected for the vertex distance; refined after fit is achieved
Evaluating Soft Contact Lens Fit	
Loose Fit	**Tight Fit**
Excessive movement	No lens movement
Poor centration; lens easily dislocates off the cornea	Centered lens
Lens-edge standoff	"Digging in" of lens edge
Blurred mires after a blink	Clear mires with blink
Fluctuating vision	Good vision initially
Continuing awareness of lens	Initial comfort, but increasing awareness of lens with continued use
Air bubbles under the lens	Limbal–scleral injection at lens edge
Adjusting Soft Contact Lens Fit	
Create a Looser Fit	**Create a Tighter Fit**
Decrease the sagittal depth	Increase the sagittal depth
Choose a flatter base curve (increase the radius of curvature)	Choose a steeper base curve (decrease the radius of curvature)
Choose a smaller diameter	Choose a larger diameter

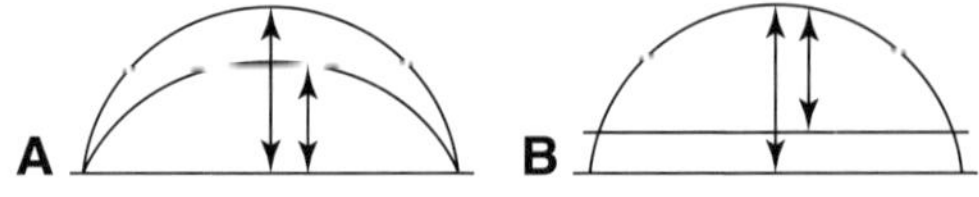

Figure 6-5 Changing the sagittal depth. **A,** Changing the base curve of a contact lens changes the sagittal depth. **B,** Changing the diameter with equal base curve also changes sagittal depth.

Table 6-6 Soft Contact Lens Parameters

Parameter	Common Abbreviation (in the United States)	Typical Range of Values
Overall diameter	OAD	12.5–16.0 mm, extended ranges available for therapeutic purposes
Base curve	BC	8.0–9.5 mm
Center thickness	CT	0.04–0.20 mm (varies with the power of the lens and is set by the manufacturer)
Prescription	RX	Sphere and astigmatism, if any, in diopters
Manufacturer	Varies	Company name and lens style

Corneal Rigid Gas-Permeable Contact Lenses

Corneal rigid gas-permeable lenses have smaller chord diameters than soft lenses and allow more circulation of fresh tears under the lenses with each blink. Central and peripheral curves, edge shape, and central thickness can be tailored for stable vision, comfort, and tear exchange. These lenses are often simply referred as "RGP lenses," not to be confused with scleral RGP lenses, which are frequently referred to simply as "scleral lenses."

Unlike a soft contact lens, an RGP lens maintains its shape when placed on the cornea, and a tear lens fills the space between the lens and the cornea. The power of the tear lens is determined by the difference between the curvature of the cornea *(K)* and that of the base curve of the contact lens (Fig 6-6). The fit is described as *apical alignment (on K)* when the base curve matches that of the cornea; *apical clearance (steeper than K)* when the base curve has a steeper fit, with a radius shorter than that of the cornea; and *apical bearing (flatter than K)* when the base curve is flatter than the cornea.

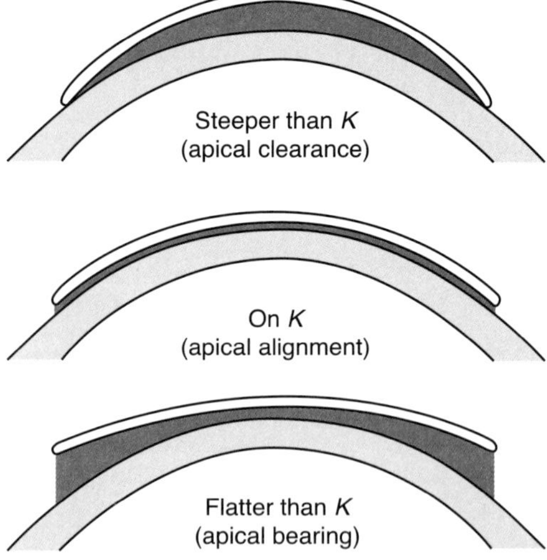

Figure 6-6 A rigid contact lens creates a tear (or fluid) lens whose power is determined by the difference between the curvature of the cornea *(K)* and that of the base curve of the contact lens. *(Courtesy of Perry Rosenthal, MD. Redrawn by Christine Gralapp.)*

To fit an RGP lens of a particular design and material, one can consult the laboratory fashioning the lens or a fitting guide for the lens, or use trial lenses. In designing the lens, consideration is given to pupil size and eyelid tension, as well as refractive error, keratometry, and possibly topography.

The most common type of RGP lens fit is an *apical alignment fit,* in which the upper edge of the lens rests under the upper eyelid (Fig 6-7). This "lid attachment" fit allows the lens to move with each blink, enhances tear exchange, and decreases lens sensation because the upper eyelid does not strike the lens edge with each blink.

Alternatively, a *central* or *interpalpebral fit* is achieved when the lens rests between the upper and lower eyelids. The diameter of the lens is smaller than with a lid-attachment fit. There may be greater lens sensation, because the eyelid strikes the lens edge with each blink. This type of fit may be preferable for patients who have hyperopia, high upper eyelids, or tight eyelids such as in some individuals of Asian descent.

To evaluate the fit of a contact lens, the clinician looks for stability of vision and appropriate lens movement. The fluorescein pattern is evaluated at the slit lamp (Fig 6-8). If there is apical clearing of the cornea, pooling or a bright green area will be observed centrally; if the RGP lens is touching the cornea, this area will appear dark. When the fit is satisfactory, overrefraction determines whether a power change is needed. Table 6-7 summarizes RGP lens parameters and the range of normal values.

Bennett ES, Henry VA. *Clinical Manual of Contact Lenses.* 4th ed. Lippincott Williams & Wilkins; 2014:133.

Tear lens power

The total power of an RGP lens includes the power of the lens itself (which can be measured with a lensmeter) *and* the power of the tear lens created by the space between the posterior surface of the lens and the anterior surface of the cornea. The power of the tear lens is approximately 0.25 D for every 0.05 mm of difference in the radius of curvature between the base curve of the contact lens and the central curvature of the cornea *(K),* and this power becomes somewhat greater for corneas steeper than 7.00 mm. Tear lenses created by rigid contact lenses with base curves that are steeper than *K* (smaller radius of curvature) have plus power, whereas tear lenses formed by base curves that are flatter than *K* (larger radius of curvature) have minus power (Figs 6-9, 6-10). Therefore, the

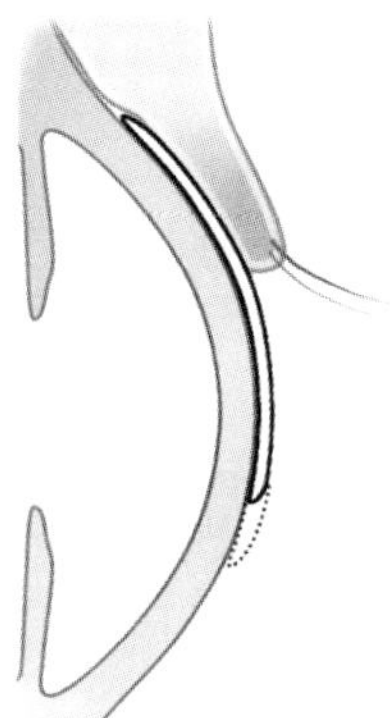

Figure 6-7 The most common and most comfortable type of rigid gas-permeable lens fit is apical alignment, in which the upper edge of the lens fits under the upper eyelid. *(Modified with permission from Albert DM, Jakobiec FA, eds.* Principles and Practice of Ophthalmology. *Saunders; 1994;5:3630. Redrawn by Christine Gralapp.)*

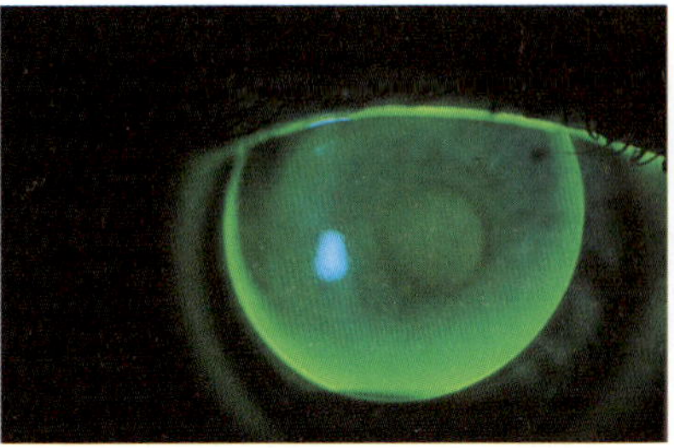

Fluorescein pattern of a good fit with minimal apical clearance

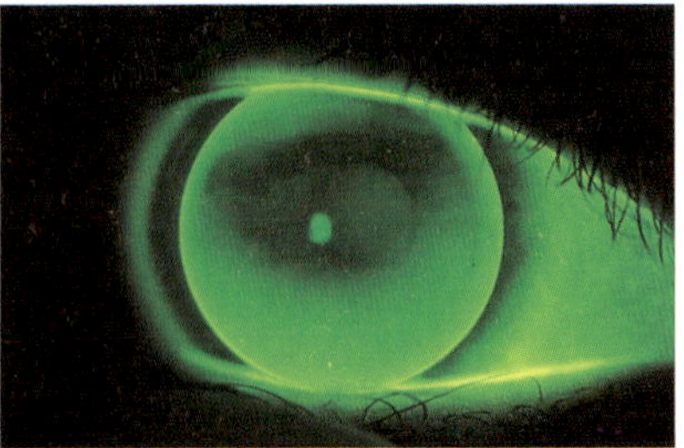

Fluorescein pattern demonstrating a flat fit

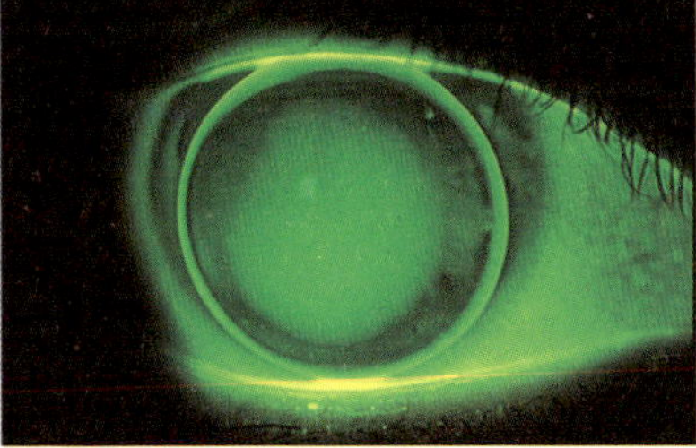

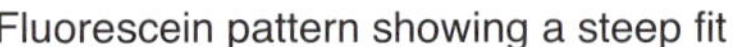

Fluorescein pattern showing a steep fit

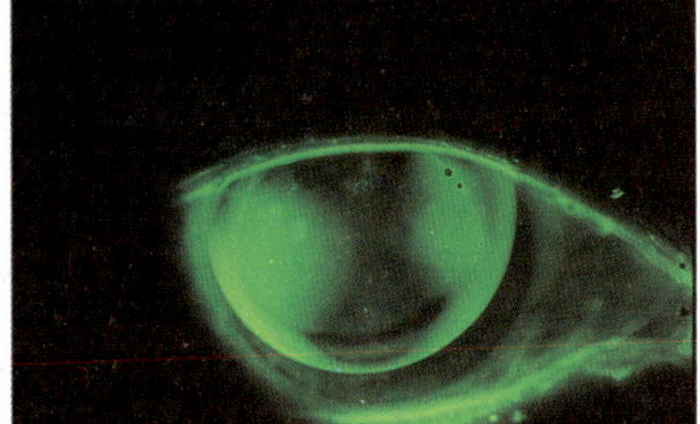

Against-the-rule astigmatic band

Figure 6-8 Examples of fluorescein patterns in contact lens fitting. *(Courtesy of Perry Rosenthal, MD.)*

Table 6-7 Corneal Rigid Gas-Permeable Lens Parameters

Parameter	Common Abbreviation (in the United States)	Range of Normal Values
Overall diameter	OAD	8.0–11.5 mm
Optic zone diameter	OZD	7.0–8.5 mm
Peripheral curve width	PCW	0.1–1.0 mm
Base curve	BC	7.0–8.5 mm
Center thickness	CT	0.08–0.30 mm
Prescription	RX	Any power required

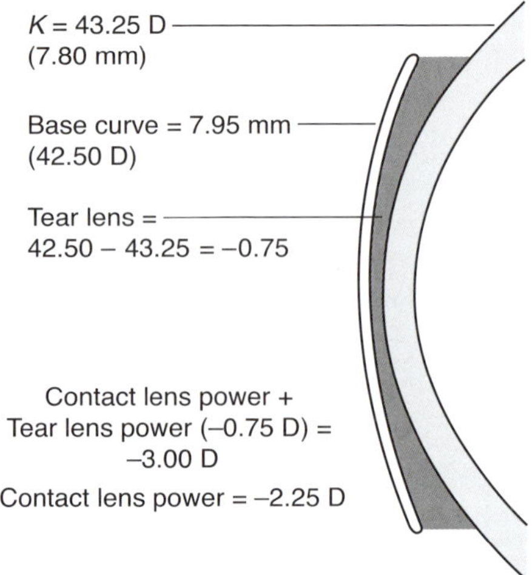

Figure 6-9 Determining the power of a contact lens using the FAP *(flatter add plus)* rule. See Clinical Example 6-3. *(Illustration developed by Thomas F. Mauger, MD.)*

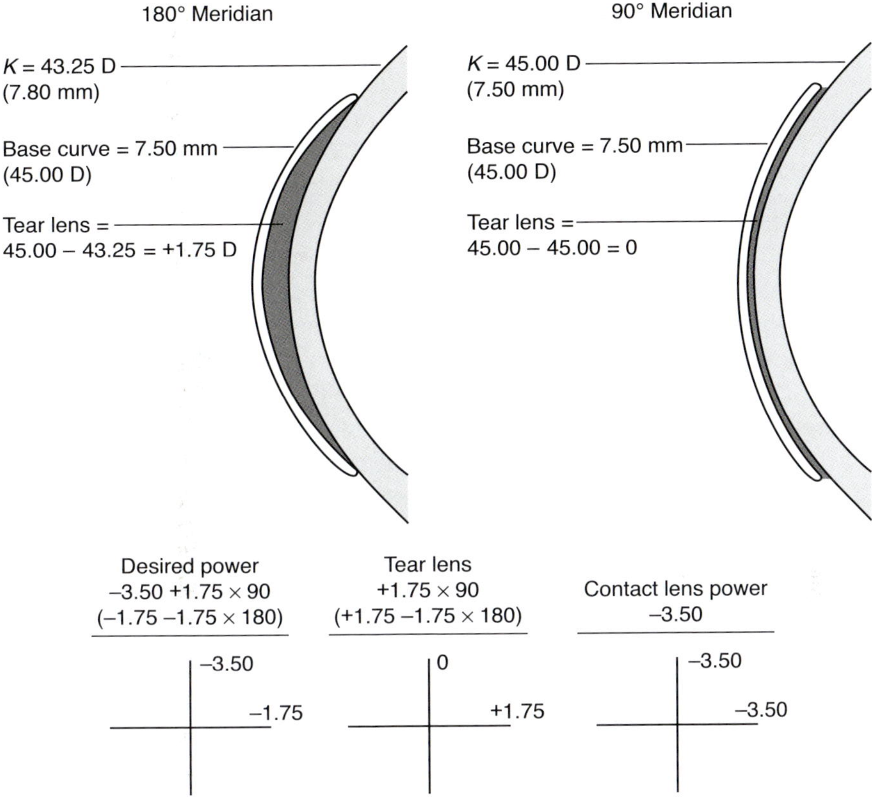

Figure 6-10 Determining the power of a contact lens using the SAM *(steeper add minus)* rule. See Clinical Example 6-4. *(Illustration developed by Thomas F. Mauger, MD.)*

power of a rigid contact lens must account for both the eye's refractive error and the power introduced by the tear lens. An easy way of remembering this is to use the rules "SAM" *(steeper add minus)* and "FAP" *(flatter add plus)*. Clinical Example 6-3 illustrates these calculations.

CLINICAL EXAMPLE 6-3

The refractive error of an eye is –3.00 D, the K *measurement is 7.80 mm (43.25 D), and the base curve chosen for the rigid contact lens is 7.95 mm (42.50 D). What is the anticipated power of the contact lens?*

The power of the resulting tear lens is –0.75 D. This power would correct –0.75 D of the refractive error. Therefore, the remaining refractive error that the contact lens is required to correct is –2.25 D (recall the FAP rule: *flatter add plus*). Conversely, if the refractive error were +3.00 D (hyperopia), then the necessary contact lens power would be +3.75 D to correct the refractive error and the –0.75 D tear lens (see Fig 6-9).

Because the refractive index of the tear lens (1.336) is almost identical to that of a cornea (1.3765), it masks the optical effect of the corneal surface. If the back surface of a contact lens is spherical, then the anterior surface of the tear lens is also spherical, regardless of the corneal topography. Thus, the tear layer created by a spherical rigid contact lens neutralizes more than 90% of regular and irregular corneal astigmatism. This principle simplifies the calculation of the tear lens power on astigmatic corneas: the powers of the steeper corneal meridians can be ignored, and only the flattest meridians need to be considered. The refractive error along the flattest meridian is represented by the spherical component of refractive errors expressed in *minus cylinder form.* For this reason, it is simpler to use the minus cylinder format when dealing with rigid contact lenses (Clinical Example 6-4). When a spherical contact lens is in place, there may still be residual astigmatism, which may be caused by the eye's natural lens and the shape of the posterior surface of the cornea. There are back-surface toric gas-permeable lenses with toric back surfaces, chosen to match the shape of the cornea; these stabilize the lens position and have spherical front surfaces. There are also bitoric RGP lenses, whose back surfaces match that of the cornea, while the toric front surfaces correct the residual refractive error (Clinical Example 6-5).

CLINICAL EXAMPLE 6-4

The refractive correction is −3.50 +1.75 × 90, and the K *measurements along the 2 principal meridians are 7.80 mm horizontal (43.25 D at 180°) and 7.50 mm vertical (45.00 D at 90°). The rigid contact lens base curve is 7.50 mm. What is the anticipated power of the contact lens?*

The refractive correction along the flattest corneal meridian (7.80 mm) is −1.75 D (convert the refractive error to minus cylinder form), and the lens has been fitted steeper than flat *K,* creating a tear lens of +1.75 D. Thus, a corresponding amount of minus power must be added (recall the SAM rule: *steeper add minus*), giving a corrective power of −3.50 D in that meridian.

The refractive correction along the steepest meridian (7.50 mm) is −3.50 D. The lens is fitted "on *K*"; therefore, no tear lens power is created. The corrective power for this meridian is also −3.50 D.

Accordingly, the power of the contact lens should be −3.50 D (see Fig 6-10).

CLINICAL EXAMPLE 6-5

A patient with a refraction of −2.00 −2.00 × 180 desires contact lens correction. The keratometry measurement is 44.00 sphere. What is the residual refractive error if this eye is fitted with a spherical RGP contact lens? A spherical soft contact lens? A toric soft contact lens?

This eye has lenticular but not corneal astigmatism. Correction with spherical soft or rigid contact lenses will result in residual astigmatism. A soft toric contact lens may be used to correct the lenticular astigmatism.

Toric Soft Contact Lenses

Perhaps one-third of contact lens wearers have at least 1.00 D of astigmatism. Up to 0.75 or 1.00 D of astigmatism will likely be masked by a spherical soft contact lens enough to offer best acuity (Table 6-8). Greater degrees of astigmatism will usually not be well corrected by spherical soft contact lenses.

Soft toric contact lenses are available in several designs. To prevent lens rotation, various techniques are used:

- adding prism ballast, that is, placing extra lens material on the bottom edge of the lens, whose weight aligns the lens
- creating thin zones, that is, making lenses with a thin zone on the top and bottom, so that eyelid pressure tends to keep the lens in the appropriate position
- truncating or removing the bottom of the lens to form a straight edge that aligns with the lower eyelid; this technique is not as commonly used

Fitting soft toric lenses is similar to fitting other soft lenses, except that lens rotation must also be evaluated. Toric lenses typically have a mark to note their 6-o'clock position. If a slit-lamp examination shows that the lens mark is consistently rotated to one side of the 6-o'clock axis, the amount of rotation should be noted, in degrees (1 clock-hour equals 30°). To adjust the prescription for lens rotation, follow the LARS rule *(left add; right subtract).* This is illustrated in Clinical Example 6-6 and Figure 6-11.

> **CLINICAL EXAMPLE 6-6**
>
> *An eye with a refraction of −3.00 −1.00 × 180 is fitted with a toric contact lens with an astigmatic axis given as 180°. Slit-lamp examination shows that the lens is well centered, but lens markings show that the 6-o'clock mark is located at the 7-o'clock position. What axis should be ordered for this eye?*
>
> Because the trial contact lens rotated 1 clock-hour, or 30°, to the left, the contact lens ordered (recall the LARS rule: *left add; right subtract*) should be 180° + 30° = 210°, which is the same as 30°, so the lens to order is −3.00 −1.00 × 30°.

Contact Lenses for Presbyopia

Presbyopia affects virtually everyone older than 40 years. Thus, as contact lens wearers age, their accommodation needs must be considered. Three options are available for these

Table 6-8 Astigmatism and Lens Fitting

Degree of Astigmatism	First Choice of Lens
Less than 1.00 D	Spherical soft or RGP lens
1.00–2.00 D	Toric soft contact or spherical RGP lens
2.00–3.00 D	Custom soft toric or spherical RGP lens
More than 3.00 D	Toric RGP or custom soft toric lens

RGP = rigid gas-permeable

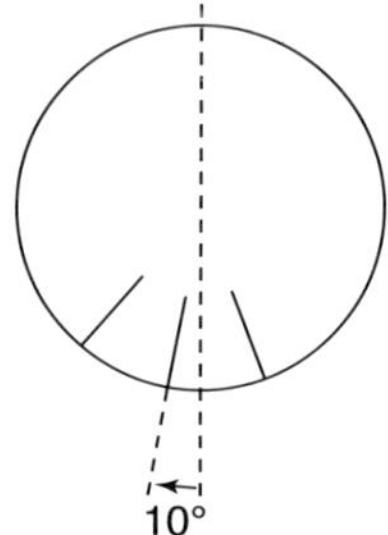

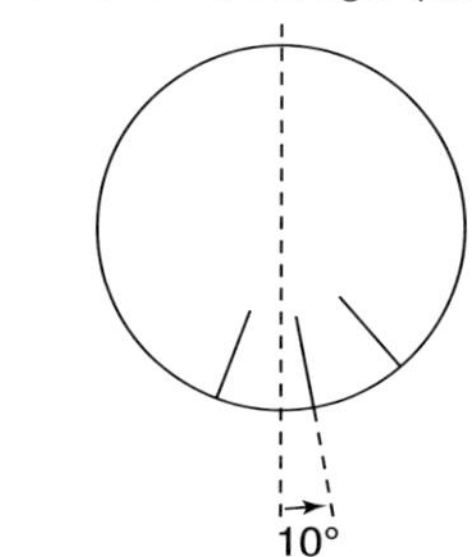

Figure 6-11 Evaluating lens rotation in fitting soft toric contact lenses using the LARS *(left add; right subtract)* rule of thumb. The spectacle prescription in this example is −2.00 −1.00 × 180°. *(Modified with permission from Key JE II, ed.* The CLAO Pocket Guide to Contact Lens Fitting. *2nd ed. Contact Lens Association of Ophthalmologists; 1998. Redrawn by Christine Gralapp.)*

patients: (1) use of reading glasses with contact lenses, (2) monovision, and (3) bifocal contact lenses.

The first option, using reading glasses over contact lenses, has the advantages of being simple, inexpensive, and effective.

The second option, monovision, involves correcting one eye for distance and the other eye for near (see BCSC Section 13, *Refractive Surgery*). Many patients are satisfied with this correction and tolerate the reduced binocular acuity and depth perception. Typically, the dominant eye is corrected for distance. For driving and other critical functions, overcorrection with glasses may be necessary. A temporary trial of monovision contact lenses is often useful for a patient who is considering a permanent monovision option with laser refractive surgery or lens implant surgery.

The third option for patients with presbyopia is to use bifocal contact lenses, either soft or RGP. There are 2 types of bifocal lenses: alternating-vision lenses and simultaneous-vision lenses. *Alternating-vision bifocal contact lenses* are similar in function to bifocal spectacles in that there are separate areas for distance and near, and that the retina receives a focused image from only 1 object plane at a time (Fig 6-12). *Segmented contact lenses* have 2 areas, top and bottom, like bifocal spectacles, whereas *concentric contact lenses* have 2 rings, 1 for far and 1 for near. For alternating-vision contact lenses, the position on the eye is critical and must change as the patient switches from distance to near viewing. The lower eyelid controls the lens position, so that as a person looks down, the lens stays up, and the eye's visual axis moves into the reading portion of the lens. The need for this "translation" of the lens in downgaze makes RGP lenses work well for these designs.

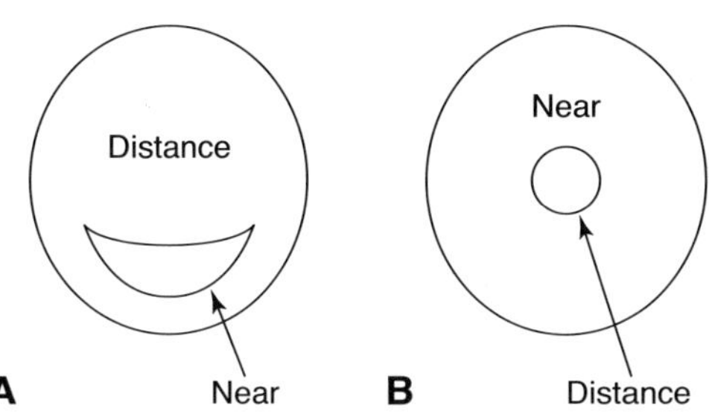

Figure 6-12 Alternating-vision bifocal contact lenses. **A,** Segmented lens. **B,** Concentric (annular) lens.

Simultaneous-vision bifocal contact lenses, generally available as soft multifocal lenses and, to a lesser extent, RGP lenses, provide the retina with focused images of near and far simultaneously. This requires the patient's brain to ignore one or the other and accept the reduction in contrast (Fig 6-13). These lenses have various optical designs, with rings of differing focal lengths to provide a bifocal or multifocal effect. The most central portion may be used for either near or distance. Another strategy is to have less add for the dominant eye, so that it has better distance vision, and more add in the nondominant eye.

Bennett, ES. Contact lens correction of presbyopia. *Clin Exp Optom.* 2008;91(3):265–278.

Keratoconus and the Abnormal Cornea

Contact lenses can provide better vision than spectacles by *masking* irregular corneal astigmatism. For mild or moderate irregularities, soft spherical, soft toric, or custom soft toric contact lenses can be used. Larger irregularities typically require an RGP lens to mask the abnormal surface; the anterior surface of the contact lens creates a smooth, spherical air–tear interface, and the tear lens fills the corneal irregularities. As is done for nonastigmatic eyes, the clinician first finds the best alignment fit and then determines the optimal power. Three-point touch can be used successfully for larger keratoconus cones to ensure lens centration and stability with slight apical and mid-peripheral touch or *bearing.* Figure 6-14 shows 3-point touch in keratoconus; the dark areas on the fluorescein

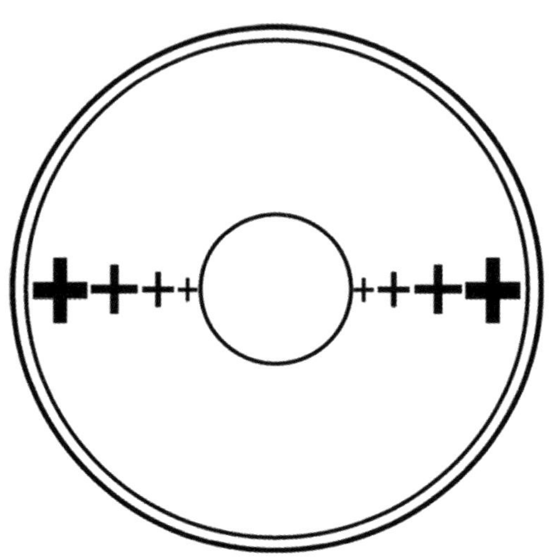

Figure 6-13 Simultaneous-vision bifocal design. *(Modified with permission from Key JE II, ed.* The CLAO Pocket Guide to Contact Lens Fitting. *2nd ed. Contact Lens Association of Ophthalmologists; 1998. Redrawn by Christine Gralapp.)*

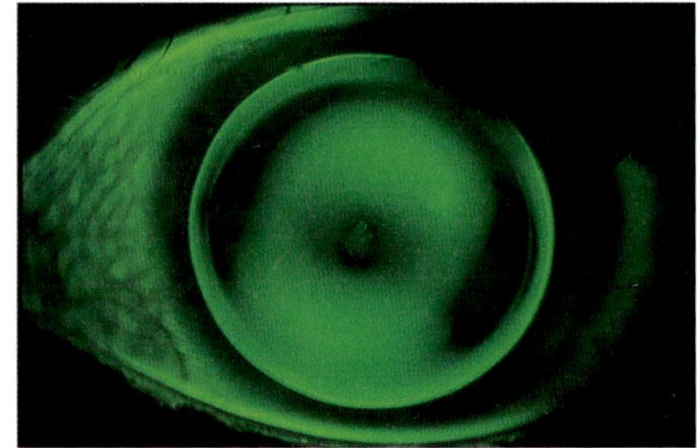

Figure 6-14 Three-point touch in keratoconus. *(Courtesy of Perry Rosenthal, MD.)*

evaluation denote apical and mid-peripheral touch. Alternatively, an apical clearance fitting technique places a lens vault slightly over the cone, which prevents the risk of contributing to apical scarring.

Specialized RGP lenses have been developed for keratoconus. Most provide a steep central posterior curve to vault over the cone and flatter peripheral curves to approximate the more normal peripheral curvature. Larger RGP contact lenses with larger optical zones (diameters >11 mm) are available for keratoconus and posttransplant fitting; they are known as intralimbic contact lenses.

A *hybrid contact lens* has a rigid center and a soft skirt. Its aim is to provide the good vision of an RGP lens and the comfort of a soft lens. A *piggyback lens system* involves the fitting of a soft contact lens with an RGP lens fitted over it. This system may allow comfort-related benefits like those offered by hybrid lenses, but with a greater choice of contact lens parameters, if the combination of lenses allows sufficient gas permeability to avoid hypoxia. *Scleral lenses* provide an increasingly popular alternative for corneas that cannot be fit with corneal gas-permeable lenses.

Finding a good fit for an abnormal cornea is well worth the determination and patience required of both fitter and patient. The lens will need refitting after any surgical intervention.

Scleral Rigid Gas-Permeable Contact Lenses

Scleral lenses have larger chord diameters than corneal RGP or soft lenses and are designed with a central optic that vaults over the cornea and a peripheral haptic that rests on the scleral surface (Fig 6-15). Standard scleral lenses have diameters of 18.10–24 mm, while smaller scleral lenses ("mini-scleral lenses") do not extend as far onto the sclera and have diameters of 15–18 mm. The space between the back of the lens and the cornea acts as a fluid reservoir. The shape of the posterior optic surface is chosen to minimize the volume of the fluid compartment while avoiding corneal contact. The posterior haptic surface is configured to minimize localized scleral compression; the transitional zone that joins the optic and haptic surfaces is designed to vault over the limbus.

These RGP lenses, with or without channels, must vent tears in and out of the fluid reservoir to prevent buildup of suction onto the cornea and allow ample circulation of fresh tears beneath the lens. Improved RGP chemistry has enabled these lenses to be well tolerated. They have 2 primary indications: (1) correcting abnormal regular and irregular

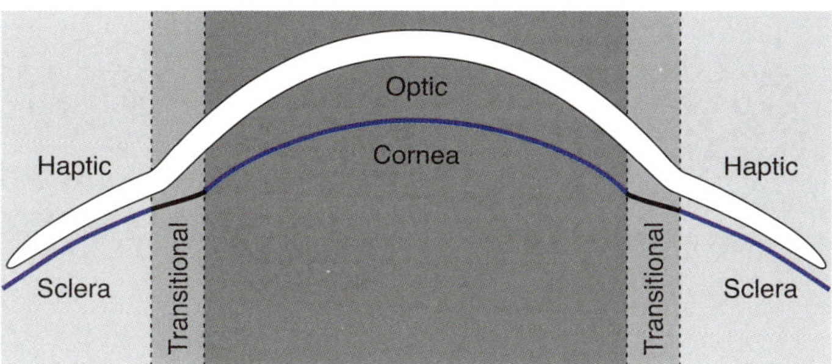

Figure 6-15 Scleral contact lens. *(Redrawn with permission from Albert DM, Jakobiec FA, eds.* Principles and Practice of Ophthalmology. *Saunders; 1994;5:3643. Redrawn by Christine Gralapp and modification redeveloped by Leon Strauss, MD, PhD.)*

astigmatism in eyes that cannot be fit with corneal contact lenses, especially for corneal ectatic disorders and following penetrating keratoplasty, and (2) managing ocular surface diseases that benefit from the constant presence of a protective, lubricating layer of oxygenated tears. See the discussion of therapeutic contact lenses in the next section.

The fitting of these lenses can be more complicated than for soft or corneal RGP lenses and typically requires special training. These lenses can be highly customizable, such as the PROSE lens (BostonSight), and can be designed based on scleral imaging or impression molds of the ocular surface. These advanced designs can be useful in patients with pingueculae, pteryia, or conjunctival blebs from glaucoma surgery that would otherwise interfere with the lens fit.

Scleral lenses can be less convenient for patients, because insertion and removal may be more difficult than with more traditional lenses. The scleral lens must be filled with preservative-free sterile saline or a special filling solution and placed on the eye such that no air bubbles form between the lens and the ocular surface; the aid of a handheld plunger or a stationary, lighted stand plunger is often necessary. Other potential issues include surface nonwetting of the lens, fogging due to the collection of debris in the fluid reservoir, conjunctival vessel impingement, and conjunctival prolapse. These lenses can also be more expensive and have more limited insurance coverage than soft or corneal RGP lenses.

Contact Lens Overrefraction

Sometimes we wish to determine the etiology of poor vision of an eye with an irregularly shaped cornea and other possible causes of decreased acuity, such as macular degeneration. Finding out whether refraction over a rigid contact lens achieves good acuity is diagnostically useful in this situation, even when actual contact lens wear is not being considered.

Therapeutic Use of Contact Lenses

Contact lenses may be used to enhance epithelial healing, prevent epithelial erosions, or control surface-generated pain. These lenses are sometimes referred to as *bandage contact lenses*. Typically, a disposable plano soft lens with high oxygen permeability is left on the eye for an extended period. Fitting principles are similar to those of other soft lenses, although for therapeutic use, a somewhat tighter fit maybe be preferable, as lens movement could further injure the healing epithelium. Some fitters prefer lenses with a high water content, but high oxygen permeability is usually the chief factor in lens selection.

Conditions and circumstances in which bandage contact lenses might be useful include

- bullous keratopathy
- recurrent erosions
- Bell palsy, exposure keratopathy
- keratitis, such as filamentary, or after chemical exposure
- corneal dystrophy with erosions
- after surgery, such as corneal transplant, laser in situ keratomileusis (LASIK), or photorefractive keratectomy (PRK)
- nonhealing epithelial defect, such as geographic herpes keratitis, slow-healing ulcer, or abrasion
- eyelid abnormalities, such as entropion, eyelid lag, or trichiasis
- bleb leak after glaucoma filtration surgery

Patients who use bandage contact lenses need to be made especially aware of the signs and symptoms of infection because their vulnerability to infection is increased due to their corneal abnormality. Some practitioners prefer to use prophylactic topical antibiotics with these lenses.

In addition to bandage contact lenses, scleral lenses are increasingly being used therapeutically to treat a variety of ocular surface disorders, including advanced dry eye disease, persistent epithelial defects, exposure keratopathy, neurotrophic keratitis, neuropathic pain, and limbal stem cell deficiency, among other conditions. Scleral lenses help by protecting the ocular surface and creating the constant presence of a lubricating layer of oxygenated tears over the cornea. These lenses can be especially helpful with complications of Stevens-Johnson syndrome, graft-vs-host disease, and ocular cicatricial pemphigoid, protecting the fragile epithelium of these corneas from the abrasive effects of keratinized eyelid margins associated with distichiasis and trichiasis and from exposure to air.

Orthokeratology and Corneal Reshaping

Orthokeratology, or corneal refractive therapy, refers to the overnight use of RGP contact lenses to temporarily mechanically reshape the cornea; its objective is that by wearing the lenses during sleep, the patient will not need to wear glasses or contacts while awake. For myopia, lenses are designed to flatten the central cornea for a period after the lenses are removed and can treat up to –6.00 D of sphere. In clinical trials, approximately one-third of patients discontinued contact lens use, and most patients (75%) experienced discomfort at some point during contact lens wear. Complications of orthokeratology include induced astigmatism, induced higher-order aberrations, recurrent erosions, and, most seriously, infectious keratitis (which can be bilateral and seems to be more common in children and teenagers than in adults).

There has been recent interest in using orthokeratology to reduce progression of myopia in children. This may be effective in children and adolescents, with a potential greater effect when initiated at an early age (6–8 years), but safety remains a concern.

Bennett ES, Henry VA. Orthokeratology. In: *Clinical Manual of Contact Lenses*. 4th ed. Lippincott Williams & Wilkins; 2019.

Van Meter WS, Musch DC, Jacobs DS, Kaufman SC, Reinhart WJ, Udell IJ; American Academy of Ophthalmology. Safety of overnight orthokeratology for myopia: a report by the American Academy of Ophthalmology. *Ophthalmology*. 2008;115(12):2301–2313.

VanderVeen DK, Kraker RT, Pineles SL, et al. Use of orthokeratology for the prevention of myopic progression in children: a report by the American Academy of Ophthalmology. *Ophthalmology*. 2019;126(4):623–636.

Custom Contact Lenses

A normal cornea is generally steepest near its geometric center; beyond the center, the surface flattens. The steep area is known as the *apical zone,* and its center is the *corneal apex.* Outside the apical zone, which is approximately 3–4 mm in diameter, the rate of peripheral flattening may vary significantly in the different corneal meridians. This variation is important, because peripheral corneal topography significantly affects the position, blink-induced excursion patterns, and, therefore, the comfort of wearing corneal contact lenses, especially gas-permeable lenses.

The availability of corneal topography and wavefront aberrometers, together with desktop graphics programs and computerized lathes, enables the preparation of individually tailored contact lenses that assist with otherwise difficult fits, such as for patients with keratoconus or trauma or after transplant surgery. There is interest in the attempt to design lenses in this way to optimize wavefront correction for normal corneas, with the caveat that contact lenses constantly change their position on the cornea. Specially painted lenses are another custom lens type and are used to reduce glare in aniridia and albinism by providing an artificial pupil.

Contact Lens Care and Solutions

Contact lenses are cleaned and disinfected after use, unless they are single-use disposable lenses that are designed to be worn only for 1 day. Lens-care systems have been developed to remove deposits and microorganisms from lenses, enhance comfort, and decrease the risk of eye infection and irritation. They include, in 1 or more bottles, cleaning, disinfection, and storage functions (Table 6-9). Enzymatic cleaners, which remove protein deposits from the lens surface, provide additional cleaning for lenses that are not replaced frequently. Alternatively, patients whose eyes form deposits can be prescribed lenses that are more frequently replaced. Serious eye infections may occur with any disinfection system, and there is more risk when patients do not follow instructions (eg, to discard and

Table 6-9 Contact Lens–Care Systems

Type	Purpose	Lens Use	Comments
Saline	Rinsing	All types	May be used with, but not instead of, disinfecting systems
Daily cleaner	Cleaning	All types	Used with some disinfecting systems
Multipurpose solution	Cleaning, disinfecting, rinsing, and storing	All types	Rubbing with a daily cleaner is usually preferred for RGP lenses
Hydrogen peroxide solution	Cleaning, disinfecting, rinsing, and storing	All types	Risk of chemical burn if instructions are not followed
Enzymatic cleaner	Removal of deposits	All types	Used to remove deposits from lenses that are not replaced frequently

replace solutions). Lens cases must be replaced every 1–3 months, unless they are treated with boiling water. Rinsing the lens or case with tap water risks contamination. If a practitioner uses trial lenses, one of the peroxide systems can be used for disinfection of soft and RGP lenses. Peroxide, however, at the concentrations used in commercially available solutions, does not kill *Acanthamoeba* species.

Several methods have been developed for disinfecting lenses, including the use of chemicals, hydrogen peroxide, and ultraviolet light exposure. Heat disinfection is no longer commonly used. The care system selected depends on the personal preference of the fitter and patient, the simplicity and convenience of use, cost, and possible allergies to solution components. Currently, multipurpose solutions are the most popular care systems in the United States.

The fitter should instruct the patient in the care and use of contact lenses:

- Clean and disinfect a lens whenever it is removed. Rubbing cleans the lens more thoroughly.
- Follow the instructions included with the lens-care system.
- Do not use tap water, saliva, home-made solutions, or any liquid not specifically formulated for use with contact lenses on the lenses.
- Do not reuse contact lens–care solutions.
- Note that swimming while wearing contact lenses increases the risk of infection.
- Do not allow the lens solution's dropper tip or bottle to be contaminated.
- Clean the contact lens case daily by rinsing it with fresh contact lens cleaning solution (not tap water) and then allowing the case to air-dry before reusing it.
- Disinfect the case with boiling water and/or replace it every 1–3 months.
- Follow the recommended lens replacement schedule.
- Seek medical assistance promptly, when indicated.

In addition to teaching appropriate contact lens and case care, the fitter should instruct the patient in proper lens insertion and removal techniques, determine a wear schedule, and decide when the lenses should be replaced. Insertion and handling techniques vary significantly among lenses; manufacturers provide written information and videos to instruct ophthalmic staff and patients in appropriate insertion and removal techniques.

Jones L, Walsh K, Willcox M, Morgan P, Nichols J. The COVID-19 pandemic: important considerations for contact lens practitioners. *Cont Lens Anterior Eye*. 2020;43(3):196–203.

Contact Lens–Related Problems and Complications

Contact lens problems can be categorized as follows: infectious, hypoxic/metabolic, toxic, mechanical, inflammatory, and dry eye (Table 6-10).

Infections

With the increased use of disposable lenses, better patient education, more convenient care systems, and the availability of more oxygen-permeable lens materials, serious eye infections from lens use have become less common. However, practitioners should be aware of unusual infections that can occur, such as *Acanthamoeba,* fungal keratitis, and *Pseudomonas* (Fig 6-16A). Diagnosis and treatment of corneal infections are covered in BCSC Section 8, *External Disease and Cornea.*

Hypoxic/Metabolic Problems

Contact lens overwear syndromes can take several forms. Hypoxia, lactate accumulation, and impaired carbon dioxide efflux are responsible for these complications.

Table 6-10 Contact Lens–Related Problems and Complications

Category	Problem or Complication
Infectious	Conjunctivitis
	Keratitis
	Bacterial infection
	Fungal infection
	Acanthamoebal infection
Hypoxic/metabolic	Metabolic epithelial damage
	Corneal neovascularization
Toxic	Punctate keratitis
	Toxic conjunctivitis
Mechanical	Corneal warpage
	Spectacle blur
	Ptosis
	Corneal abrasions
	3-o'clock and 9-o'clock staining
Inflammatory	Contact lens–induced keratoconjunctivitis (CLIK)
	Allergic reactions
	Giant papillary conjunctivitis (GPC)
	Sterile infiltrates
Dry eye	Punctate keratitis
	Keratitis sicca

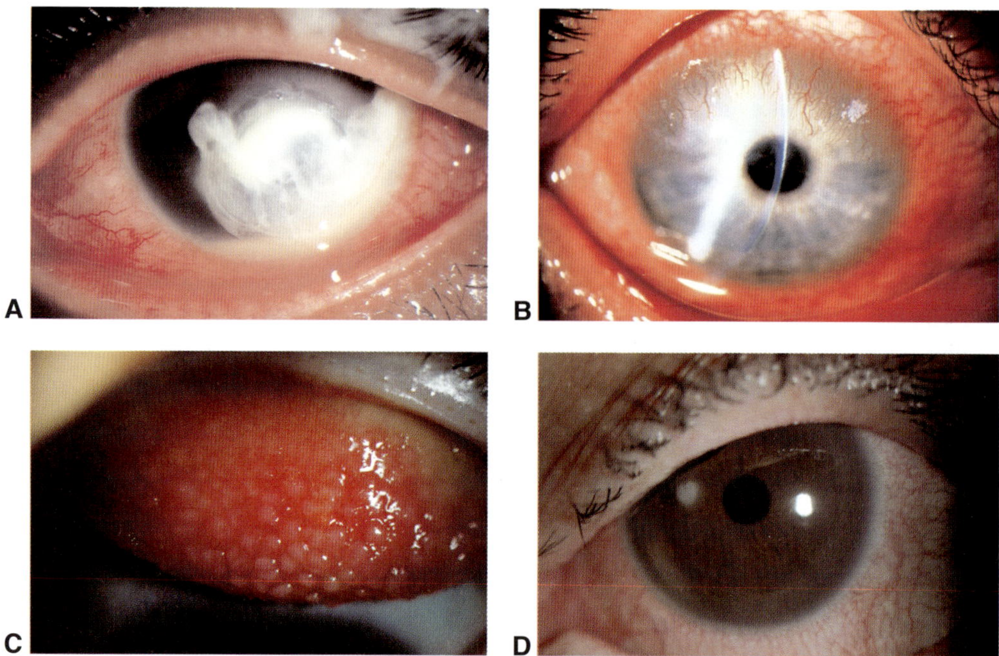

Figure 6-16 Contact lens complications. **A,** *Pseudomonas* corneal ulcer. **B,** Corneal neovascularization (vascular pannus). **C,** Giant papillary conjunctivitis. **D,** Sterile corneal infiltrates. *(Part B courtesy of Kirk R. Wilhelmus, MD, PhD. Parts C and D courtesy of Deborah S. Jacobs, MD.)*

Central epithelial edema (Sattler veil) may present after many hours of wear, more commonly with hard contact lenses. This epithelial edema causes blurred vision that may persist for many hours or, in rare instances, progress to acute epithelial necrosis.

Microcystic epitheliopathy, another condition caused by impaired metabolism in the corneal epithelium, shows fine epithelial cysts, which are most easily observed with retroillumination. This condition is more common with extended-wear contact lenses. The cysts may be either asymptomatic or cause recurrent brief episodes of pain and epiphora. It takes up to 6 weeks following discontinuation of contact lens wear for the cysts to resolve. In some cases, this epitheliopathy may have a dendritic appearance.

Corneal neovascularization (Fig 6-16B) is usually a sign of hypoxia. Refitting with lenses made of a material with higher oxygen permeability or lenses that fit more loosely, decreasing the number of hours of wear time per day, or switching to disposable lenses can prevent further progression. If neovascularization is extensive, it can lead to corneal scarring and lipid deposition or intracorneal hemorrhage. Superficial pannus is rarely associated with RGP contact lens wear; it is encountered more frequently in patients who use extended-wear or disposable soft lenses and replace them less frequently than is recommended. This type of neovascularization is probably caused by hypoxia and chronic trauma to the limbus. Other causes of pannus, such as staphylococcal and chlamydial keratoconjunctivitis, should be considered in the presence of accompanying signs that suggest them.

Deep stromal neovascularization has been associated with extended-wear contact lenses, especially in aphakia. This condition is not usually symptomatic unless there is secondary lipid deposition. Deep neovascularization of the cornea is often irreversible and is best managed by discontinuing contact lens wear.

Toxicity

Punctate keratitis

Punctate keratitis may be related to poor contact lens fit, toxic reaction to contact lens solutions, or dry eye.

Toxic conjunctivitis

Conjunctival injection, epithelial staining, punctate epithelial keratopathy, erosions, microcysts, and limbal stem cell deficiency are all potential findings of conjunctival or corneal toxicity that arise from contact lens solutions. Any of the proteolytic enzymes or chemicals used for cleaning contact lenses or the soaking solution, which contains preservatives, may be the culprit. Cleaning and disinfecting agents can cause an immediate, painful epitheliopathy.

Mechanical Problems

Corneal warpage

Change in corneal shape from contact lens use occurs with both soft and RGP lenses, but it is more commonly associated with hard lenses. Most warpage resolves after the patient discontinues wearing the lens, but the time to resolution can vary significantly. To monitor corneal shape on an ongoing basis, the clinician can follow keratometry or corneal topography and manifest refraction as part of the contact lens follow-up examinations. The common term *spectacle blur* misleadingly suggests that these changes are somehow due to a problem with the spectacle correction. If there is more than a little fluctuation of refractive error, the contact lens fit should be reevaluated.

Ptosis

Ptosis related to dehiscence of the levator aponeurosis has been associated with long-term use of RGP lenses.

Corneal abrasions

Corneal abrasions can result from foreign bodies under a lens, poor insertion or removal technique, or a damaged contact lens. Most clinicians treat abrasions with topical antibiotics and try to avoid patching, particularly in the context of contact lens wear, to reduce the likelihood of infection.

3-o'clock and 9-o'clock staining

This specific superficial punctate keratitis staining pattern may be observed in RGP contact lens users, especially with interpalpebral fit; it is probably related to poor wetting (Fig 6-17). Paralimbal staining is characteristic of low-fitting lenses and is associated with an abortive reflex-blink pattern, insufficient lens movement, inadequate tear meniscus, and a thick peripheral lens profile. Refitting the lens or regular use of rewetting drops may help.

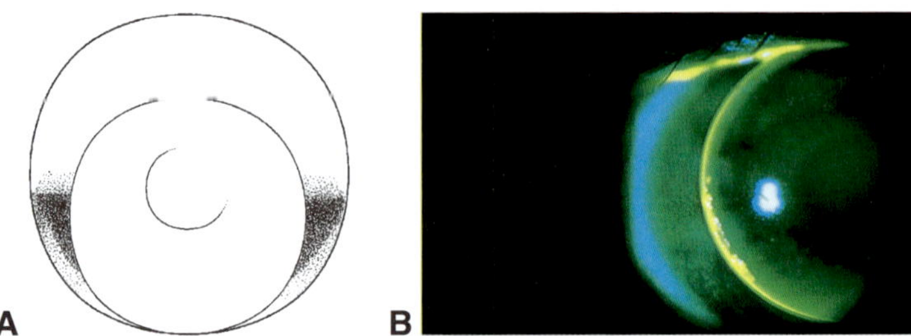

Figure 6-17 Three-o'clock and 9-o'clock corneal staining. **A,** Inferior corneal desiccation of the tear film. **B,** Peripheral corneal desiccation. *(Part B courtesy of Perry Rosenthal, MD.)*

Inflammation

Contact lens–induced keratoconjunctivitis

Contact lens–induced keratoconjunctivitis (CLIK) can be ascribed to allergy, dry eye, infection, and deposits on lenses. Patients with ocular prostheses and exposed monofilament sutures have similar reactions. Findings suggest a combined mechanical and immune-mediated pathophysiology.

Allergic reactions

Preservative chemicals can produce a type IV delayed hypersensitivity response, resulting in conjunctivitis, keratitis, coarse epithelial and subepithelial opacities, and superior limbic keratoconjunctivitis. This condition has become less common, probably because of the replacement of thimerosal by other preservatives in contact lens solutions and the introduction of disposable contact lenses.

Giant papillary conjunctivitis

Giant papillary conjunctivitis (GPC) (Fig 6-16C) tends to develop more frequently with use of extended-wear soft contact lenses, dry eye, and meibomian gland dysfunction. It may also be induced by other irritants, such as loose sutures or prosthetics. Symptoms include contact lens intolerance, itching, excessive mucus discharge, and blurred vision with mucus coating the contact lens, contact lens decentration, and conjunctival redness. Sometimes, there may be bloody tears and ptosis secondary to inflammation of the superior tarsal conjunctiva.

The signs of GPC consist of hyperemia, thickening, and abnormally large papillae (diameter >0.3 mm) of the superior tarsal conjunctiva due to disruption of the anchoring septae. In some cases, the giant papillae cover the entire central tarsus from the posterior eyelid margin to the upper border of the tarsal plate; involvement in other cases may be less extensive. Long-standing or involuted giant papillae on the superior tarsus may resemble follicles. The symptoms of GPC generally resolve when contact lens wear is discontinued. The tarsal conjunctival hyperemia and thickening may resolve in several weeks, but papillae or dome-shaped scars on the superior tarsus can persist for years.

If GPC persists, the clinician should consider changing the lens to a different polymer or to daily wear disposable lenses. Some patients prefer low-water-content lenses. In persistent cases, consider fitting the patient with RGP contact lenses, which are associated with a lower incidence of GPC, or discontinuing contact lens wear.

Many practitioners recommend discontinuing lens wear for 2–3 weeks while treatment is initiated. Mast-cell stabilizer/antihistamine topical medications are used for mild GPC. Topical corticosteroids may be used for several weeks for these or more advanced cases, with appropriate monitoring of the increased long-term risks of infection, elevated intraocular pressure, and cataract formation. Topical cyclosporine and tacrolimus may be helpful in some cases. In the most severe cases, it may be necessary to discontinue contact lens wear.

Sterile infiltrates

Typically, sterile infiltrates are observed in the peripheral cornea. They occur more often in younger patients. Often there is more than one spot, the infiltrates are relatively small, and the epithelium over the area is intact (Fig 6-16D). Discontinuing lens use can usually solve the problem quickly, but clinicians often prescribe an antibiotic, even though cultures tend to show no growth. Increased bacterial bioburden has been found on these lenses.

Dry Eye

Patients with severe dry eye probably are not good candidates for contact lens use. However, patients with moderate to mild dry eye may do well with contact lenses. Some soft lenses are marketed for patients with dry eye; lenses often have lower water content and better wettability, and are thicker than average. They may be made of material that is less prone to lens deposit formation.

Some patients may succeed in contact lens wear with the placement of punctal plugs. Occasionally, the signs and symptoms of dry eye result from incomplete or infrequent blinking (fewer than 12 times per minute). Scleral lenses are used for some cases of severe dry eye.

Over-the-Counter Contact Lenses

Contact lenses should not be sold over the counter without being fitted by someone qualified to do so. Unfortunately, this continues to occur despite a federal statute stating that contact lens sellers cannot provide contact lenses to customers without a valid prescription. Colored contacts, circle lenses, and other decorative and costume contact lenses are often advertised like toys, and consumers may not understand the risks of using unprescribed lenses.

Cosmetic contact lenses: potential threat to vision health. Joint statement by the American Academy of Optometry and American Academy of Ophthalmology. October 2018. Accessed November 22, 2021. https://www.aao.org/education/clinical-statement/cosmetic-contact-lenses-potential-threat-to-vision

Federal Law and Contact Lenses

The Federal Fairness to Contact Lens Consumers Act (PL 108-164) "increases consumers' ability to shop around when buying contact lenses." The patient must be given, without having to ask, a copy of the prescription. If the patient calls in contact lens parameters to a seller, and the seller leaves a message for the prescriber, it is considered "verified" if the prescriber doesn't reply within 8 business hours, Monday through Friday, except federal holidays. Although the fit of a rigid lens may depend on the laboratory's machinery and modifications the practitioner may have made, these lenses are not excluded from this law, which also forbids the prescriber from asking the patient to sign a waiver of responsibility for the prescription. State laws may also address these issues.

Contact lens law is clarified by EU court. EUbusiness. Accessed November 22, 2021. www.eubusiness.com/topics/eulaw/lens.01/

Federal Trade Commission. The contact lens rule: a guide for prescribers and sellers. June 2020. Accessed November 1, 2022. www.ftc.gov/business-guidance/resources/contact-lens-rule-guide-prescribers-sellers

Chapter Exercises

Questions

6.1. A 40-year-old patient is prescribed single-vision glasses −6.00 D OU and also fitted with contact lenses −5.50 D OU. He calls to say that he has trouble reading when wearing the contacts. What is the most likely explanation?
   a. The contact lenses are "overminused."
   b. With the contacts, he is losing near effectivity, which the glasses give him.
   c. Looking through the contacts causes base-in prism, making it difficult for the eyes to converge.
   d. The contacts have plus-powered tear lenses, which increase accommodative demand.

6.2. A patient tore her soft contact lens, and it has caused a corneal abrasion. What is the next step?
   a. Put in a fresh lens, which will have a bandage effect, while the abrasion heals.
   b. Put in a fresh lens and use topical antibiotics for several days.
   c. Pressure-patch the eye with antibiotic and see the patient the next day.
   d. Do not use a contact lens; use lubrication and perhaps antibiotic drops.

6.3. A trial soft contact lens moves excessively with eyelid blinks. Which of the following would decrease lens movement?
   a. flattening the base curve while maintaining the diameter
   b. decreasing the diameter while maintaining the base curve
   c. increasing the power of the contact lens
   d. steepening the base curve while maintaining the diameter
   e. flattening the base curve and decreasing the diameter

6.4. You fit a patient who has −3.50 D of myopia with an RGP contact lens that is flatter than *K*. If the patient's average *K* reading is 7.80 mm and you fit a lens with a base curve of 8.00 mm, what is the shape of the tear lens?
   a. plano
   b. teardrop
   c. concave
   d. convex

6.5. For the patient in question 6.4, which power RGP lens should you order?
   a. −2.00 D
   b. −2.50 D
   c. −3.50 D
   d. −4.00 D

6.6. You fit a toric soft contact lens on a patient with a refractive error of −2.50 −1.50 × 175. The trial lens centers well, but the lens mark at the 6-o'clock position appears to rest at the 5-o'clock position when the lens is placed on the patient's eye. What power contact lens should you order?
   a. −2.50 −1.50 × 175
   b. −2.50 −1.50 × 145
   c. −2.50 −1.50 × 55
   d. −2.50 −1.00 × 175

Answers

6.1. **b.** The near effectivity of the glasses decreases accommodative demand, making it easier to read than when the myopia is corrected at the cornea by the contact lenses. The glasses have their optical centers placed for distance viewing. Converging to read induces base-in prism, so that less convergence is required to look at near objects when the patient wears the glasses. If the contacts are rigid, and thus form a plus-powered tear lens, they will blur distance vision and aid reading vision, unless the power of the lenses is properly adjusted by over-refracting with the lenses in place. The contact lens has slightly less power than the spectacle lens because of the difference in vertex distance (see Table 6-4).

6.2. **d.** With contact lens involvement, we are more concerned than otherwise about infection. Avoid patching, and use bandage contact lenses with caution; instead consider lubrication and topical antibiotics, and see the patient soon for follow-up evaluation.

6.3. **d.** Increasing the sagittal depth of the contact lens tightens the fit and decreases lens movement, which may be achieved through steepening (decreasing) the base curve or increasing the diameter of the contact lens. Flattening (increasing) the base curve or decreasing the diameter of the lens decreases sagittal depth and increases the movement of the lens on the cornea. The power of the contact lens should not affect the fitting relationships.

6.4. **c.** The tear lens is formed by the posterior surface of the contact lens and the anterior surface of the cornea. If these 2 curvatures are the same, as with a soft lens, the tear lens is plano. If they are different (as is typical of RGP lenses), a plus or minus tear lens forms. In this case, the contact lens is flatter than *K*, so the tear lens is negative, or concave, in shape.

6.5. **b.** For every 0.05-mm radius-of-curvature difference between the base curve and *K*, the induced power of the tear film is 0.25 D. The power of the concave tear lens in this case is −1.00 D. The power of the RGP contact lens you should order is −3.50 D − (−1.00 D) = −2.50 D. An easy way to remember this formula is to use the following rule: SAM = *steeper add minus*, and FAP = *flatter add plus*.

6.6. **b.** The amount and direction of rotation should be observed. In this case, they are, respectively, 1 clock-hour and rotation to the right. Each clock-hour represents 30° (360°/12 = 30°), so the adjustment should be 30°. Because the rotation is to the right, you should order a contact lens with axis 145° instead of 175°—that is, −2.50 D −1.50 × 145. An easy rule to remember is "LARS": *left add, right subtract.*

CHAPTER 7

Intraocular Lenses

This chapter includes related videos, which can be accessed by scanning the QR codes provided in the text or going to www.aao.org/bcscvideo_section03.

Highlights

- Intraocular lens (IOL) design influences the development of posterior capsular opacity, and the presence of an IOL influences the likelihood of retinal detachment.
- Eyes that have undergone refractive surgery require different calculation methods than surgically naïve eyes.
- The presence of silicone oil in the eye necessitates adjustments to biometry. If silicone oil is to remain in the eye, adjustment to the refractive target is necessary.
- Small angular misalignments of toric lenses can produce substantial reductions in net astigmatic correction.
- Modulation transfer function (MTF) curves are a good tool for evaluating different sorts of multifocal IOLs.

Glossary

Dysphotopsias Various light-related visual disturbances, typically in the temporal visual field, encountered by pseudophakic (and phakic) patients. Positive dysphotopsias are characterized by brightness, streaks, and rays emanating from a central point source of light, sometimes with a diffuse, hazy glare. Negative dysphotopsias are characterized by subjective darkness or shadowing.

Effective lens position An estimation of the distance at which the principal plane of the IOL will be situated behind the cornea. Derived from biometric measurement of the eye used in IOL power calculation.

Modulation transfer function A measure of optical performance that describes contrast degradation of a sinusoidal pattern as it passes through the optical system as well as the cutoff spatial frequency beyond which fine detail will not be resolved. Often used in discussion of wavefront aberrations.

Monovision A refractive strategy for the selection of contact lens or IOL powers such that 1 eye has better distance vision and the other eye has better near vision.

Introduction

It is difficult to imagine a time without intraocular lenses (IOLs). Yet, it is well within the lives of many of the readers of this volume that IOL insertion did not necessarily follow extraction of the cataractous lens. Although Sir Harold Ridley devised the earliest IOLs in the 1940s, IOL implantation did not become common practice for another 30 years.

Aphakia is sufficiently visually impairing to give one pause before undergoing cataract extraction. Not only does the condition require heavy spectacles that alter one's appearance by magnifying the wearer's eyes to any observer, but, in the absence of contact lens wear, *monocular* aphakia is essentially untreatable because of the aniseikonia such spectacles would induce.

The widespread adoption of IOLs in the 1970s removed much of the disincentive to cataract surgery. In 1968, hospital admissions in the United Kingdom for cataract surgery totaled only 62 per 100,000 people. By 2004, that number had grown tenfold to 637. Certainly, cataract surgery has seen great advancements in technique and equipment, but none of these is as significant to the patient as the development of the IOL.

Progress in the accuracy of IOL biometry, new IOL designs, and the concomitant rise in patients' refractive expectations has brought emphasis to the optics of IOLs. This chapter focuses on the optical considerations relevant to IOLs. For information on the history and development of IOLs, and more surgical information with respect to IOLs, see BCSC Section 11, *Lens and Cataract.*

In the 1970s, surgeons implanting IOLs included those who used *intracapsular cataract extraction (ICCE)* and those who used *small-incision phacoemulsification (phaco).* The IOL optic was made from polymethylmethacrylate (PMMA), with supporting haptics of metal, polypropylene, or PMMA. The rigidity of these materials required that a small phaco incision be enlarged for IOL insertion. However, following the introduction of a foldable optic (made from silicone) in the late 1980s, enlargement was no longer required, and the combination of phaco and IOL implantation was widely adopted.

The basic lens designs currently in use are differentiated by the plane in which the lens is placed (posterior chamber or anterior chamber) and by the tissue supporting the lens (capsule/ciliary sulcus or chamber angle). Figure 7-1 illustrates the major types of IOLs and optics.

The effect of lens material on factors such as *posterior capsular opacification (PCO)* has been investigated. Earlier studies suggested that IOLs made from acrylic are associated with lower rates of PCO than are those made from silicone or PMMA. However, more recent studies suggest that lens edge design is a more important factor in PCO than is lens material, as Kenneth Hoffer proposed in 1979 in the lens edge barrier theory. An IOL with an annular, ridged edge or a square, truncated edge creates a barrier effect at the optic edge, exerting a 69% increase in pressure of the IOL edge against the posterior capsule. This reduces cell migration (shown in Figure 7-2 as "pearls") behind the optic and thus reduces PCO (Figs 7-2, 7-3, 7-4). The ridge concept led to the development of partial-ridge and meniscus IOLs, which were used for a time, and the sharp-edge designs now in use.

Plano and even negative-power IOLs are available for patients with very high myopia. The presence of even a plano IOL helps maintain the structural integrity of the anterior segment and decreases the incidence of posterior capsular opacity compared to simply leaving

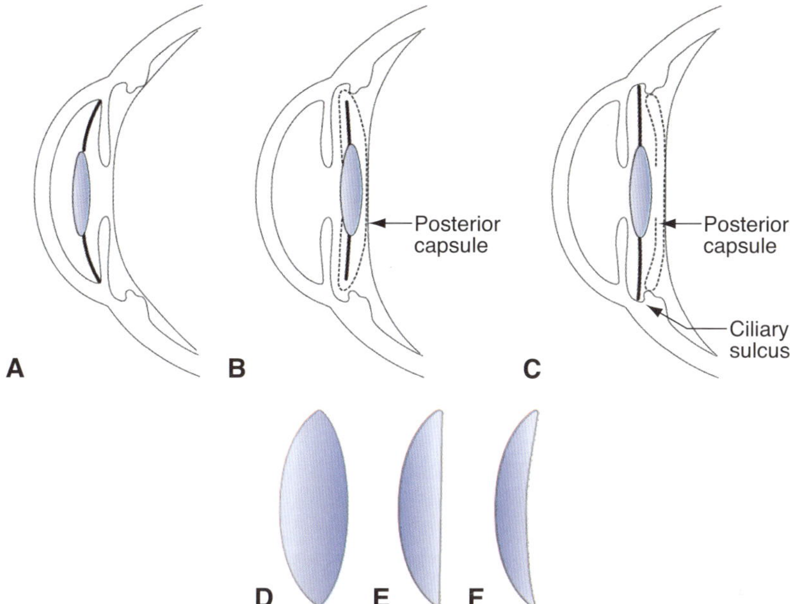

Figure 7-1 The major types of intraocular lenses (IOLs) and optics. **A,** Anterior chamber lens. **B,** Posterior chamber lens in the capsular bag. **C,** Posterior chamber lens in the ciliary sulcus. **D,** Biconvex optic. **E,** Planoconvex optic. **F,** Meniscus optic. *(Redrawn by C. H. Wooley.)*

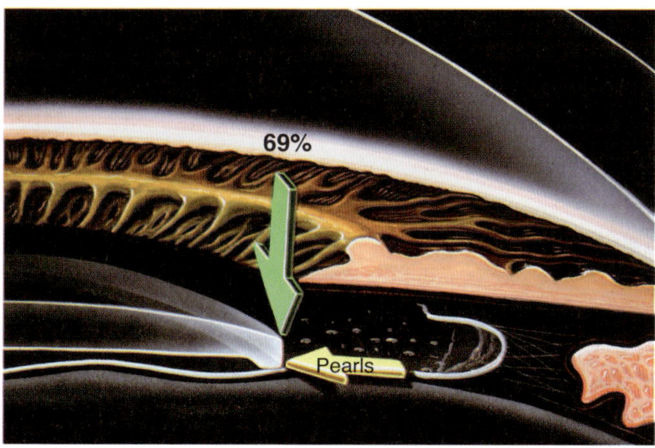

Figure 7-2 Schematic illustrating the concept of a 69% increase in pressure *(green arrow)* at the edge of an intraocular lens. *(Courtesy of Kenneth J. Hoffer, MD.)*

the eye aphakic. Moreover, yttrium-aluminum-garnet (YAG) capsulotomy in aphakic eyes is associated with a higher incidence of retinal detachment than in eyes with IOLs.

"Piggyback" lenses (ie, 2 IOLs in 1 eye; biphakia), implanted either simultaneously or sequentially, may be used when the postoperative IOL power is incorrect or when the needed IOL power is higher than what is commercially available. Minus-power IOLs can

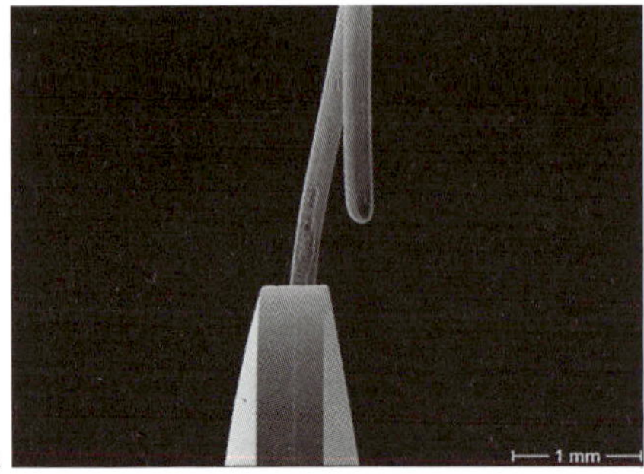

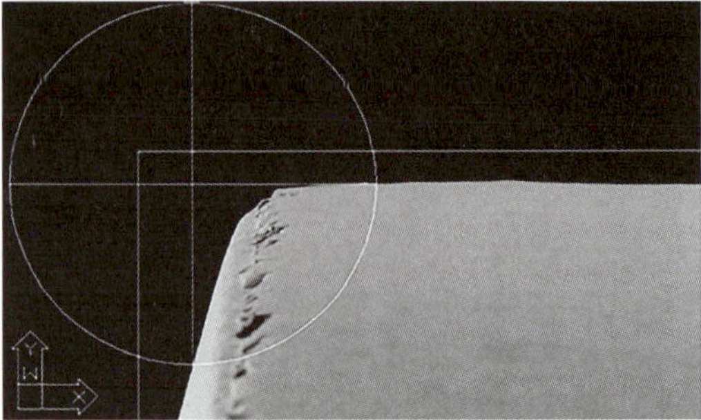

Figure 7-3 The actual geometry of the "square" posterior optic edge depends on the configuration of the optic and the IOL power. **A,** Scanning electron micrograph (SEM) shows the IOL at 25× magnification, with the posterior edge on the left. **B,** SEM shows the junction of the posterior surface with the lateral edge of the optic at 1000× magnification. Increasing the power of the IOL on the posterior surface increases the curvature of that surface and increases the obtuse angle of the intersecting surfaces. *(Courtesy of Werner L, Müller M. Evaluating and defining the sharpness of intraocular lenses: microedge structure of commercially available square-edged hydrophobic lenses.* J Cataract Refract Surg. *2008:34(2):310-317.)*

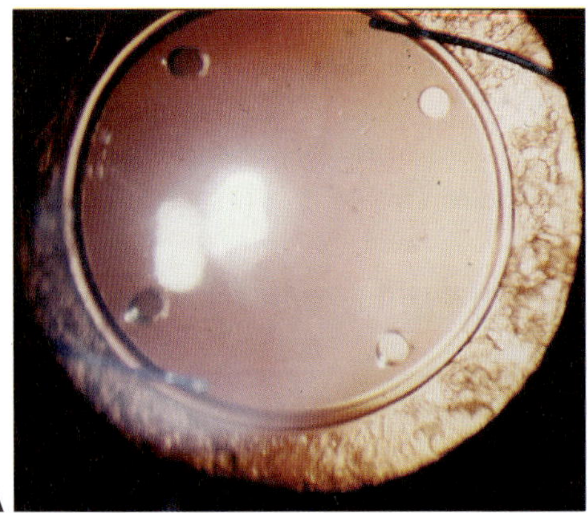

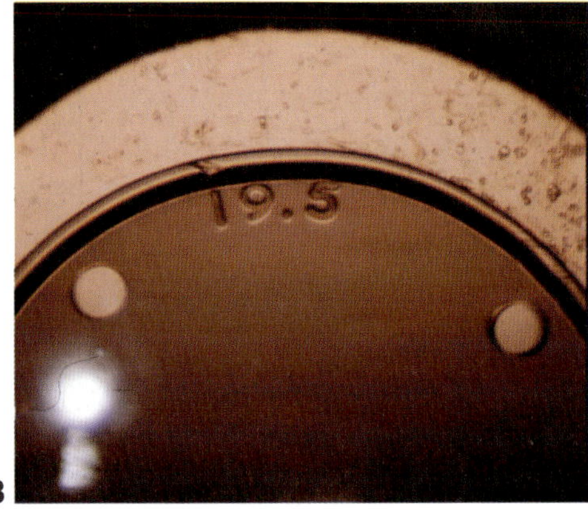

Figure 7-4 Increasing the pressure at the edge of an intraocular lens leads to a blockage of migration of cells from the periphery to the central posterior capsule. **A,** Opacification of the lens capsule peripheral to the optic edge. **B,** Part A at higher magnification. *(Courtesy of Kenneth J. Hoffer, MD.)*

be used to correct extreme myopia and (as piggybacks) to correct IOL power errors. Interlenticular fibrosis may occur after placement of a piggyback lens arrangement. To the extent that this fibrosis may displace or tilt the piggyback IOL, it will change the refractive effect of the IOL and result in ametropia.

Current IOLs are foldable, injectable, aspheric, sharp edged, and single piece (or 3 piece), and they have higher refractive indices; together, these features allow for implantation through smaller incisions than were used for the earlier designs.

Apple DJ. Influence of intraocular lens material and design on postoperative intracapsular cellular reactivity. *Trans Am Ophthalmol Soc.* 2000;98:257–283.

Badr IA, Hussain HM, Jabak M, Wagoner MD. Extracapsular cataract extraction with or without posterior chamber intraocular lenses in eyes with cataract and high myopia. *Ophthalmology.* 1995;102(8):1139–1143.

Behrendt S, Giess L, Duncker G. Incidence of retinal detachment after treatment with the Nd:YAG laser. *Fortschr Ophthalmol.* 1991;88(6):809–811.
Boyce JF, Bhermi GS, Spalton DJ, El-Osta AR. Mathematical modeling of the forces between an intraocular lens and the capsule. *J Cataract Refract Surg.* 2002;28(10):1853–1859.
Hoffer KJ. Hoffer barrier ridge concept [letter]. *J Cataract Refract Surg.* 2007;33(7):1142–1143; author reply 1143.
Keenan T, Rosen P, Yeates D, Goldacre M. Time trends and geographical variation in cataract surgery rates in England: study of surgical workload. *Br J Ophthalmol.* 2007;91(7):901–904.
Nagamoto T, Fujiwara T. Inhibition of lens epithelial cell migration at the intraocular lens optic edge: role of capsule bending and contact pressure. *J Cataract Refract Surg.* 2003; 29(8):1605–1612.

Optical Considerations for Intraocular Lenses

Intraocular Lens Power Calculation

In IOL power calculation, a formula is used that requires accurate biometric measurements of the eye, the visual *axial length (AL),* and the *central corneal power (K).* The desired "target" postoperative refraction and the effective position of the IOL *(effective lens position [ELP])* are added to these factors for use in power calculation. Some surgeons target a slightly myopic result, which allows for some degree of near vision and reduces the possibility of a postoperative hyperopic refractive surprise.

Power prediction formulas

Intraocular lens power prediction formulas are divided into 3 overlapping categories: regression formulas, theoretical formulas, and artificial intelligence formulas. Regression formulas are those that model empiric data by means of a mathematical strategy such as linear regression. The best known regression formulas are the SRK formulas (Sanders, Retzlaff, Kraff [SRK] formulas I and II). Popular in the 1980s, regression formulas were simple to employ but performed poorly, particularly for short and long axial lengths.

In the 1990s, regression formulas were largely supplanted by more accurate theoretical formulas based on ray-tracing calculations. These calculations took the Gullstrand model eye (see Chapter 3) as a starting point and treated the IOL as an idealized thin lens.

An example of a simple geometric optics–based theoretical formula for IOL power calculation is shown below. The pseudophakic eye can be modeled as a 2-element optical system (Fig 7-5). Using Gaussian reduction equations (see Chapter 1), the IOL power that produces emmetropia may be given by

$$P = \frac{n_V}{AL - C} - \frac{K}{1 - K \times \frac{C}{n_A}}$$

where

P = power of the target IOL (in diopters [D])
n_V = index of refraction of the vitreous

AL = visual axial length (in meters)
$C = ELP$ (in meters), the distance from the anterior corneal surface to the principal plane of the IOL
K = average dioptric power of the central cornea
n_A = index of refraction of the aqueous

Further advances to theoretical IOL calculation formulas aimed to refine the effective lens position (ELP) by incorporating additional biometric parameters. Depending upon the formula employed, theoretical formulas require, in addition to axial length and keratometry, anterior chamber depth, lens thickness, white-to-white measure (nasal-temporal limbus to limbus), and even patient age. The surgeon must be aware that dense corneal arcus may be misinterpreted by the biometer as the corneal limbus; if this occurs, the inaccurately small white-to-white measure obtained will produce a faulty *ELP*, and thus an inaccurate IOL calculation.

The 2010s saw a return to empiric data modeling reminiscent of early regression formulas. New, sophisticated artificial intelligence (AI) techniques allowed the modeling of empiric data rather than simple linear regression. The most popular of these early AI formulas was the Hill Radial Basis Function formula (Hill RBF). The Hill RBF employs a machine-learning technique and is especially adept at IOL calculation for eyes of unusual axial length. The performance of the Hill RBF rivals the outcomes achieved with newer theoretical formulas, such as the Barrett Universal II.

The latest and, at the time of publishing, best-performing IOL formulas combine both theoretical and AI approaches. The Kane formula, developed in 2017, combines all 3 approaches of regression, theoretical optics, and AI based upon 30,000 empiric data points, and is a highly accurate means of IOL calculation.

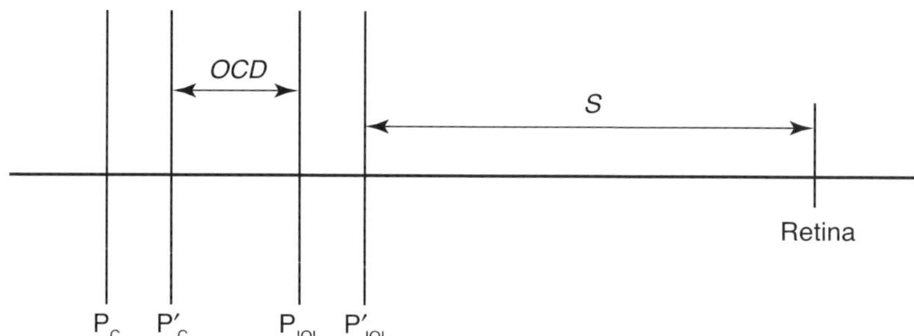

Figure 7-5 Schematic eye. P_C and P'_C are the front and back principal planes of the cornea, respectively. Similarly, P_{IOL} and P'_{IOL} are the front and back principal planes of the intraocular lens (IOL). *OCD* = optical chapter depth and represents a mathematical construct of this simplified model and is not identical to the anatomical anterior chamber depth; *S* = distance between back principal plane of the IOL and retina. (Drawing is not to scale.) *(Redrawn by C. H. Wooley.)*

Biometric formula requirements

Axial length The *AL* is the most important factor in these formulas. A 1-mm error in *AL* measurement results in a refractive error of approximately 2.35 D in a 23.5-mm eye. The refractive error declines to only 1.75 D/mm in a 30-mm eye but rises to 3.75 D/mm in a

20-mm eye. Therefore, accuracy in *AL* measurement is more important in short eyes than in long eyes.

ULTRASONIC MEASUREMENT OF AXIAL LENGTH When *A-scan ultrasonography* is used to measure *AL*, the practitioner either assumes a constant ultrasound velocity through the entire eye or measures each of the various ocular structures at its individual velocity. A-scans measure not distance but rather the time required for a sound pulse to travel from the cornea to the retina and back again. Sound travels faster through the crystalline lens and the cornea (1641 m/s) than it does through aqueous and vitreous (1532 m/s). Even within the lens itself, the speed of sound can vary in different layers and is altered by nuclear sclerosis.

The average velocity through a phakic eye of normal length is 1555 m/s; however, it rises to 1560 m/s for a short (20-mm) eye and drops to 1550 m/s for a long (30-mm) eye. This variation is due to the presence of the crystalline lens; 1554 m/s is an accurate value for an aphakic eye of any length.

The following formula can be used to easily correct any *AL* measured with an incorrect average velocity:

$$AL_C = AL_M \times \frac{V_C}{V_M}$$

where AL_C is the *AL* value at the correct velocity, AL_M is the resultant *AL* value at the incorrect velocity, V_C is the correct velocity, and V_M is the incorrect velocity.

In eyes with *AL* values greater than 25 mm, *staphyloma* should be suspected, especially when numerous disparate readings are obtained. Such errors occur because the macula is located either at the deepest part of the staphyloma or very near it, "on the side of the hill." To measure such eyes and obtain the true measurement to the fovea, the patient must fixate on the light in the center of the A-scan probe. If such a lighted probe is unavailable or if the patient is unable to fixate upon it, the clinician must use a *B-scan technique*. Optical methods (eg, IOLMaster, Lenstar) are very useful in these cases (see the following section, "Optical Measurement of Axial Length").

When ultrasonography is used to measure the *AL* in a *biphakic* eye (ie, a phakic IOL in a phakic eye), it is difficult to eliminate the effect of the sound velocity through the implanted phakic lens. To correct for this potential error, one can use the following published formula:

$$AL_{corrected} = AL_{1555} + C \times T$$

where

AL_{1555} = the measured *AL* of the eye at a sound velocity of 1555 m/s
C = the material-specific correction factor, which is +0.42 for PMMA, −0.59 for silicone, +0.11 for Collamer, and +0.23 for acrylic
T = the central thickness of the implanted phakic IOL

Published tables list the central thickness of phakic IOLs available on the market (for each dioptric power). The least degree of error (in terms of *AL* error) is associated with use of a very thin myopic Collamer lens, and the greatest amount of error is associated with use of a thick hyperopic silicone lens.

The primary A-scan techniques—*applanation* (contact) and *immersion* (noncontact)—often give different results (Figs 7-6, 7-7). Although the immersion method is accepted as the more accurate of the 2 techniques, it is more difficult to perform and less widely employed than the applanation method. The applanation method is susceptible to artificially shortened *AL* measurement because of inadvertent corneal indentation.

OPTICAL MEASUREMENT OF AXIAL LENGTH Optical biometry uses a partial coherence laser for *AL* measurement (Fig 7-8). In a manner analogous to ultrasonography, an optical biometer indirectly measures the time required for infrared light to travel to the retina. Because light travels at too high a speed to be measured directly, light interference methodology (interferometry) is used to determine the transit time and thus the *AL*. This technique does not require contact with the globe, so corneal compression artifacts are eliminated. The optical biometer was developed such that its readings would be equivalent to those of the immersion ultrasound technique. Because this device requires the patient to fixate on a target, the length measured is the path the light takes to the fovea: the "visual" *AL*. The ocular media must be clear enough to allow voluntary fixation and light transmission. Thus, in the 5%–8% of cataract patients with dense cataracts (especially posterior subcapsular cataracts), ultrasound biometry is still necessary. Compared with ultrasonography, this technique provides more accurate, reproducible *AL* measurements. In addition, optical measurement is ideal in 2 clinical situations that are difficult to achieve using ultrasonography: eyes with staphyloma and eyes filled with silicone oil, although such measurements require adjustment.

If removal of the silicone oil is not intended, additional optical accommodations must be made. Because of the element of reduced vergence (see Chapter 1) introduced by a medium of a different refractive index, IOL power must be increased to achieve the intended refractive target. This problem is further compounded by the decreased refractive power achieved at the interface between the posterior surface of the IOL and the silicone oil. When these elements are not considered, Grinbaum and colleagues demonstrated that patients exhibit a mean postoperative hyperopic surprise of close to 4.00 D. This hyperopic shift may be minimized by avoiding the use of IOLs with convex posterior surfaces.

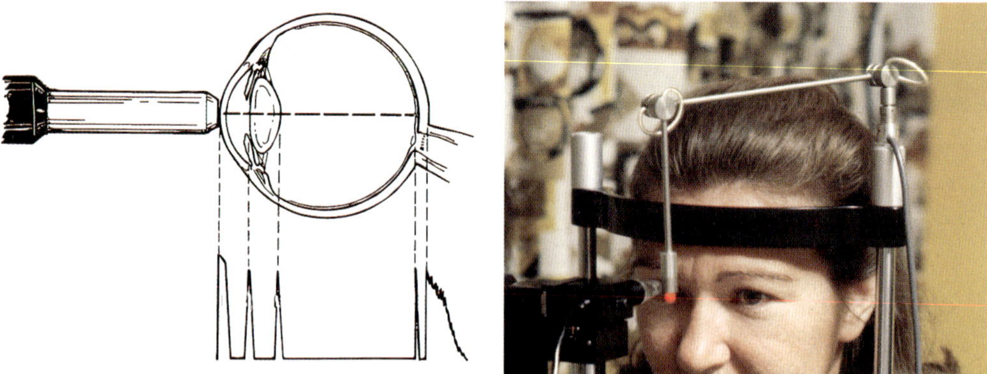

Figure 7-6 In applanation ultrasonography, the probe must contact the cornea, which causes corneal depression and shortening of the axial length reading. *(Courtesy of Kenneth J. Hoffer, MD.)*

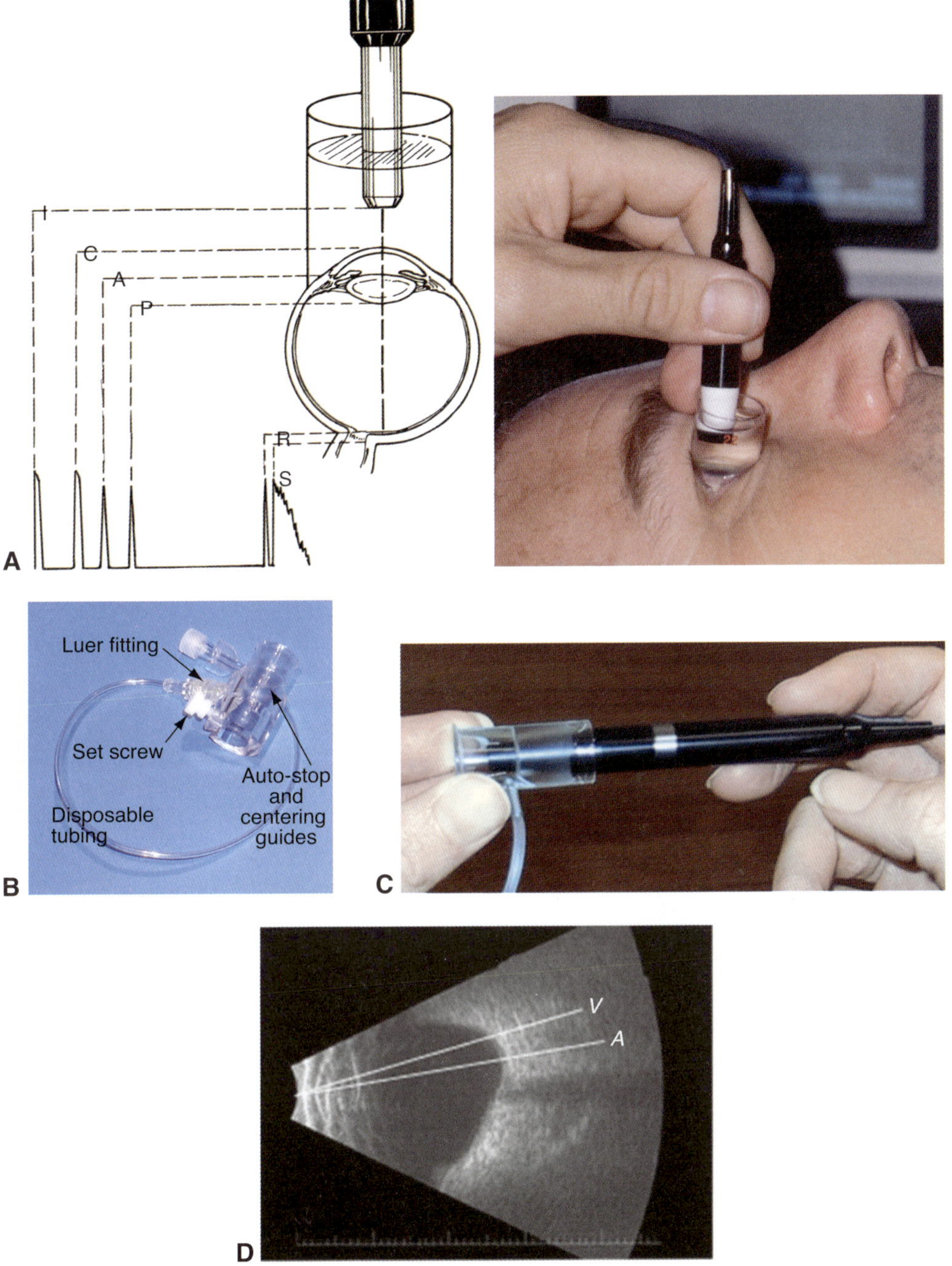

Figure 7-7 Ultrasonography techniques. **A,** In immersion ultrasonography, the probe is immersed in the solution; it does not touch the cornea. **B,** Prager shell for immersion A-scan. **C,** Ultrasound probe and Kohn shell. **D,** B-scan of an eye with staphyloma, showing the difference between the anatomical length *(A)* and the visual length *(V)*. *(Courtesy of Kenneth J. Hoffer, MD.)*

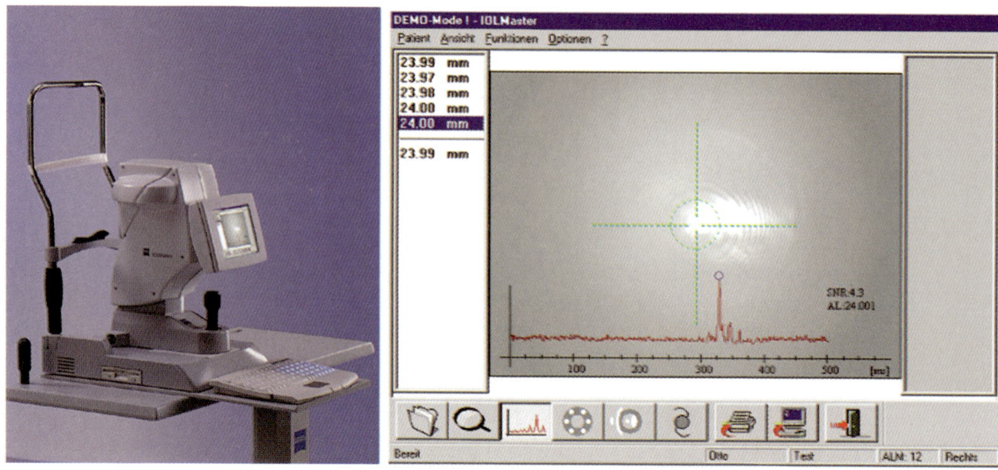

Figure 7-8 An optical biometer *(left)* and view of the instrument's axial length screen *(right)*. *(Courtesy of Kenneth J. Hoffer, MD.)*

Dong J, Tang M, Zhang Y, et al. Comparison of anterior segment biometric measurements between Pentacam HR and IOLMaster in normal and high myopic eyes. *PLoS One.* 2015;10(11):e0143110.

Freeman G, Pesudovs K. The impact of cataract severity on measurement acquisition with the IOLMaster. *Acta Ophthalmol Scand.* 2005;83(4):439–442.

Grinbaum A, Treister G, Moisseiev J. Predicted and actual refraction after intraocular lens implantation in eyes with silicone oil. *J Cataract Refract Surg.* 1996;22(6):726–729.

Corneal power The central corneal power, *K*, is the second most important factor in the calculation formula; a 1.00 D error in corneal power causes a 1.00 D postoperative refractive error. Corneal power can be estimated by keratometry or corneal topography, neither of which measures corneal power directly. The standard manual keratometer (Fig 7-9) measures only a small central portion (3.2-mm diameter ring) of the cornea and views the cornea as a convex mirror. The corneal radius of curvature can be calculated from the size of the reflected image. Both front and back corneal surfaces contribute to corneal power, but the keratometer power "reading" is based on measurement of the radius of curvature of only the front surface and assumptions about the posterior surface.

Conventional Placido disk corneal topographers provide measurement over a larger area of the corneal surface. However, like keratometers, these corneal topographers are limited to measurement of the anterior curvature of the cornea. Scheimpflug camera devices measure both the anterior and posterior curvatures and can provide optical pachymetry values as well. Originally employed in the 19th century to correct for distortion in military aerial photographs, the Scheimpflug principle allows for the isolation of an oblique focal plane through an object. By rotating one or more Scheimpflug cameras about a cornea, 3-dimensional data are captured (see Chapter 9).

Special attention must be paid to contact lens wearers. Contact lens wear can transiently mold the cornea and result in inaccurate keratometry measurements. This molding can influence both astigmatic measurement as well as spherical power. A 2018 study

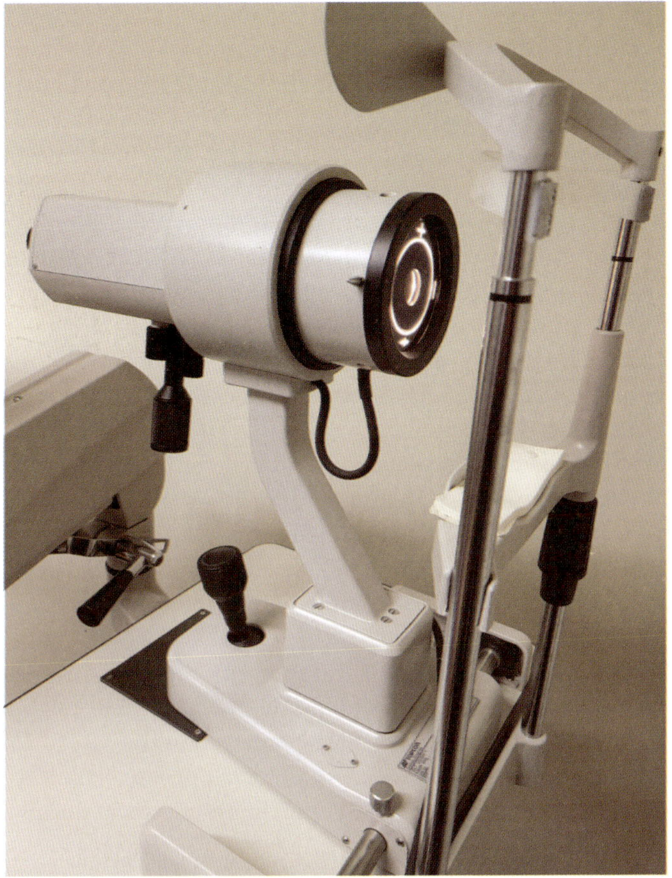

Figure 7-9 Manual keratometer. *(Courtesy of Joshua Young, MD.)*

demonstrated that a contact lens wear hiatus before biometery resulted in a different spherical IOL power in more than half of the participating patients.

Effective lens position All theoretical formulas require an estimation of the distance at which the principal plane of the IOL will be situated behind the cornea—a factor now known as the *ELP.* Initially, most IOLs were either anterior chamber or prepupillary IOLs. Thus, in the original theoretical formulas, this factor was called the *anterior chamber depth (ACD),* and it was a constant value (usually 2.8 or 3.5 mm). This value became incorporated in the *A* constant of the regression formulas of the 1980s.

In 1983, using pachymetry studies of posterior chamber IOLs as a basis, Hoffer introduced an *ACD* prediction formula for posterior chamber lenses that was based on the eye's *AL:*

$$ACD = 0.293 \times AL - 2.92$$

Effective lens position is a mathematical construct that is valuable for calculating IOL power. However, it must be remembered that *ELP* is simply a mathematical parameter and does not actually describe the real anatomical position of either the IOL or the patient's crystalline lens. The purpose of this parameter is to improve the accuracy of IOL calculation and not to describe the patient's anatomy, and so the noncorrespondence of *ELP* to anatomical lens position is not of clinical relevance when employing these formulas.

The most accurate way to measure the preoperative *ACD* or the postoperative *ELP* is by optical means, using scanning slit topography, Scheimpflug imaging, or optical interferometry. Ultrasonography is usually less precise and provides a shorter reading.

Most formulas use only one constant, such as the *ACD*, the *A* constant, or the *surgeon factor (SF)*. The *A* constant, developed as a result of regression formulas, was widely used in the 1980s, so much so that manufacturers assigned each lens design a specific *A* constant, as well as an *ACD* value. Even though regression formulas (eg, the SRK formula) are no longer recommended and rarely used for IOL calculation, the *A* constants are still provided for this purpose.

It is prudent to calculate the power of an alternate IOL before surgery. If not calculated in advance, the power of an IOL intended for bag placement can be decreased for sulcus placement with subtraction depending on the IOL power (Table 7-1). Reduction of IOL power is not necessary if the surgeon places a 3-piece IOL such that the haptics are in the sulcus and the optic is "buttonholed" into the capsular bag ("optic capture" technique).

Careful attention to avoiding IOL tilt is important, especially in cases of sutured-in IOLs. Such tilt will induce astigmatism of oblique incidence. For plus-power IOLs, the induced astigmatism will be of with-the-rule orientation in the case of a lens tilted about the horizontal axis and against-the-rule astigmatism in the case of an IOL tilted about the vertical axis. The opposite holds true for the much less common minus-powered IOLs.

Li X, Zhou Y, Young CA, Chen A, Jin G, Zheng D. Comparison of a new anterior segment optical coherence tomography and Oculus Pentacam for measurement of anterior chamber depth and corneal thickness. *Ann Transl Med.* 2020;8(14):857.

Millar ER, Allen D, Steel DH. Effect of anterior capsulorhexis optic capture of a sulcus-fixated intraocular lens on refractive outcomes. *J Cataract Refract Surg.* 2013;39(6):841–844.

Savini G, Hoffer KJ, Lombardo M, Serrao S, Schiano-Lomoriello D, Ducoli P. Influence of the effective lens position, as predicted by axial length and keratometry, on the near add power of multifocal intraocular lenses. *J Cataract Refract Surg.* 2016;42(1):44–49.

Formula choice

The initial decision the surgeon must face is whether to use a formula built into the biometer or whether to use an internet or software calculator. Although internet-based tools

Table 7-1 IOL Power Adjustment for Sulcus Placement

IOL Power Calculated for In-the-Bag Placement	Power Adjustment for Sulcus Placement
+28.50 D to +30.00 D	Subtract 1.50 D
+17.50 D to +28.00 D	Subtract 1.00 D
+9.50 D to +17.00 D	Subtract 0.50 D
+5.00 D to +9.00 D	No change

may be more accurate, they are vulnerable to transcription errors; when the practitioner views the results, attention must be paid that biometry values have been entered correctly. Earlier theoretical formulas tended to perform best within certain ranges of axial lengths. Newer theoretical formulas, such as Barrett Universal II; AI-based formulas such as Hill RBF; and hybrid theoretical-AI formulas, such as Kane, demonstrate excellent performance over a wide range of axial lengths.

The choice of formula is, of course, up to the surgeon, but whatever the method, every effort should be made to ensure that the biometry is as accurate as possible. The operating surgeon should review preoperative *AL* values and *K* readings. If a reading is suspect because it lies outside normal limits, biometry should be repeated during or immediately after the initial reading. Similarly, it is prudent to measure both eyes and recheck the readings if there is a large discrepancy between the 2 eyes. Great care should be taken in the measurement of eyes that have undergone previous refractive surgery (corneal procedures or placement of a phakic IOL) as well as those that have undergone an encircling band procedure for repair of retinal detachment.

Abulafia A, Barrett GD, Rotenberg M, et al. Intraocular lens power calculation for eyes with an axial length greater than 26.0 mm: comparison of formulas and methods. *J Cataract Refract Surg.* 2015;41(3):548–556.

Aristodemou P, Knox Cartwright NE, Sparrow JM, Johnston RL. Formula choice: Hoffer Q, Holladay 1, or SRK/T and refractive outcomes in 8108 eyes after cataract surgery with biometry by partial coherence interferometry. *J Cataract Refract Surg.* 2011;37(1):63–71.

Cooke DL, Cooke TL. Comparison of 9 intraocular lens power calculation formulas. *J Cataract Refract Surg.* 2016;42(8):1157–1164.

Intraocular Lens Power Calculation After Corneal Refractive Surgery

Intraocular lens power calculation is a problem in eyes that have undergone *radial keratotomy (RK)* or laser corneal refractive procedures. The difficulty stems from 3 sources of errors: (1) instrument error, (2) index of refraction error, and (3) formula error.

Instrument Error

Instrument error was first described by Douglas Koch in 1989. The instruments used by ophthalmologists to measure corneal power (keratometers and corneal topographers) cannot obtain accurate measurements in eyes that have undergone corneal refractive surgery. These instruments often miss the central, flatter zone of effective corneal power. The flatter the cornea is, the larger the zone of measurement is, and the greater the error. Placido disk topography is susceptible to similar errors and usually overestimates the central corneal power, leading to a postoperative hyperopic refractive surprise in myopic eyes. Emerging technologies based on direct anatomical analysis of the cornea (Scheimpflug and computer modeling techniques) may offer a truer measure of corneal central power.

Index of Refraction Error

The assumed index of refraction (IR) of the normal cornea is based on the relationship between the anterior and posterior corneal curvatures. This relationship changes in eyes treated with ablative laser procedures. Ophthalmologists long believed that IR error did not occur in eyes that have undergone RK; this misconception leads to an overestimation of the corneal power by approximately 1.00 D for every 7.00 D of correction obtained and results in hyperopic refractive surprise. A recent study showed that in eyes treated with RK, there is greater flattening of the posterior curvature than of the anterior curvature. Both manual keratometers and computerized corneal topographers that measure only the front surface curvature convert the radius of curvature *(r)* obtained to diopters (D), usually by using an IR value of 1.3375. The following formula can be used to convert diopters to radius:

$$r = \frac{337.5}{\mathrm{D}}$$

To convert *r* to D, use

$$\mathrm{D} = \frac{337.5}{r}$$

Formula Error

Flatter-than-normal *K* values for eyes that have undergone myopic refractive surgery tend to cause errors in *ELP* because the anterior chamber dimensions do not actually change in these eyes commensurately with ablation-induced flattening. These *ELP* errors also tend to result in hyperopic refractive surprise.

Power Calculation Methods for Eyes After a Keratorefractive Procedure

The double-*K* method uses the pre-LASIK corneal power (or, if unknown, 43.50 D) to calculate the *ELP*, and the post-LASIK (much flatter) corneal power to calculate the IOL power. These calculations can be performed automatically with computer programs.

The double-*K* method is only 1 of more than 20 methods proposed over the years either to calculate the true corneal power or to adjust the calculated IOL power to account for the errors discussed in the preceding sections. Some methods require knowledge of pre–refractive surgery values such as refractive error and *K* reading. A definitive strategy has not been determined, and clinical context often dictates the best approach. Generally, formulas can be divided into 3 categories: those that require historical data, such as the corneal-bypass and double-*K* formulas; those that do not require historical data but rely upon a specific biometrical device, such as a particular corneal topographer or Scheimpflug device; and those that require only generically measured biometry.

While methods for IOL power calculation remain imperfect for keratorefractive patients generally, those who have undergone hyperopic ablation are at a particular disadvantage.

Perhaps in the future there will be a more satisfactory method of measuring true corneal power by use of topography and advanced measuring techniques. In the meantime, this remains a fluid field. The American Academy of Cataract and Refractive Surgery maintains a useful resource of multiple current postrefractive formulas on their website, ASCRS.org.

Abulafia A, Hill WE, Koch DD, Wang L, Barrett GD. Accuracy of the Barrett True-K formula for intraocular lens power prediction after laser in situ keratomileusis or photorefractive keratectomy for myopia. *J Cataract Refract Surg.* 2016;42(3):363–369.

Alió JL, Abdelghany AA, Abdou AA, Maldonado MJ. Cataract surgery on the previous corneal refractive surgery patient. *Surv Ophthalmol.* 2016;61(6):769–777.

Francone A, Lemanski N, Charles M, et al. Retrospective comparative analysis of intraocular lens calculation formulas after hyperopic refractive surgery. *PLoS One.* 2019;14(11):e0224981.

Koch DD, Liu JF, Hyde LL, Rock RL, Emery JM. Refractive complications of cataract surgery after radial keratotomy. *Am J Ophthalmol.* 1989;108(6):676–682.

Meyer JJ, Kim MJ, Kim T. Effects of contact lens wear on biometry measurements for intraocular lens calculations. *Eye Contact Lens.* 2018;44(Suppl 1):S255–S258.

Wang L, Koch DD. Intraocular lens power calculations in eyes with previous corneal refractive surgery: review and expert opinion. *Ophthalmology.* 2020;128(11):e121–e131.

Special Consideration: Postoperative Refractive Surprise in Patients Who Have Undergone Myopic Keratorefractive Correction

- Keratometers fail to measure the flattest portion of the cornea. This overestimation of corneal power will result in a hyperopic refractive surprise.
- Keratometers and computerized corneal topographers underestimate the relative contribution of the posterior cornea and therefore overestimate the net corneal refractive index and overall corneal refractive power. This overestimation of corneal power will result in a hyperopic refractive surprise.
- Standard IOL formulas estimate the *ELP* to be too anterior and therefore overestimate the refractive contribution of the IOL. This overestimation of IOL refractive contribution will result in a hyperopic refractive surprise.

Intraocular Lens Power in Corneal Transplant Eyes

Both Descemet stripping endothelial keratoplasty (DSAEK) and Descemet membrane endothelial keratoplasty (DMEK) procedures consist of implantation of additional tissue to the posterior surface of the host cornea. Both procedures change the relationship of the anterior corneal curvature to the posterior curvature in a manner that, if ignored, will yield a hyperopic result if IOL calculation is based solely upon keratometry. Posterior corneal topography can mitigate this hyperopic tendency. Note, however, that cataract surgery often precedes endothelial keratoplasty; if endothelial keratoplasty is likely to follow cataract extraction, a slightly myopic target of –1.50 D to –0.70 D should be chosen.

It is difficult to predict the ultimate power of the cornea after the eye has undergone penetrating keratoplasty. Thus, in 1987 Hoffer recommended that the surgeon wait for the corneal transplant to heal completely before implanting an IOL. The current safety of intraocular surgery allows for such a double-procedure approach in all but the rarest cases.

If simultaneous IOL implantation and corneal transplant are necessary, surgeons may use either the *K* reading of the fellow eye or the average postoperative *K* value of a previous series of transplants, but substantial unintended postoperative refractive errors are common. Viestenz and colleagues have introduced a multiple regression technique, but even employing this, they obtained post–suture removal refractive outcomes of −1.39 ± 2.86 D.

Alnawaiseh M, Zumhagen L, Rosentreter A, Eter N. Intraocular lens power calculation using standard formulas and ray tracing after DMEK in patients with Fuchs endothelial dystrophy. *BMC Ophthalmol.* 2017;17(1):152.

Flowers CW, McLeod SD, McDonnell PJ, Irvine JA, Smith RE. Evaluation of intraocular lens power calculation formulas in the triple procedure. *J Cataract Refract Surg.* 1996;22(1):116–122.

Geggel HS. Intraocular lens implantation after penetrating keratoplasty. Improved unaided visual acuity, astigmatism, and safety in patients with combined corneal disease and cataract. *Ophthalmology.* 1990;97(11):1460–1467.

Hoffer KJ. Triple procedure for intraocular lens exchange. *Arch Ophthalmol.* 1987;105(5): 609–610.

Viestenz A, Seitz B, Langenbucher A. Intraocular lens power prediction for triple procedures in Fuchs' dystrophy using multiple regression analysis. *Acta Ophthalmol Scand.* 2005;83(3): 312–315.

Xu K, Qi H, Peng R, et al. Keratometric measurements and IOL calculations in pseudophakic post-DSAEK patients. *BMC Ophthalmol.* 2018;18(1):268.

Silicone Oil Eyes

Ophthalmologists considering IOL implantation in eyes filled with silicone oil encounter 2 major problems. The first is obtaining an accurate *AL* measurement with the ultrasonic biometer. Recall that this instrument measures the transit time of the ultrasound pulse and, using estimated ultrasound velocities through the various ocular media, calculates the axial length of the eye. This concept must be taken into consideration when velocities differ from the norm, for example, when silicone oil fills the posterior segment (980 m/s for silicone oil vs 1532 m/s for vitreous). Use of optical biometry to measure *AL* solves this problem somewhat. It is recommended that retinal surgeons perform an optical or immersion *AL* measurement before silicone oil placement, but doing so is not common practice. The second problem is that, because the refractive index of silicone oil is greater than that of the vitreous humor, the oil filling the vitreous cavity reduces the optical power of the posterior surface of the IOL in the eye when a biconvex IOL is implanted. This problem must be counteracted by an increase in IOL power of 3.00–5.00 D.

Suk KK, Smiddy WE, Shi W. Refractive outcomes after silicone oil removal and intraocular lens implantation. *Retina.* 2013;33(3):634–641.

Symes RJ. Accurate biometry in silicone oil–filled eyes. *Eye (Lond).* 2013;27(6):778–779.

Pediatric Eyes

Several issues make IOL power selection for children much more complex than for adults. The first challenge is obtaining accurate *AL* and corneal measurements, which is usually performed when the child is under general anesthesia. The second issue is that, because shorter *AL* causes greater IOL power errors, the small size of a child's eye compounds power calculation errors, particularly if the child is very young. The third problem is selecting an appropriate target IOL power, one that will not only provide adequate visual acuity to prevent amblyopia but also allow adequate vision with the expected growth of the eye after the IOL implantation.

Readers are referred to Section 6, *Pediatric Ophthalmology and Strabismus,* for additional information.

Hoffer KJ, Aramberri J, Haigis W, Norrby S, Olsen T, Shammas HJ; IOL Power Club Executive Committee. The final frontier: pediatric intraocular lens power. *Am J Ophthalmol.* 2012;154(1):1–2.e1.

O'Hara MA. Pediatric intraocular lens power calculations. *Curr Opin Ophthalmol.* 2012;23(5):388–393.

Image Magnification

Image magnification of as much as 20%–35% is the major disadvantage of aphakic spectacles. Contact lenses magnify images by only 7%–12%, whereas IOLs magnify images by 4% or less. An IOL implanted in the posterior chamber produces less image magnification than does an IOL in the anterior chamber. The issue of magnification is further complicated by the correction of residual postsurgical refractive errors. A Galilean telescope effect is created when spectacles are worn over pseudophakic eyes. Clinically, each diopter of spectacle overcorrection at a vertex of 12 mm causes a 2% magnification or minification (for plus or minus lenses, respectively). Thus, a pseudophakic patient with a posterior chamber IOL and a residual refractive error of −1.00 D would have 2% magnification from the IOL and 2% minification from the spectacle lens, resulting in little change in image size.

Aniseikonia is defined as a difference in image size between the 2 eyes; it can cause disturbances in stereopsis. Generally, a person can tolerate spherical aniseikonia of 5%–8%. In clinical practice, aniseikonia is rarely a significant problem; however, it should be considered in patients with unexplained vision symptoms.

Gobin L, Rozema JJ, Tassignon MJ. Predicting refractive aniseikonia after cataract surgery in anisometropia. *J Cataract Refract Surg.* 2008;34(8):1353–1361.

Lens-Related Vision Disturbances

The presence of IOLs may cause numerous optical phenomena. Various light-related visual phenomena encountered by pseudophakic (and phakic) patients are termed *dysphotopsias.* These phenomena are divided into positive and negative dysphotopsias, which primarily occur in the patient's temporal visual field and in photopic conditions. Positive dysphotopsias are characterized by brightness, streaks, and rays emanating from a central point source of light, sometimes with a diffuse, hazy glare. Negative dysphotopsias are characterized by subjective darkness or shadowing and are associated with a small pupil, a distance between the pupil and the IOL of 0.06 mm or greater, and a nasal location of the pupil relative to the optical axis. Such optical phenomena may be related to light reflection and refraction oblique to the surface of the IOL. High-index acrylic lenses with square or truncated edges produce a more intense edge glare (Fig 7-10A). These phenomena may also be due to internal re-reflection within the IOL itself; such re-reflection is more likely to occur with materials that have a higher refractive index, such as acrylic (Fig 7-10B). With a less steeply curved anterior surface, the lens may be more likely to have internal reflections that are directed toward the fovea and are therefore more distracting (Fig 7-10 C, D).

Davison JA. Positive and negative dysphotopsia in patients with acrylic intraocular lenses. *J Cataract Refract Surg.* 2000;26(9):1346–1355.

Erie JC, Bandhauer MH. Intraocular lens surfaces and their relationship to postoperative glare. *J Cataract Refract Surg.* 2003;29(2):336–341.

Franchini A, Gallarati BZ, Vaccari E. Computerized analysis of the effects of intraocular lens edge design on the quality of vision in pseudophakic patients. *J Cataract Refract Surg.* 2003;29(2):342–347.

Henderson BA, Geneva II. Negative dysphotopsia: a perfect storm. *J Cataract Refract Surg.* 2015;41(10):2291–2312.

Holladay JT, Zhao H, Reisin CR. Negative dysphotopsia: the enigmatic penumbra. *J Cataract Refract Surg.* 2012;38(7):1251–1265.

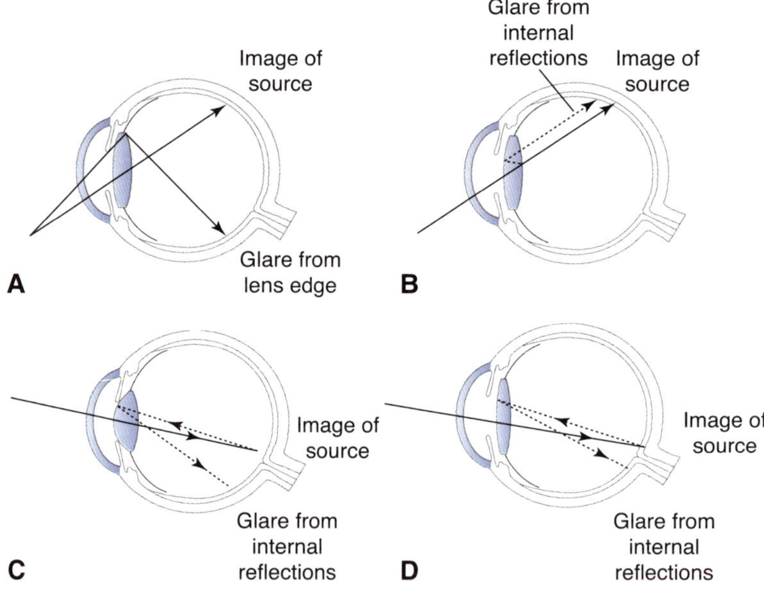

Figure 7-10 Lens-related vision disturbances. IOLs are not drawn to scale. **A,** Light striking the edge of the IOL may be reflected to another site on the retina, resulting in dysphotopsias. These problems arise less often with smoother-edged IOLs. **B,** Light may be internally re-reflected within an IOL, producing an undesirable second image or halo. Such re-reflection may be more likely to occur as the index of refraction of the IOL increases. **C,** Light may reflect back from the surface of the retina and reach the anterior surface of the IOL. The IOL acts as a concave mirror, reflecting back a dysphotopsic image. When the anterior surface of the IOL is more curved, the annoying image is displaced relatively far from the fovea. **D,** When the anterior IOL surface is less steeply curved, the annoying image appears closer to the true image and is likely to be more distracting. *(Redrawn by C. H. Wooley.)*

Nonspherical Optics

IOLs with more complex optical designs are now available. It may be possible to offset the positive spherical aberration of the cornea in a pseudophakic patient by implanting an IOL with the appropriate negative asphericity on its anterior surface. An IOL with a *toric* surface may be used to correct astigmatism. As a toric lens rotates from the optimal desired angular orientation, the benefit of the toric correction diminishes. Misalignment of a toric lens may occur because of excyclotorsion or incyclotorsion of the eye as the patient moves from a vertical position to a recumbent position during surgery. Therefore, it is important to mark the eye for purposes of orientation while the patient is standing or sitting up. For the same reason, optical registration systems obtain their orientation data while the patient is sitting up. A misalignment of only 10° of a properly powered toric IOL reduces its efficacy by 30%, and a misalignment of more than 30° off-axis increases the residual astigmatism of an eye; if it is 90° off-axis, the residual astigmatism doubles. Fortunately, some benefit remains even with lesser degrees of axis error, although the axis of residual cylinder changes. Newer designs are more stable than earlier ones.

Toric IOLs do not correct lenticular astigmatism; moreover, they correct only that portion of corneal astigmatism that is regular. Although toric IOLs may hold benefit for patients with irregular, nonorthogonal, asymmetric, or unstable astigmatism, as may occur with keratoconus, caution should be exercised with the degree of astigmatic correction attempted.

Researchers have developed an IOL in which the optical power can be altered by laser after lens implantation. Similarly, a laser system in development may alter the optical power of a conventional acrylic lens after implantation. These technologies would be useful for correcting both IOL power calculation errors and residual astigmatism.

Mester U, Dillinger P, Anterist N. Impact of a modified optic design on visual function: clinical comparative study. *J Cataract Refract Surg.* 2003;29(4):652–660.

Sahler R, Bille JF, Enright S, Chhoeung S, Chan K. Creation of a refractive lens within an existing intraocular lens using a femtosecond laser. *J Cataract Refract Surg.* 2016;42(8):1207–1215.

Multifocal Intraocular Lenses

Conventional IOLs are *monofocal* and correct the refractive ametropia associated with removal of the crystalline lens. Because a standard IOL has no accommodative power, it provides a clear focus for visual targets at a single distance only. However, the improved visual acuity resulting from IOL implantation may allow a patient to see with acceptable clarity over a range of distances. If the patient is left with a residual refractive error of simple myopic astigmatism, the ability to see with acceptable clarity over a range of distances may be further augmented. In this situation, 1 endpoint of the astigmatic conoid of Sturm corresponds to the distance focus and the other endpoint represents myopia and, thus, a near focus; satisfactory clarity of vision may be possible if the object in view is focused between these 2 endpoints. In bilateral, asymmetric, and oblique myopic astigmatism, the blurred axis images are ignored and the clearest axis images are chosen to form 1 clear image for distance vision; the opposite images are selected for near vision. Thus, even standard IOLs may provide some degree of depth of focus and "bifocal" capabilities.

An alternate approach to this problem is to correct 1 eye for distance and the other for near vision; this approach is called *monovision*—this approach is also used with contact lenses. Nevertheless, the vision of most patients who receive IOLs is corrected for distance, and the recipients wear reading glasses as needed.

Multifocal IOLs are designed to improve both near and distance vision to decrease patients' dependence on glasses. With a multifocal IOL, the correcting lens is placed in a fixed location within the eye, and the patient cannot voluntarily change the focus. Because object rays encounter both the distance and near portions of the optic, both near and far images are presented to the eye at the same time. The brain then processes the clearest image, ignoring the other(s). Most patients, but not all, can adapt to the use of multifocal IOLs.

The performance of certain types of IOLs is greatly impaired by decentration if the visual axis does not pass through the center of the IOL. On the 1 hand, the use of modern surgical techniques generally results in adequate lens centration. Pupil size, on the other hand, is an active variable, but it can be employed in some situations to improve multifocal function. Other disadvantages of multifocal IOLs are image degradation, "ghost" images (or *monocular diplopia*), decreased contrast sensitivity, and reduced performance in lower light (eg, decreased night vision); these phenomena are discussed in Videos 7-1 and 7-2. These potential problems make multifocal IOLs less desirable for use in eyes with established or impending macular disease.

Accuracy of IOL power calculation is very important for multifocal IOLs because their purpose is to reduce the patient's dependence on glasses. Postoperative astigmatism should be low, given that visual acuity and contrast sensitivity are degraded with greater degrees of residual astigmatism.

VIDEO 7-1 Multifocal IOLs.
Courtesy of Mark Packer, MD.

VIDEO 7-2 The optical cost of multifocal IOLs.
Animation developed by Joshua A. Young, MD.

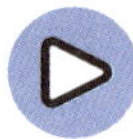

Types of Multifocal Intraocular Lenses

The intraocular lens correction of presbyopia is not comparable to the normal accommodation of a young person. The strategies employed in these IOLs involve trade-offs between visual function and quality of vision. The distinguishing feature between different multifocal lens designs is the way in which this trade-off is made.

Early presbyopia-correcting intraocular lenses were based upon refractive multifocal designs. The first bifocal IOL implanted in a human was a split bifocal invented by Hoffer in 1982 and was implanted in a patient in Santa Monica, California, in 1990. In this simple design, which functioned independently of pupil size, half the optic was focused for distance vision and the other half for near vision (Fig 7-11A). This design was reintroduced in 2010 as the Lentis Mplus (Oculentis). Of course, as with contact lenses, the direction of gaze does not influence the portion of the intraocular lens through which the patient looks. Since the intraocular lens moves with the eye, the image cast on the retina is the product of both the distance and near optical portions of the lens.

Multifocal intraocular lenses gained early popularity with the introduction of refractive designs consisting of multiple concentric annuli. Each annulus would bring into focus either distance or near objects (Fig 7-11B). An example of this design, the AMO

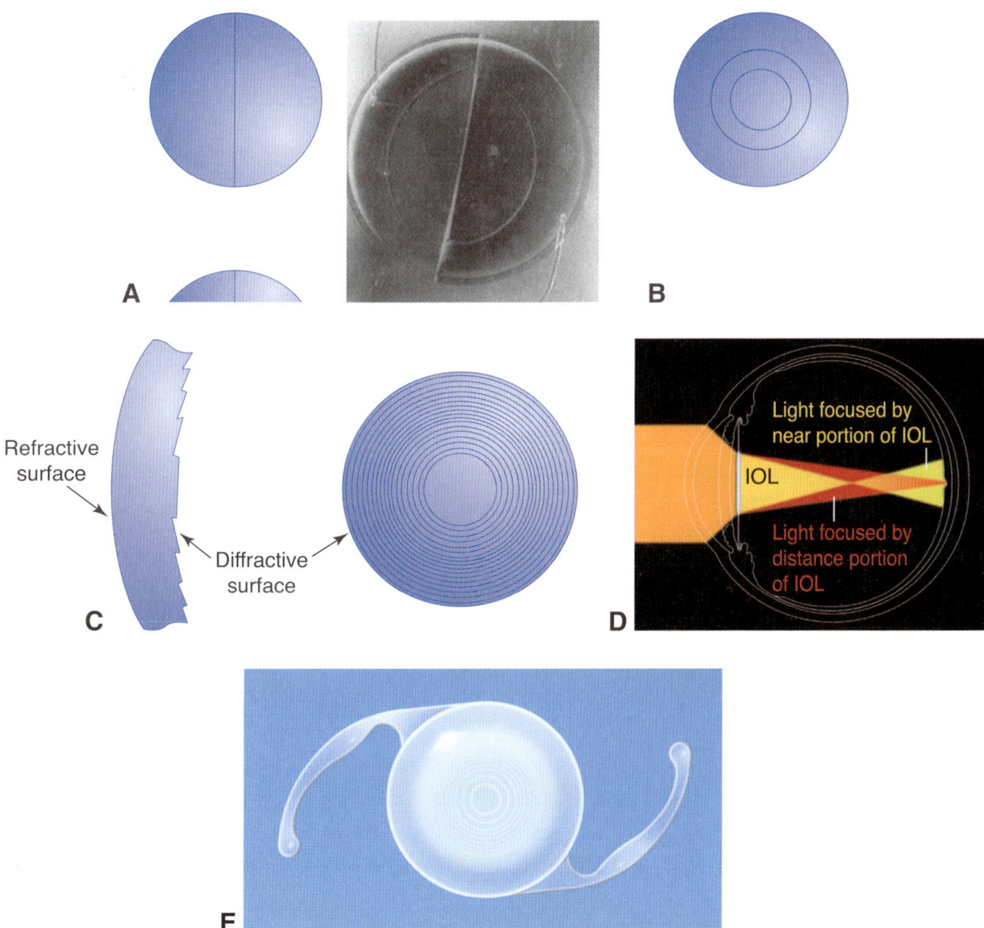

Figure 7-11 Multifocal IOLs. **A,** Hoffer split bifocal IOL *(left)* and an early photograph of a lens implanted in a patient *(right)*. **B,** Three-zone multifocal design. **C,** Diffractive multifocal IOL; the cross section of the central portion is magnified. (The depth of the grooves is exaggerated.) Note that the diffractive element may be on the anterior or posterior aspect of the optic. **D,** Diffractive optics of a multifocal (bifocal) IOL. Note the unfocused light rays hitting the retina, which can contribute to dysphotopsias. **E,** Multifocal IOL. *(Part A photograph courtesy of Kenneth J. Hoffer, MD; part A, B, C illustrations redrawn by C. H. Wooley; part D and E illustrations courtesy of Mark Miller.)*

ReZoom, had a distance zone in the center surrounded by a near annulus and then distance and near annuli, for a total of 6 alternating zones. Although it transmitted rays of light to the retina without any loss, the effectiveness of this design was highly dependent upon pupil size, as a very small pupil would render only distance rays in focus on the retina.

Subsequent multifocal IOL designs introduced a diffractive element, on either the back or front surface of the IOL (Fig 7-11C, D, and E). This diffractive add captures a portion of the incoming rays to produce an image on the retina for near objects. The advantage of this optical strategy is that it is far less pupil-dependent than purely refractive designs. A disadvantage of this strategy is that a portion of the incoming rays of light are lost to destructive interference and are not available for producing either near or distance images.

The design of the diffractive element varies by IOL model. Some lenses have relatively high adds to improve acuity at reading distance, while others have adds appropriate for intermediate or computer distance. In addition to differing in the power of the add, multifocal IOL designs also differ in the percentage of incoming rays diverted to near rather than to distance vision. Some designs devote as much as 50% of rays to produce near vision, while others designate as little as 35%. The implications of these choices are discussed in greater detail below. Although presbyopia-correcting IOLs comprise less than 10% of the US IOL market, there is every reason to believe that these premium lenses will become more important.

Truly accommodating IOLs that can yield the level of accommodation equal to that of the prepresbyopic eye are eagerly hoped for, but no such lenses are currently available. The United States Food and Drug Administration (FDA) has approved 1 design that has shown some degree of accommodation, and other designs are awaiting FDA approval. However, currently, there is no clinical evidence that "accommodating" IOLs change axial position in the eye during near-vision tasks.

Clinical Results of Multifocal Intraocular Lenses

Some multifocal IOLs are designed to perform better for near vision; others, for intermediate. The performance targets of different multifocal IOLs are discussed in the following section, Modulation Transfer Function.

The best-corrected visual acuity (also called *corrected distance visual acuity*) may be worse with a multifocal IOL than with a monofocal IOL and this disparity is even greater in low-light situations. However, the need for additional spectacle correction for near vision is greatly reduced in patients with multifocal IOLs. Some patients are quite pleased with multifocal IOLs; others request their removal and replacement with monofocal IOLs. Interestingly, patients with a multifocal IOL in 1 eye and a monofocal IOL in the other often seem to be less tolerant of the multifocal IOLs than are patients with bilateral multifocal IOLs.

Patient selection is crucial for successful adaptation to multifocal IOLs. Patients must be willing to accept the trade-off—particularly in low-light situations—between decreased performance for distance vision (and for near vision, compared with that of a monofocal

IOL and reading glasses) and the possibility of seeing well enough at all distances to be able to dispense with spectacles altogether. Patients with low contrast-sensitivity function potential, such as those affected by glaucoma, retinal dystrophies, macular disease, and advanced age, should be considered poor candidates for multifocal IOL implantation.

Altinkurt E, Muftuoglu O. Comparison of three different diffractive multifocal intraocular lenses with a +2.5, +3.0, and +3.75 diopter addition power. *Saudi J Ophthalmol.* 2019;33(4): 353–362.

Cumming JS, Colvard DM, Dell SJ, et al. Clinical evaluation of the Crystalens AT-45 accommodating intraocular lens: results of the U.S. Food and Drug Administration clinical trial. *J Cataract Refract Surg.* 2006;32(5):812–825.

Dhital A, Spalton DJ, Gala KB. Comparison of near vision, intraocular lens movement, and depth of focus with accommodating and monofocal intraocular lenses. *J Cataract Refract Surg.* 2013;39(12):1872–1878.

Findl O, Kiss B, Petternel V, et al. Intraocular lens movement caused by ciliary muscle contraction. *J Cataract Refract Surg.* 2003;29(4):669–676.

Kohl JC, Werner L, Ford JR, et al. Long-term uveal and capsular biocompatibility of a new accommodating intraocular lens. *J Cataract Refract Surg.* 2014;40(12):2113–2119.

Langenbucher A, Huber S, Nguyen NX, Seitz B, Gusek-Schneider GC, Küchle M. Measurement of accommodation after implantation of an accommodating posterior chamber intraocular lens. *J Cataract Refract Surg.* 2003;29(4):677–685.

Matthews MW, Eggleston HC, Hilmas GE. Development of a repeatedly adjustable intraocular lens. *J Cataract Refract Surg.* 2003;29(11):2204–2210.

Matthews MW, Eggleston HC, Pekarek SD, Hilmas GE. Magnetically adjustable intraocular lens. *J Cataract Refract Surg.* 2003;29(11):2211–2216.

Sachdev GS, Sachdev M. Optimizing outcomes with multifocal intraocular lenses. *Indian J Ophthalmol.* 2017;65(12):1294–1300.

Modulation Transfer Function

In order to understand the trade-offs between different multifocal lens designs, an objective measure must be employed. This objective measure is the modulation transfer function (MTF), which describes the contrast of sinusoidal patterns as they pass through an optical system. The MTF is mathematically related to the point spread function, a parameter used when discussing wavefront aberrations. In the context of IOLs, the MTF describes contrast degradation as images are processed by the pseudophakic eye as well as the cutoff spatial frequency beyond which fine detail will not be resolved. MTF data are generally presented in the form of a graph in which the MTF for a particular wavelength and spatial frequency is shown over diopters of defocus or over distance. A reasonable simplification would be to understand these graphs as describing an IOL's performance over a range of distances. MTF patterns are specific to both the spatial frequency of the sinusoidal pattern (eg, the number of light and dark bands per centimeter) and to the pupil size.

It is important for the surgeon to be able to evaluate differences in IOL designs by their respective MTF curves. Bifocal IOLs demonstrate 2 distinct peaks in their MTF curves, 1 at distance and 1 at a near focal point that differs depending on IOL design. Trifocal IOLs demonstrate 3 peaks of varying heights.

The area under the MTF curve represents the total light employed in imaging. This is always less than the total amount of light entering the eye because of absorption and, in the case of diffractive IOLs, destructive interference. The area under the MTF curve can be thought of as a photon budget; different IOLs spend this budget differently. Bifocal IOLs with higher near peaks can only improve MTF at near at the expense of distance MTF. This is clearly demonstrated in the comparison of the MTF curves of a monofocal, a low-add bifocal, and a high-add bifocal IOL (Fig 7-12). It should be apparent that none of the multifocal IOLs has a distance vision peak as high as that of the monofocal IOL. This decrease in MTF is illustrated visually in the degradation of contrast for higher spatial frequencies with USAF (United States Air Force) target images (Fig 7-13).

MTF is useful for comparing conventional multifocal IOLs to extended-depth-of-focus (EDOF) lenses. A common feature of bifocal and trifocal IOLs is the very low MTF between the focal peaks, representing poor visual performance between the distance and near peaks. The MTF curves of EDOF lenses do not have a precipitous drop between peaks and therefore demonstrate better performance at focal lengths between distance and near (see Fig 7-12). However, it is important to remember that the total area under the MTF curve is not increased in EDOF lenses and that the improvement in intermediate vision necessarily comes at the expense of performance at the peak focal distances.

Artigas JM, Menezo JL, Peris C, Felipe A, Díaz-Llopis M. Image quality with multifocal intraocular lenses and the effect of pupil size: comparison of refractive and hybrid refractive-diffractive designs. *J Cataract Refract Surg.* 2007;33(12):2111–2117.

Carson D, Hill WE, Hong X, Karakelle M. Optical bench performance of AcrySof® IQ ReSTOR®, AT LISA®tri, and FineVision® intraocular lenses. *Clin Ophthalmol.* 2014;8: 2105–2113.

Esteve-Taboada JJ, Domínguez-Vicent A, Del Águila-Carrasco AJ, Ferrer-Blasco T, Montés-Micó R. Effect of large apertures on the optical quality of three multifocal lenses. *J Refract Surg.* 2015;31(10):666–676.

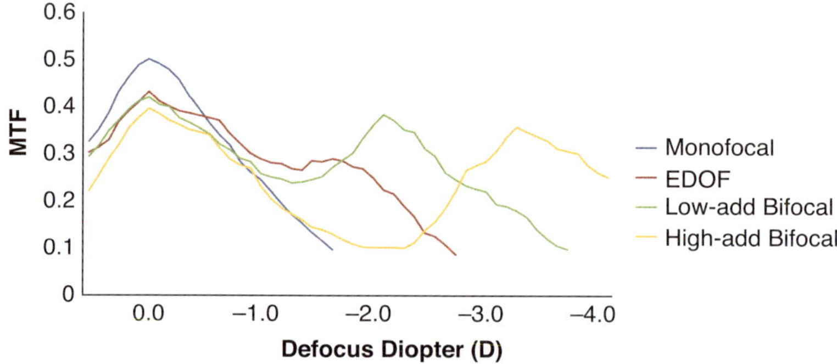

Figure 7-12 Through-focus modulation transfer function (MTF) of 4 different IOLs. This measurement was done for a 3-mm artificial pupil and a spatial frequency of 14.81 cycles/degree. EDOF = extended depth of focus. *Yoo YS, Whang WJ, Byun Ys, et al. Through-focus optical bench performance of extended-depth-of-focus and bifocal intraocular lenses compared to a monofocal lens.* J Refract Surg. *2018;34(4):236–243. doi:10.3928/1081597X-20180206-04. Reprinted with permission from SLACK Incorporated.*

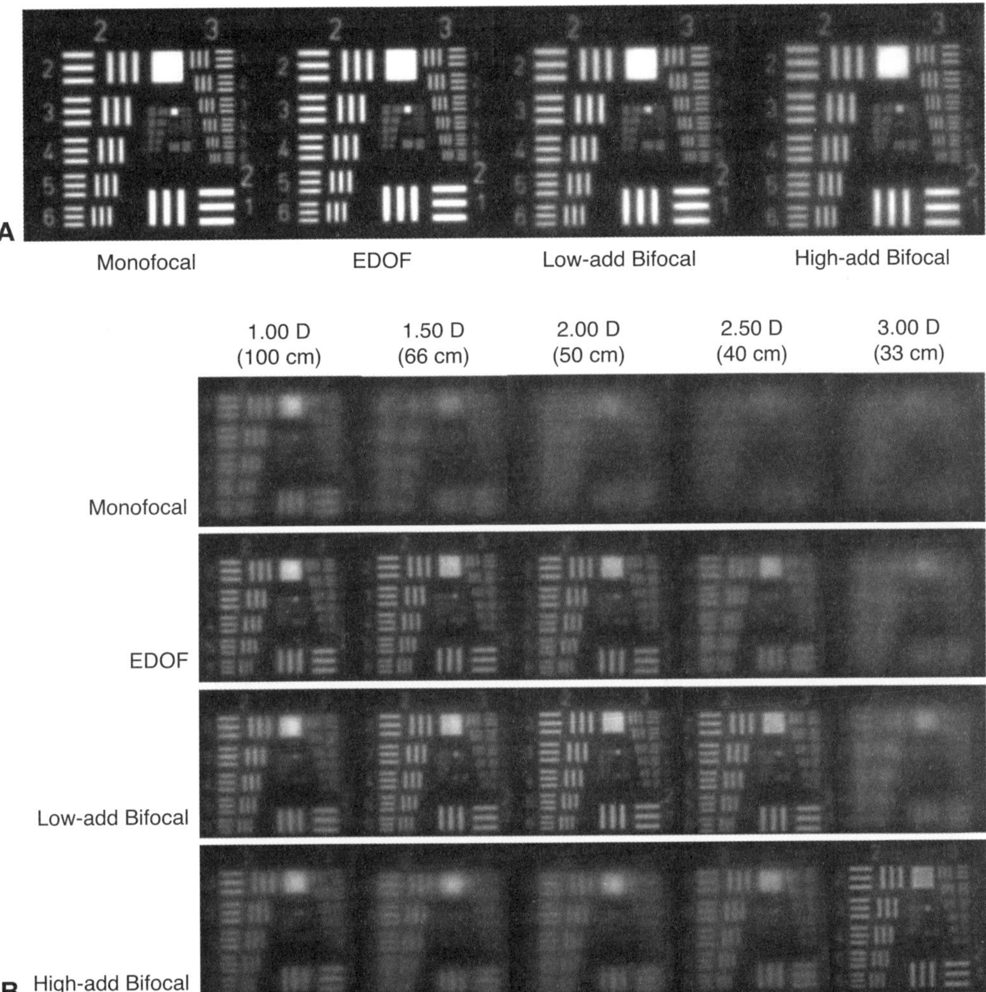

Figure 7-13 Representative 1951 United States Air Force (USAF) target images for the 4 different intraocular lenses. **A,** Imaged at far distance. **B,** Imaged between intermediate and near distance with 0.50 diopters (D) of defocus. All images were measured using a 3-mm artificial pupil. The far distance was defined as the camera position at which the image quality of the bar in the USAF target, corresponding to 20/20 Snellen visual acuity, was peak. EDOF = extended depth of focus. *Yoo YS, Whang WJ, Byun Ys, et al. Through-focus optical bench performance of extended-depth-of-focus and bifocal intraocular lenses compared to a monofocal lens.* J Refract Surg. *2018;34(4):236–243. doi:10.3928/1081597X-20180206-04 Reprinted with permission from SLACK Incorporated.*

Intraocular Lens Standards

The American National Standards Institute (ANSI) and the International Standards Organization (ISO) set standards for IOLs. Among these standards is one for IOL power labeling; it requires that IOLs with powers labeled as less than 25.00 D be within ±0.40 D of the labeled power and have no axial-power variations of more than 0.25 D. IOLs labeled 25.00–30.00 D must be within ±0.50 D of the labeled power, and those labeled greater than 30.00 D must be within ±1.00 D. Most ophthalmologists are unaware of this wide range allowed for the labeling of high-power IOLs. Although controversial, attempts are being made to narrow this allowed range so that all IOL powers would be within ±0.25 D of the labeled powers. Actual mislabeling of IOL power is rare but still occurs.

In addition to the labeling standards, the ANSI, ISO, and FDA have set various other IOL standards for *optical performance,* a term that refers broadly to the image quality produced by an IOL. Lenses are also tested for biocompatibility, the absence of cytotoxicity of their material, the presence of any additives (such as ultraviolet filters), genotoxicity, and photostability, as well as for their safety with YAG lasers. There are also standards for spectral transmission. Physical standards exist to ensure adherence to the labeled optic diameter, haptic angulation, strength, and mechanical fatigability of the components, as well as to ensure sterility and safety during injection.

Chapter Exercises

Questions

7.1. *Error in sound velocity.* An ophthalmologist discovers that a measured axial length (*AL*) was taken using an incorrect *AL*. What should be the next course of action?
   a. The patient should be scheduled for a return visit and the ultrasound repeated using the correct sound velocity.
   b. A simple correction factor can be added algebraically to the incorrect *AL* value.
   c. The incorrect *AL* is likely due to an incorrect velocity. The incorrect *AL* can be corrected by dividing the *AL* by the incorrect velocity and multiplying by the correct velocity.
   d. The sound velocity is so negligible that it does not need to be corrected.

7.2. The optical performance of monofocal, bifocal, and extended-depth-of-focus (EDOF) IOLs necessarily differ in which way?
   a. the acuities they produce at distance
   b. the chromatic aberration induced
   c. the contrast degradation induced at distance
   d. the degree of accommodation each exhibits *(ELP)*

7.3. Which statement is the most characteristic of multifocal IOLs?
   a. They offer increased image clarity and contrast for both near and far viewing.
   b. They are independent of pupil size if they are well centered.
   c. They offer a trade-off between decreased image quality and increased depth of focus.
   d. They are indicated for all patients.

7.4. Which statement applies to piggyback IOLs?
   a. Piggyback IOLs modify the vergence of light entering the eye after it exits the incorrectly powered primary IOL.
   b. Piggyback IOLs can be used in a second operation only if the original IOL power was too low and additional dioptric strength is indicated.

c. A piggyback IOL may be useful after removal of an incorrectly powered IOL.
d. Piggyback IOLs may be less necessary as standard IOL power ranges increase.

7.5. What is the most relevant statement with respect to biometric formulas for IOL calculation?
a. The *AL* is the least important factor in the formula.
b. The refractive error resulting from an error in *AL* measurement is more consequential in long eyes than in short eyes.
c. Accuracy in *AL* measurement is relatively more important in short eyes than in long eyes.
d. During ultrasonic measurement of *AL* (A-scan), sound travels faster through the aqueous and vitreous than through the crystalline lens and cornea. Therefore, there is a need to adjust the *AL* "measurement" by correcting for the incorrect velocity of sound.
e. The velocity of sound in an aphakic eye varies significantly between short and long eyes.

Answers

7.1. **c.** The formula to correct the *AL* is

$$AL_C = AL_M \times \frac{V_C}{V_M}$$

where AL_C is the *AL* value at the correct velocity, AL_M is the resultant *AL* value at the incorrect velocity, V_C is the correct velocity, and V_M is the incorrect velocity. This correction eliminates the need for the patient to undergo the procedure again. There is no factor that can be added to the *AL* to correct such an error, and the error is not negligible and thus cannot be ignored.

7.2. **c.** Multifocal IOLs, including bifocal and EDOF IOLs, necessarily trade contrast performance at distance for multifocality. Although distance acuity may be degraded in dim light in multifocal IOLs, acuity may be excellent at distance in all lenses. It is important to understand that acuity is not identical to optical performance.

7.3. **c.** Multifocal IOLs present both near and distant foci to the retina at the same time. This leads to an unavoidable decrease in image quality and contrast sensitivity, particularly at low levels of illumination. Pupil size may be a factor, particularly with certain types of multifocal IOLs.

7.4. **d.** Piggyback IOLs have been used to reach a total dioptric power that was unavailable in a single lens. As IOLs are becoming available in a wider range of powers, however, it is less likely that a piggyback IOL will be needed to reach an unusually high or low power. Piggyback IOLs are placed anterior to the primary lens and thus modify the light vergence before the light reaches the primary IOL. These IOLs may be used to correct inaccurate primary IOLs in a second operation if the original IOL power was too low or too high. They are not used after removal of an incorrectly powered IOL—"piggyback" implies that a second IOL is present in the eye.

7.5. **c.** Note the following comments for each option:

a. The *AL* is the *most* important factor in the formula.

b. The refractive error resulting from an error in *AL* measurement is more consequential in *short* eyes than in long eyes.

c. Accuracy in *AL* measurement is relatively more important in short eyes than in long eyes. *Correct answer.*

d. During ultrasonic measurement of *AL* (A-scan), sound travels faster through the *crystalline lens and cornea* than through the aqueous and vitreous. Therefore, there is a need to adjust the *AL* "measurement" by correcting for the incorrect velocity of sound.

e. The velocity of sound in an aphakic eye varies *insignificantly* between short and long eyes (ie, it is almost comparable).

CHAPTER 8

Optical Considerations in Keratorefractive Surgery

Highlights

- The normal human cornea has a prolate shape that reduces spherical aberration.
- Keratorefractive surgical procedures modulate the shape of the cornea to reduce refractive error but can induce irregular astigmatism.
- New algorithms for excimer procedures have dramatically decreased the incidence and severity of night-vision problems.
- The diagnosis of irregular astigmatism is made by meeting clinical and imaging criteria: loss of spectacle-aided best-corrected vision but preservation of vision with the use of a rigid contact lens, coupled with topographic corneal irregularity.
- Irregular astigmatism can frequently be understood in terms of basic aberration types, of which as few as 5 are of clinical interest. Aberrations are also described in terms of Zernike polynomials.

Glossary

Angle kappa Angle between the pupillary axis and the visual axis.

Irregular astigmatism In practice, astigmatism that decreases spectacle-aided best-corrected vision but is improved with the use of a rigid gas-permeable lens and shows topographic corneal irregularity.

Oblate A spheroidal shape whereby the curvature is flattest centrally and gradually steepens toward the periphery. An oblate shape is similar to that of a grapefruit: a sphere flattened at the poles.

Prolate A spheroidal shape whereby the curvature is steepest centrally and gradually flattens toward the periphery. A prolate shape is similar to that of the pole of an egg.

Q factor Value of the difference in corneal asphericity between peripheral and central rays.

Spherical aberration Higher-order aberration in which paraxial rays focus in a different plane than peripheral rays.

Wavefront analysis Method to describe irregular astigmatism quantitatively, most frequently with Zernike polynomials.

Introduction

This chapter provides an overview of the optical considerations specific to keratorefractive surgery. Refractive surgical procedures performed with the intent to reduce refractive errors can be categorized as *corneal* (keratorefractive) or *intraocular.*

Keratorefractive surgery can be divided into surface ablation procedures, "flap" or "cap" procedures, incisional procedures, and surgical-addition procedures. Surface ablation procedures include photorefractive keratectomy (PRK), laser subepithelial keratomileusis (LASEK), and epithelial laser in situ keratomileusis (epi-LASIK). Flap/cap procedures include laser in situ keratomileusis (LASIK) and small-incision lenticule extraction (SMILE). Incisional procedures include radial keratotomy (RK), astigmatic keratotomy (AK), and limbal relaxing incisions (LRIs). Surgical-addition procedures include implantation of intracorneal ring segments and corneal inlays. Other keratorefractive procedures include laser thermal keratoplasty (LTK) and radiofrequency conductive keratoplasty (CK). Intraocular refractive procedures include implantation of a phakic intraocular lens (IOL) or a piggyback lens, and cataract and clear lens extraction with implantation of a monofocal, toric, multifocal, or accommodative IOL.

Although these refractive surgical techniques alter the optical properties of the eye, keratorefractive surgery is generally more likely than lenticular refractive surgery to induce optical aberrations. This chapter discusses only keratorefractive procedures and their optical considerations. For a discussion of optical considerations in lenticular refractive surgery, see BCSC Section 11, *Lens and Cataract.*

Various optical considerations are relevant to refractive surgery, both in screening patients for candidacy and in evaluating patients with vision complaints after surgery. Screening is discussed in more detail in BCSC Section 13, *Refractive Surgery.* This chapter addresses optical considerations related to the change in corneal shape after keratorefractive surgery, issues concerning the angle kappa and pupil size, and the various causes of irregular astigmatism.

Corneal Shape

A basic premise of refractive surgery is that the cornea's optical properties are intimately related to its shape. Consequently, manipulation of the corneal shape changes the eye's refractive status. Although this assumption is true, the relationship between corneal shape and the cornea's optical properties is more complex than is generally appreciated.

The normal human cornea has a prolate shape (Fig 8-1), similar to that of the pole of an egg. The curvature of the human eye is steepest in the central cornea and gradually

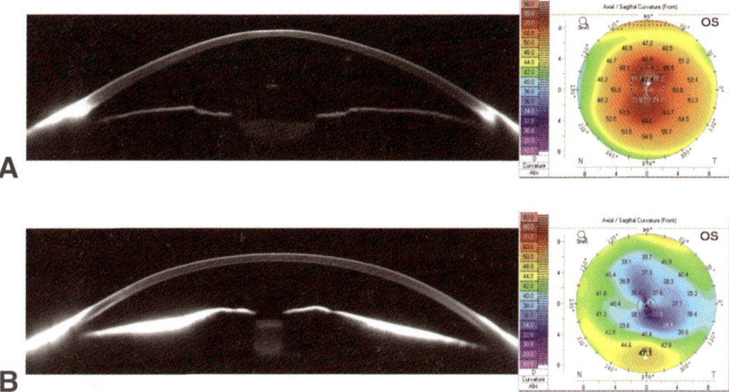

Figure 8-1 Prolate and oblate corneas. **A,** Scheimpflug image and axial map of a patient with a hyperprolate cornea due to keratoconus ($Q = -2.21$). **B,** Scheimpflug image and axial map of a patient with an oblate cornea after myopic LASIK ($Q = +1.20$). *(Courtesy of Tyler Oostra, MD.)*

flattens toward the periphery. This configuration reduces the optical problems associated with simple spherical refracting surfaces, which produce a nearer point of focus for peripheral rays than for paraxial rays—a refractive condition known as *spherical aberration* (see Figs 1-26 and 1-29). *Corneal asphericity,* the relative difference between the peripheral and central cornea, is represented by the Q factor. In an ideal visual system, the curvature at the center of the cornea would be steeper than at the periphery (ie, the cornea would be prolate), and the Q factor would have a value close to –0.50; at this value of negative Q, the degree of spherical aberration would approach zero. However, in the normal human eye, because of the junction between the cornea and the sclera, the Q factor has an average value of –0.26, allowing for a smooth transition at the limbus. The human visual system, therefore, suffers from minor spherical aberrations, which increase with increasing pupil size. It is important to note that, while related, spherical aberration and corneal asphericity are not the same thing. Whereas spherical aberration measures the effect of the optical system on incoming light and is measured in microns, corneal asphericity describes the shape of the refractive surface and the measured Q factor has no units.

Ablative procedures, incisional procedures, and intracorneal rings change the natural shape of the cornea to reduce refractive error. Keratometry readings conducted in eyes before they undergo keratorefractive surgery typically range from 38.00 D to 48.00 D. When refractive surgical procedures are being considered, it is important to avoid changes that may result in excessively flat (<33.00 D) or excessively steep (>50.00 D) corneal powers, which decrease vision quality and increase aberrations. A 0.80 D change in keratometry value *(K)* corresponds to approximately a 1.00 D change in refraction for myopic ablations. The following equation is often used to predict corneal curvature after myopic keratorefractive surgery:

$$K_{postop} = K_{preop} + (0.8 \cdot RE)$$

where K_{preop} and K_{postop} are preoperative and postoperative K readings, respectively, and RE is the refractive error to be corrected at the corneal plane. For example, if a patient's preoperative keratometry readings are 45.00 D (steepest meridian) and 43.00 D (flattest meridian), then the average *K* value is 44.00 D. If the amount of refractive correction at the corneal plane is −8.50 D, then the predicted average postoperative *K* reading is 44.00 + (0.8 × −8.50) = 37.20 D, which is acceptable. For hyperopic ablations, a 1.00 D change in *K* corresponds to approximately a 1.00 D change in refraction.

The ratio of dioptric change in keratometry to dioptric change in refractive error is approximately 0.8:1 due to the change in posterior corneal surface power after excimer ablation. The anterior corneal surface produces most of the eye's refractive power. In the Gullstrand model eye (see Table 3-1), the anterior corneal surface has a power of +48.80 D and the posterior corneal surface has a power of −5.80 D, so the overall corneal refractive power is +43.00 D. It is important to note that standard corneal topography instruments and keratometers do not measure corneal power precisely because they do not assess the posterior corneal surface. Instead, these instruments estimate total corneal power by assuming a constant relationship between the anterior and posterior corneal surfaces, which is represented in the standard keratometric index that these instruments use (1.3375) in place of the actual refractive index of the cornea (1.376). This relationship is disrupted with surgical removal or surgical addition procedures, causing the standard keratometric index no longer to be valid. For example, after myopic excimer surgery, the anterior corneal curvature is flattened. At the same time, the posterior corneal surface remains unchanged or, owing to the reduction in corneal pachymetry and weakening of the cornea, the posterior corneal surface may become slightly steeper than the preoperative posterior corneal curvature, increasing its negative power.

The removal of even a small amount of tissue (eg, a few microns) during keratorefractive surgery may cause a substantial change in refraction (Fig 8-2). The Munnerlyn

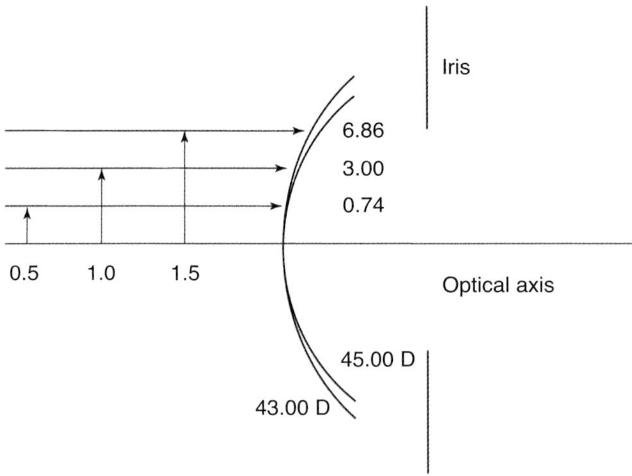

Figure 8-2 Comparison of a 43.00 D cornea with a 45.00 D cornea. Numbers below the vertical arrows indicate distance from the optical axis in millimeters; numbers to the right of the horizontal arrows indicate the separation between the corneas in microns. A typical pupil size of 3.0 mm is indicated. A typical red blood cell has a diameter of 7 µm. Within the pupillary space (ie, the optical zone of the cornea), the separation between the corneas is less than the diameter of a red blood cell. *(Courtesy of Edmond H. Thall, MD. Modified by C. H. Wooley.)*

formula approximates the depth of the ablation based on the optical zone and the refractive correction:

$$t = \frac{S^2 D}{3}$$

where t is the depth of the central ablation in microns, S is the diameter of the optical zone in millimeters, and D is the degree of refractive correction in diopters. See Appendix 8-1 for the derivation of this formula. For commonly used optical zones (~6.5 mm), the Munnerlyn formula shows that approximately 15 microns are removed for each diopter of correction.

An ideal LASIK ablation or PRK removes tissue resembling a positive meniscus in corrections of myopia (Fig 8-3A) and a negative meniscus with no tissue removed centrally in simple corrections of hyperopia (Fig 8-3B). Intracorneal rings flatten the corneal surface to correct myopia, while arcuate incisional procedures cause localized flattening to reduce myopic astigmatism. LTK and CK cause focal stromal contraction and central steepening

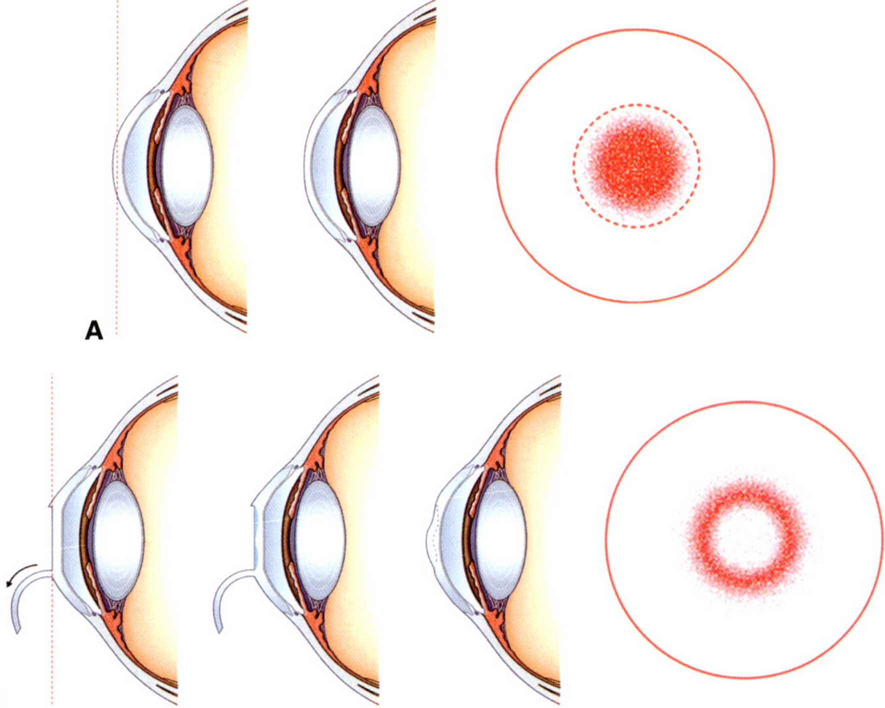

Figure 8-3 Myopic photorefractive keratectomy (PRK) and hyperopic laser in situ keratomileusis (LASIK). **A,** Schematic illustration of myopic PRK. The shaded area refers to the location of tissue subtraction. More stromal tissue is removed in the central than in the paracentral region (which resembles a positive meniscus). **B,** Schematic illustration of hyperopic LASIK. A superficial corneal flap is raised. The shaded area refers to the location of tissue subtraction (which resembles a negative meniscus with no tissue removed centrally) under the thin flap. After treatment, the flap is repositioned. *(Used with permission from Poothullil AM, Azar DT. Terminology, classification, and history of refractive surgery. In: Azar DT, ed. Gatinel D, Hoang-Xuan T, associate eds.* Refractive Surgery. *2nd ed. Elsevier-Mosby; 2007:5–6. Figs 1–4, 1–5.)*

to correct hyperopia. Finally, pinhole corneal inlays do not change the shape of the cornea but increase depth of focus on the retina by decreasing the size of the entrance pupil.

Angle Kappa

As discussed in Chapter 3, the pupillary axis is the imaginary line that is perpendicular to the corneal surface and passes through the midpoint of the entrance pupil (see Fig 3-3). The visual axis is the imaginary line that connects the point of fixation to the fovea. The angle kappa (κ) is imagined as the angle between the pupillary axis and the visual axis (the visual axis intersects the corneal surface very near the corneal apex in a regular cornea) and is estimated by observing the difference between the apparent center of the pupil and the penlight reflex during monocular fixation of the light source; a large angle kappa results from a significant difference between them. If the angle kappa is large, centering an excimer ablation over the geometric center of the cornea will effectively result in a decentered ablation and induce significant higher-order aberrations, most notably coma. This can be particularly problematic in a hyperopic correction, in which a large angle kappa can result in a refractively significant "second corneal apex," causing monocular diplopia and decreased quality of vision. A large angle kappa must be identified before surgery to reduce the likelihood of a poor visual outcome.

While angle kappa is a useful construct, in practice it is inconsistently defined and difficult to accurately measure. (See Chapter 3.) Accordingly, chord mu (μ), also called the Chang-Waring chord, has been proposed as a more clearly defined and easily measurable quantity that is representative of angle kappa. It is defined as the displacement between the subject-fixated coaxially sighted corneal light reflex and the entrance pupil center. Many corneal topographers and optical biometers can precisely measure chord mu or similar representative values of angle kappa.

Chang DH, Waring GO. The subject-fixated coaxially sighted corneal light reflex: a clinical marker for centration of refractive treatments and devices. *Am J Ophthalmol.* 2014;158(5): 863–874.

Pupil Size

Measurement of pupil size has been an important factor in preoperative evaluations, prompted by observations that some patients with large pupils (>8 mm) reported difficulties with night vision after undergoing keratorefractive surgery as a result of induced higher-order aberrations, mainly increased spherical aberration. Typical symptoms included the appearance of glare, starbursts, and halos; decreased contrast sensitivity; and poor overall quality of vision. Night-vision problems tended to occur in patients with both large pupils and small treatment zones (≤6 mm). The algorithms used in third-generation lasers (wavefront-guided and wavefront-optimized ablations), however, incorporate larger optical and transition zones to reduce higher-order aberrations, enabling surgeons to perform refractive procedures on patients with larger pupils. Use of these algorithms has dramatically decreased the incidence and severity of night-vision problems.

Many surgeons use default ablation zones during excimer procedures. The accepted standard transition zone between ablated and unablated cornea is 0.5–1.0 mm larger than the pupil; use of this zone helps minimize night-vision problems. To conserve corneal tissue, smaller optical zones are typically used in higher myopic corrections. In patients who require such corrections, the incidence of night-vision problems increases in part because of the mismatch between the size of the pupil and that of the optical zone. Modern transition zones aim to minimize this mismatch.

Patients with extremely large pupils (≥8 mm), especially in mesopic and scotopic light conditions, should be identified and counseled about the potential for increased risk of complications. Spherical aberration may be increased in these patients. Clinical management of postoperative night-vision problems includes the use of a miotic such as brimonidine (0.2%) or pilocarpine (0.5%–1%).

Chan A, Manche EE. Effect of preoperative pupil size on quality of vision after wavefront-guided LASIK. *Ophthalmology.* 2011;118(4):736–741.

Myung D, Schallhorn S, Manche EE. Pupil size and LASIK: a review. *J Refract Surg.* 2013;29(11):734–741.

Irregular Astigmatism

Refractive surgeons benefit from having a thorough understanding of irregular astigmatism, for 3 reasons. First, recognizing irregular astigmatism preoperatively is important in determining if an individual is a suitable candidate for keratorefractive surgery. Second, keratorefractive surgery may lead to visually significant irregular astigmatism in a small percentage of cases. Third, keratorefractive surgery may also be able to treat it. The treatment of postoperative irregular corneal astigmatism is a substantial challenge in refractive surgery.

The diagnosis of irregular astigmatism is made with both clinical and imaging criteria: loss of spectacle-aided best-corrected vision but preservation of vision with the use of a rigid gas-permeable contact lens, coupled with topographic corneal irregularity. An important sign of postsurgical irregular astigmatism is a refraction that is inconsistent with the uncorrected visual acuity. For example, consider a patient who has −3.50 D myopia with essentially no astigmatism before the operation. After keratorefractive surgery, the patient has an uncorrected visual acuity of 20/25 but a refraction of +2.00 −3.00 × 60. Ordinarily, such a refraction would be inconsistent with an uncorrected visual acuity of 20/25, but it can occur in patients who have irregular astigmatism after keratorefractive surgery.

Another important sign is the difficulty of determining axis location during manifest refraction in patients with a high degree of astigmatism. Normally, determining the correcting cylinder axis accurately in a patient with significant cylinder is easy; however, patients with irregular astigmatism after keratorefractive surgery often have difficulty choosing an axis. Automated refractors may identify high degrees of astigmatism that are rejected by patients during manifest refraction. Because their astigmatism is irregular (and thus has no definite axis), these patients may achieve almost the same visual acuity with high powers of cylinder at various axes. Streak retinoscopy often demonstrates irregular "scissoring" in patients with irregular astigmatism.

Typically, a limbal relaxing incision will decrease regular astigmatism while maintaining the spherical equivalent (coupling); however, results of astigmatic enhancements can be unpredictable for patients with irregular astigmatism. In such cases, the astigmatic enhancement may cause the axis to change dramatically without substantially reducing cylinder power.

Irregular astigmatism can be described in much the same way as is regular astigmatism. We think of regular astigmatism as a cylinder superimposed on a sphere. Irregular astigmatism, then, can be thought of as additional shapes superimposed on cylinders and spheres. This corneal irregularity can be measured and quantified by wavefront analysis.

Application of Wavefront Analysis in Irregular Astigmatism

For irregular astigmatism to be studied effectively, it must be described quantitatively. Wavefront analysis is an effective method for such descriptions of irregular astigmatism. An understanding of irregular astigmatism and wavefront analysis begins with stigmatic imaging. A stigmatic imaging system brings all the rays from a single object point to a perfect point focus. According to the Fermat principle, a stigmatic focus is possible only when the time required for light to travel from an object point to an image point is identical for all the possible paths that the light may take. (See the section Aberrations in Chapter 1 of this volume.)

An analogy to a footrace is helpful. Suppose that several runners simultaneously depart from an object point (A). Each runner follows a different path, represented by a ray. In this case, all the runners travel at the same speed on the ground, but slow down when running through water. Similarly, light rays will travel at the same speed in air but slow down in the lens. If all the runners reach the image point (B) simultaneously, the "image" is stigmatic. If the rays do not meet at point B, then the "image" is astigmatic.

Wavefront analysis is based on the Fermat principle. Construct a circular arc centered on the paraxial image point and intersecting the center of the exit pupil (Fig 8-4A). This arc is called the *reference sphere.* We may consider the analogy of a footrace, but now think of the reference sphere (rather than a point) as the finish line. If the image is stigmatic, all runners starting from a single point will cross the reference sphere simultaneously. If the image is astigmatic, the runners will cross the reference sphere at slightly different times (Fig 8-4B). The *geometric wavefront* is analogous to a photo finish of the race. It represents the position of each runner shortly after the fastest runner crosses the finish line. The *wavefront aberration* of each runner is the time at which the runner finishes minus the time of the fastest runner. In other words, it is the difference between the reference sphere and the wavefront. When the focus is stigmatic, the reference sphere and the wavefront coincide so that the wavefront aberration is zero. Another useful depiction of the higher-order aberrations is by means of the point spread function, the distribution of light in the image plane from a point source (Fig 8-5).

Myopia, hyperopia, and regular astigmatism can be expressed as wavefront aberrations. Myopia produces an aberration that optical engineers call *positive defocus.* Hyperopia is called *negative defocus.* Regular (cylindrical) astigmatism produces a wavefront aberration that resembles a saddle. Defocus (myopia and hyperopia) and regular astigmatism constitute the lower-order aberrations. Wavefront aberrations are also a function of pupil position. For example, coma is a partial deflection of spherical aberration. Figure 8-6 shows some typical wavefront aberrations.

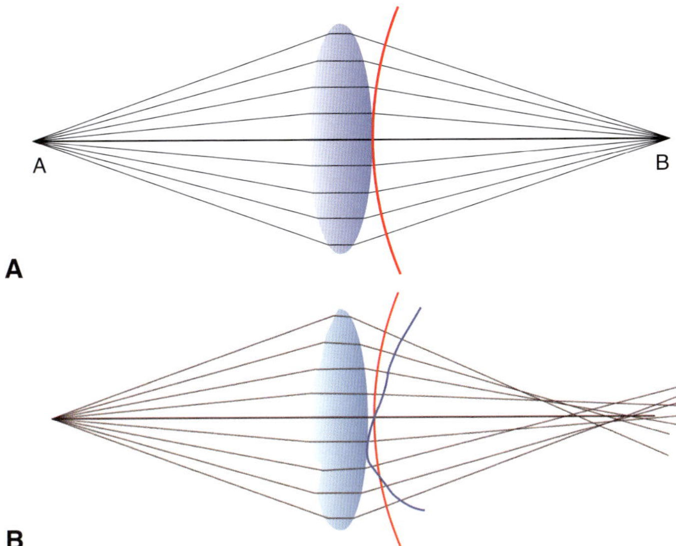

Figure 8-4 Wavefront analysis. **A,** The reference sphere (in red) is represented in 2 dimensions by a circular arc centered on point B and drawn through the center of the exit pupil of the lens. If the image is stigmatic, all light from point A crosses the reference sphere simultaneously. **B,** When the image is astigmatic, light rays from the object point simultaneously cross the wavefront (in blue), not the reference sphere. *(Courtesy of Edmond H. Thall, MD. Part B modified by C. H. Wooley.)*

Keratorefractive surgery for myopia using surgical removal procedures reduces spherical refractive error and regular astigmatism, but it does so at the expense of increasing spherical aberration and irregular astigmatism. The cornea subsequently becomes less prolate, and its shape resembles an egg lying on its side. The central cornea becomes flatter than the periphery and results in an increase in the spherical aberration of the treated zone. Generally, keratorefractive surgery moves the location of the best focus closer to the retina but, at the same time, makes the focus less stigmatic. Such irregular astigmatism leads to decreased contrast sensitivity and underlies many visual complaints after refractive surgery, such as glare and halos in mesopic light conditions.

When peripheral rays focus in front of more central rays, the effect is termed *spherical aberration*. Clinically, spherical aberration is one of the main causes of night myopia following LASIK and PRK. After keratorefractive surgery, corneas that become more oblate (after myopic correction) will induce more-positive spherical aberration, while those that become more prolate (after hyperopic correction) will induce more-negative spherical aberration.

Another important aberration is *coma*. In this aberration, rays at one edge of the pupil cross the reference sphere first; rays at the opposite edge of the pupil cross last. The effect is that the image of each object point resembles a comet with a tail (one meaning of *coma* is "comet"). It is commonly observed in the aiming beam during retinal laser photocoagulation; if the ophthalmologist tilts the lens too far off-axis, the aiming beam spot becomes coma shaped. Coma also arises in patients with decentered keratorefractive ablation or keratoconus. These situations may be treatable with intrastromal rings.

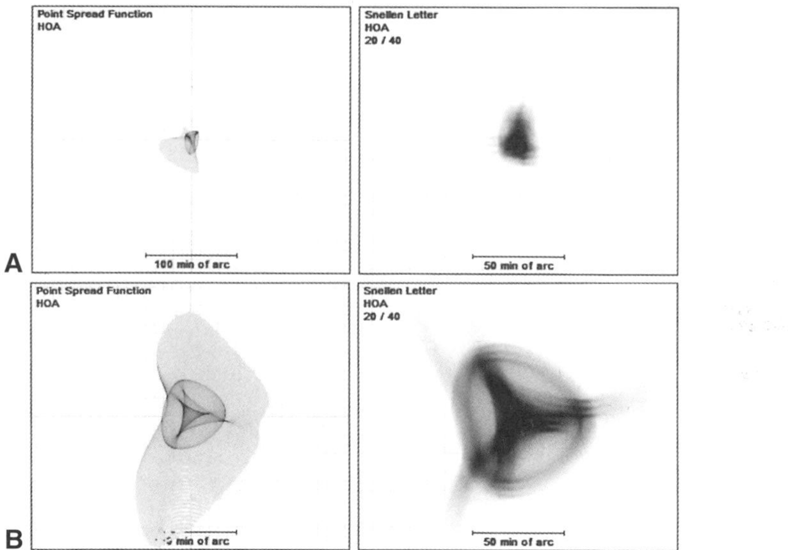

Figure 8-5 Examples of the effects of coma **(A)** and trefoil **(B)** on the point spread functions of a light source. *(Courtesy of Ming Wang, MD.)*

Higher-order aberrations tend to be less significant than lower-order aberrations, but the higher-order ones may worsen in diseased or surgically altered eyes. For example, if interrupted sutures are used to sew in a corneal graft during corneal transplant, they will produce higher-order trefoil or tetrafoil aberrations. These can then be addressed with suture removal, suture addition, or AK. Also, in the manufacture of IOLs, the lens blank is sometimes improperly positioned on the lathe; such improper positioning can also produce higher-order aberrations.

Wavefront aberrations can be represented in different ways. One approach is to show them as 3-dimensional shapes. Another is to represent them as contour plots. Irregular astigmatism can be described as a combination of a few basic shapes, just as conventional refractive error represents a combination of a sphere and a cylinder.

Currently, wavefront aberrations are specified by *Zernike polynomials,* which are the mathematical formulas used to describe wavefront surfaces. *Wavefront aberration surfaces* are graphs generated by using Zernike polynomials. There are several techniques for measuring wavefront aberrations clinically. The most popular is based on the *Hartmann-Shack wavefront sensor,* which uses a low-power laser beam focused on the retina. A point on the retina then acts as a point source. In a perfect eye, all the rays would emerge in parallel and the wavefront would be a flat plane; however, in most eyes, the wavefront is not flat. Within the sensor is a grid of small lenses (lenslet array) that samples parts of the wavefront. The images formed are focused onto a charge-coupled device chip, and the degree of deviation of the focused images from the expected focal points determines the aberration and thus the wavefront error (eg, see Fig 9-8).

For a more detailed discussion of the topics covered in this subsection, see BCSC Section 13, *Refractive Surgery.*

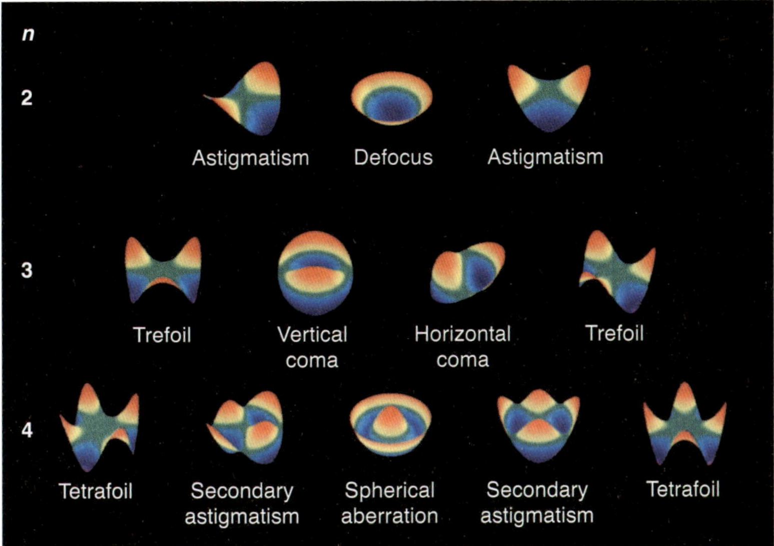

Figure 8-6 Second-, third-, and fourth-order wavefront aberrations (indicated by *n* values 2, 3, and 4, respectively) are most pertinent to refractive surgery. *(Reproduced with permission from Applegate RA. Glenn Fry Award Lecture 2002: wavefront sensing, ideal corrections, and visual performance.* Optom Vis Sci. *2004;81[3]:169.)*

Causes of Irregular Astigmatism

Irregular astigmatism may be present before keratorefractive surgery; it may be caused by the surgery; or it may develop postoperatively. Preoperative causes include keratoconus, pellucid marginal degeneration, contact lens warpage, significant dry eye, corneal injury, microbial keratitis, and epithelial basement membrane dystrophy (Fig 8-7). All these conditions should be identified before surgery. Common intraoperative causes include decentered ablations and central islands, and, less commonly, poor laser optics, nonuniform stromal bed hydration, and LASIK flap complications (a thin, torn, irregular, incomplete, or buttonhole flap; folds or striae of the flap; and epithelial defects). Postoperative causes of irregular astigmatism include flap displacement, diffuse lamellar keratitis and its sequelae, flap striae, posterior corneal ectasia, irregular wound healing, dry eye, and flap edema.

Schallhorn SC, Farjo AA, Huang D, et al. Wavefront-guided LASIK for the correction of primary myopia and astigmatism: a report by the American Academy of Ophthalmology. *Ophthalmology*. 2008;115(7):1249–1261.

Conclusion

Understanding and incorporating optical considerations into the treatment of patients undergoing keratorefractive surgery is important to enhance the visual results. Patient dissatisfaction after surgery, albeit rare, often stems from the subjective loss of visual acuity or quality, the source of which can usually be identified through a sound understanding of how keratorefractive surgery alters the optics of the eye. A good understanding of

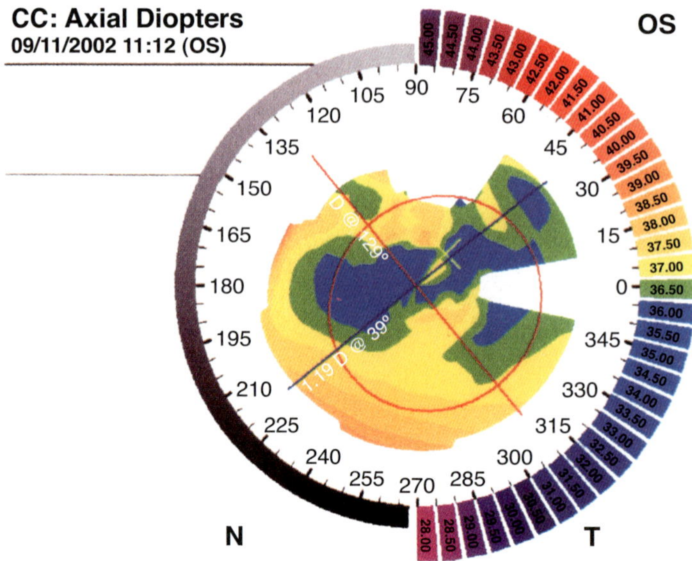

Figure 8-7 Irregular astigmatism in a corneal topographic map of the left eye of a patient with significant epithelial basement membrane dystrophy. The patient experienced glare and a general decline in quality of vision. Simulated *K* shows the flattest meridian at 39° and the steeper meridian at 129°. N = nasal; T = temporal. *(Courtesy of Ming Wang, MD.)*

key parameters such as corneal shape, pupil size, the ocular surface, spherical and astigmatic errors, higher-order aberrations, laser centration and the angle kappa, and irregular corneal astigmatism can help optimize visual outcomes for keratorefractive surgery.

Appendix 8-1

Derivation of the Munnerlyn Formula

The sagittal depth of a circle can be calculated using the formula:

$$R - \sqrt{R^2 - (S/2)^2}$$

where R is the radius of the circle and S is the chord length.

Consider Figure 8-A1, in which the smaller circle represents the preoperative cornea and the larger circle, with an increased radius of curvature, represents the postoperative cornea after myopic ablation. The shaded area represents the ablated tissue. The diameter of the optical zone of the ablation is equivalent to the chord length of the circles, S, as shown. Using the above formula, we can calculate the central ablation thickness, t, as a difference between the sagittal depths of the 2 circles, t_1 and t_2:

$$t = t_1 - t_2 = R_1 - \sqrt{R_1^2 - (S/2)^2} - R_2 + \sqrt{R_2^2 - (S/2)^2} \qquad (1)$$

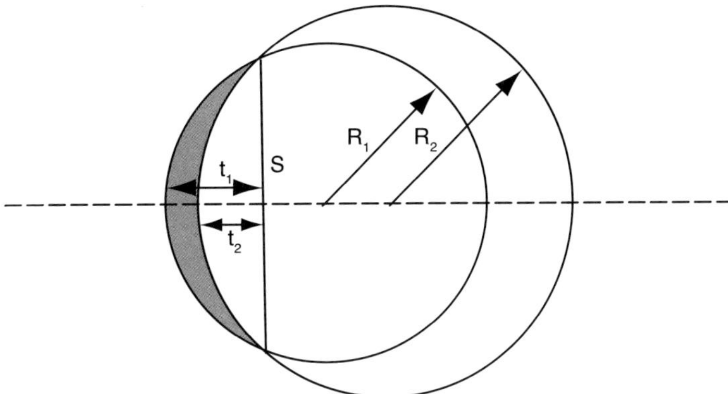

Figure 8-A1 Geometry for deriving the Munnerlyn formula. *(Illustration developed by Tyler Oostra, MD.)*

The square root term can be represented by a power series:

$$\sqrt{R^2-(S/2)^2}=R-\frac{S^2}{8R}-\frac{S^4}{128R^3}-\frac{S^6}{1024R^5}-\cdots$$

For small values of S relative to R, as in our case, the first 2 terms are a reasonable approximation. Thus Equation (1) becomes:

$$t\approx R_1-\left(R_1-\frac{S^2}{8R_1}\right)-R_2+\left(R_2-\frac{S^2}{8R_2}\right)=\frac{S^2}{8R_1}-\frac{S^2}{8R_2}=\frac{S^2}{8}\left(\frac{1}{R_1}-\frac{1}{R_2}\right) \quad (2)$$

Using the thin lens approximation of the lensmaker's equation, we can calculate the power of the ablative correction, D, as:

$$D=(n-1)\left(\frac{1}{R_2}-\frac{1}{R_1}\right) \quad (3)$$

We can then use Equation (3) to simplify Equation (2) to:

$$t\approx-\frac{S^2D}{8(n-1)}$$

This is the Munnerlyn formula as originally published in 1988. It is frequently simplified further by using a value of 1.377 for n, in which case $(n-1)\approx 3/8$, and denoting D as positive rather than negative for myopic ablations and thus dropping the negative sign:

$$t\approx\frac{S^2D}{3}$$

Munnerlyn CR, Koons SJ, Marshall J. Photorefractive keratectomy: a technique for laser refractive surgery. *J Cataract Refract Surg.* 1988;14(1):46–52.

Chapter Exercises

Questions

8.1. The Munnerlyn formula approximates the depth of excimer laser tissue ablation:

$$t = \frac{S^2 D}{3}$$

where t is the central ablation depth in micrometers, S is the diameter of the optical zone in millimeters, and D is the degree of refractive correction in diopters. For a LASIK patient with a refractive correction of −6.00 −6.00 × 90 and a central corneal thickness of 520 µm, and for whom the LASIK flap thickness is 120 µm, an extremely conservative surgeon would not want to have a residual stromal bed (RSB) thickness of less than 300 µm. According to the Munnerlyn formula, what is the largest optical zone diameter that can be used for this treatment?

8.2. For the situation described in Question 8.1, what is the largest optical zone diameter that can be used if PRK, rather than LASIK, is planned? Assume an epithelium thickness of 58 µm and an RSB thickness of 300 µm.

8.3. A patient with a preoperative manifest refraction of −3.50 D, normal keratometry *(K)* readings, and a pachymetry measurement of 550 µm undergoes keratorefractive surgery. Three months postoperatively, the patient has an uncorrected visual acuity of 20/30 with a refraction of +2.00 −3.00 × 60 associated with postsurgical irregular astigmatism. What are the important signs that will aid in reaching a diagnosis?

a. difficulty in determining axis location during manifest refraction
b. discrepancy between automated refraction and manifest refraction
c. no improvement or change in visual acuity with large powers of cylinder at markedly different axes
d. all of the above

8.4. Corneal asphericity is represented by Q value. A spherical cornea with asphericity of $Q = 0$ is associated with

a. better visual acuity than a prolate cornea
b. improved optics if keratorefractive surgery results in postoperative $Q = -0.3$
c. improved optics if keratorefractive surgery results in postoperative $Q = 0$
d. improved optics if keratorefractive surgery results in postoperative $Q = +0.3$

8.5. A patient undergoing an evaluation for refractive surgery has K readings of 46.00 D/42.00 D. If LASIK were performed, what are the largest hyperopic and myopic spherical corrections tolerable?

a. +5.00 D, −11.25 D
b. +3.00 D, −11.25 D
c. +3.00 D, −6.25 D
d. +5.00 D, −7.00 D

Answers

8.1. Pachymetry value = t + LASIK flap thickness + RSB thickness = t + 120 μm + 300 μm. This implies that $t = 100$ μm. Then, $t = 100 = S^2 \times D/3$, where $D = 12$, the maximum refractive component necessary to correct along the steep meridian, which implies that $S^2 = 25$. Therefore, $S = 5$ mm; that is, the largest diameter that can be used for LASIK treatment in this situation by this surgeon is 5 mm.

8.2. Pachymetry value = t + epithelium thickness + RSB thickness. This implies that $t = 520$ μm − 58 μm − 300 μm = 162 μm. Because $t = S^2 \times 12/3$, this implies that $S^2 = 162/4 = 40.5$; thus, $S = 6.4$ mm, the largest diameter that can be used for PRK treatment in this situation by this surgeon.

8.3. **d.** all of the above.

8.4. **b.** improved optics if keratorefractive surgery results in postoperative $Q = -0.3$

8.5. **a.** +8.75 D, −11.25 D. The postoperative K readings should be less than 50.00 D and more than 33.00 D to avoid an excessively steep or flat cornea, which can decrease visual quality and increase aberrations. The formula for keratometry change is approximately = 0.8 × refractive change. Here, the refractive change = (50 − 46)/0.8 = +5.00 D and (33 − 42)/0.8 = −11.25 D based on maximum steepening of the steep axis and maximum flattening of the flat axis.

CHAPTER 9

Optical Instruments

Highlights

- Optical instruments that assist in refraction and topography include the lensmeter, autorefractor, keratometer, corneal topographer, and wavefront aberrometer.
- The slit-lamp biomicroscope and ophthalmoscope are important instruments used in daily clinical practice; with the aid of several attachments and auxiliary lenses, the slit lamp allows diverse examination techniques (including applanation tonometry) for both the anterior and posterior segments.
- Technological advances in scanning laser ophthalmoscopy and optical coherence tomography, in particular the development of adaptive optics, allow for the delineation of anatomical structures of the eye with greater detail.

Glossary

Adaptive optics A technique to compensate for irregularities (wavefront distortions) caused by imperfections (optical aberrations) in the ocular media, in particular in the cornea and crystalline lens, when the ocular fundus is imaged.

Autorefractor An automated system that uses a source of light reflected off of the retina to reveal the eye's refractive characteristics.

Corneal topography system An automated system that produces a detailed map of the corneal surface. It is most useful for evaluation of corneal astigmatism, preoperative assessment for refractive surgery, assessment after corneal transplant surgery, and evaluation of patients with known or suspected keratoconus.

Direct ophthalmoscope A handheld instrument used to examine the posterior segment (using the optics of the patient's eye as a simple magnifier) and to assess the red reflex.

Indirect ophthalmoscope A device, worn on the head, that is used for posterior segment examination in conjunction with auxiliary handheld diagnostic condensing lenses.

Instrument myopia The tendency of the eye to accommodate when a person looks into instruments.

Keratometer A device used to approximate the refracting power of the cornea by determining the curvature of the central anterior corneal surface. It is typically used when fitting a patient for contact lenses and to diagnose disorders such as keratoconus.

Lensmeter A device that measures the power of spectacles or contact lenses.

Optical coherence tomography (OCT) A system based on low-coherence interferometry and that uses interference of broadband or tunable coherent light to provide a high-resolution cross-sectional image of the retina or cornea.

Ray-deflection principle A method employed in autorefractors and aberrometers that infers the eye's refractive error. A stationary source of light "floods" the eye, and the light that emerges from the eye is then isolated into multiple beams; the deflection or deviation of each light beam is then compared with its ideal reference position.

Scanning laser ophthalmoscope A device that functions as both an ophthalmoscope and a fundus camera but requires significantly less light than those conventional flood-illumination systems, thanks to the use of a highly concentrated beam from a laser that is rapidly moved across the retina and illuminates only a small spot at a time.

Scheimpflug camera A device based on the *Scheimpflug principle* that images the anterior segment. A camera rotates perpendicular to a source of illumination, such as a slit beam of light incident on the cornea; this configuration corrects for the nonplanar shape of the cornea and thus results in distortion-free cross sections.

Scheiner principle A method for detecting refractive errors using a double-pinhole aperture placed before the eye. Through such an aperture, an emmetropic eye forms a single-point image of a distant point source on the retina; an ametropic eye forms a double image on the retina.

Slit-lamp biomicroscope A stereoscopic microscope mounted on a common pivot with an adjustable slit illuminator, commonly called the *slit lamp*. The slit-lamp biomicroscope permits magnified examination of the eye, using various kinds of illumination. It is primarily used to perform anterior segment examinations. Several attachments for the slit lamp extend its use beyond these examination techniques, such as auxiliary lenses for slit-lamp examination of the retina.

Specular microscope A device used to visualize and evaluate the corneal endothelium. Contact specular microscopy allows for higher magnifications than slit-lamp biomicroscopy, demonstrates cell morphology, and calculates endothelial cell density.

Tonometer A device used to measure intraocular pressure. In Goldmann applanation tonometry specifically, performed with an attachment to the slit lamp, intraocular pressure is inferred from the amount of force required to flatten a circular region of 3.06 mm in diameter on the cornea.

Introduction

This chapter discusses the basic principles and underlying concepts of various optical instruments that are commonly used to examine the eye. The discussion includes some recent technological developments.

Refraction and Topography

Lensmeter

Manual lensmeter

The lensmeter measures the power of a spectacle or contact lens. It uses a fixed lens positioned a focal length away from the spectacle plane at the tip of the nose cone (Fig 9-1), by which the vergence induced in the spectacle plane becomes linearly related to moving a target.

In the lensmeter, an illuminated target is moved, varying the vergence at the tip of the nose cone, until it becomes focused on the reticle of a telescope. The target is focused only when parallel rays are entering the telescope (ie, when the light entering has zero vergence), which indicates that the "unknown" lens is exactly neutralizing the vergence that is exiting the nose cone. The actual power of the lens can then be read from a dioptric scale, which is the opposite of the power emerging from the nose cone.

The addition of the telescope facilitates the detection of zero vergence. This is because the telescope magnifies vergence by the square of the power of the telescope, which enables the examiner to detect very small deviations from zero vergence without having

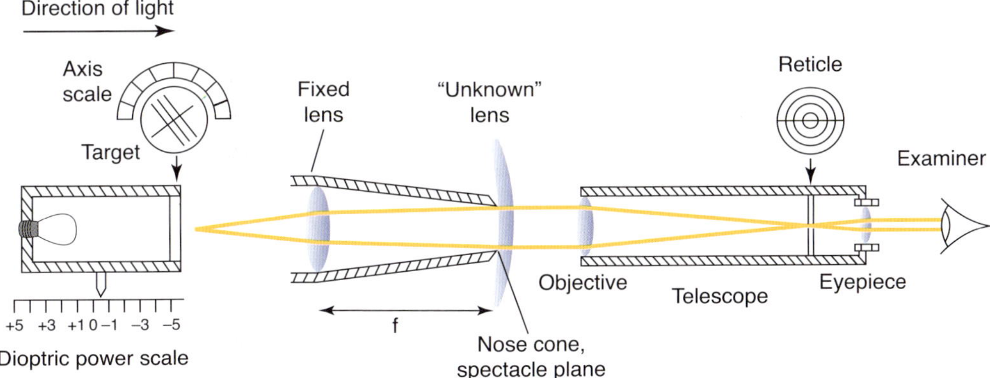

Figure 9-1 The lensmeter. An illuminated target is moved, varying the vergence at the tip of the nose cone, until it becomes focused on the reticle of a telescope. This is the case when the "unknown" spectacle lens is exactly neutralizing the vergence that is coming out of the nose cone. The light will then emerge from the spectacle lens with zero vergence (ie, collimated), and the target will be seen in sharp focus by the observer. The telescope magnifies vergence by the square of its power and thus facilitates the detection of zero vergence, increasing the precision of the measurement and reducing the effect of the observer's accommodation or refractive error. *(Reproduced from Guyton DL, et al.* Ophthalmic Optics and Clinical Refraction. *Prism Press; 1999. Illustration modified by Kristina Irsch, PhD.)*

their uncorrected refractive error cause significant error in the measurement. For best accuracy, the eyepiece can be adjusted beforehand, by focusing it on a reticle located inside the telescope, which eliminates any residual effect from the examiner's refractive error.

Note that the true power of a lens cannot be measured with the lensmeter, as this would require measurement from the lens's principal planes rather than from the lens's surface. To measure the distance correction using a lensmeter, the spectacle lens is placed on the nose cone with the temples turned away from the examiner, so that the nose cone is against the back surface, because spectacle lenses are designated by their back vertex power (ie, the reciprocal of their back focal length).

The target usually has a set of lines (eg, the American cross-line target as depicted in Fig 9-2) that permits the observer to determine whether the lens has cylindrical power. In

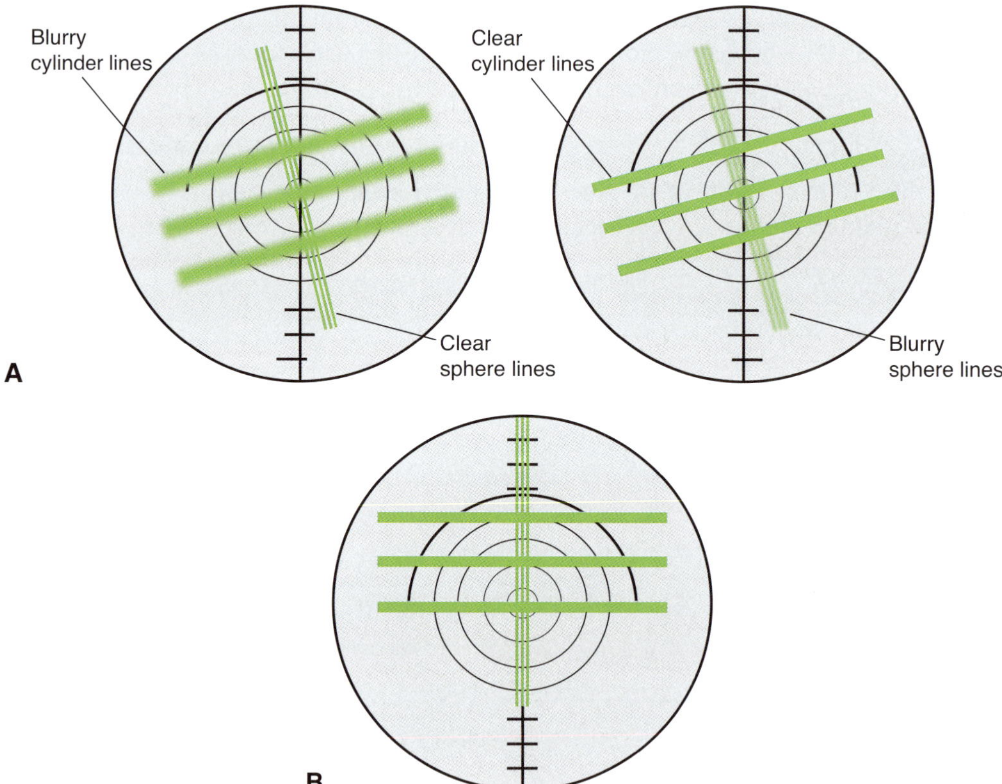

Figure 9-2 Illustration of view inside the lensmeter. **A,** In the measurement of cylindrical power, the cross-line target is rotated, via the axis wheel, so that the lines are continuous and do not appear "broken"; continuous lines indicate the correct axis of the cylinder. The cross-line target is also moved forward or backward, via the power wheel, until 1 set of lines is clear *(left).* It is then moved forward or backward until the perpendicular set of lines is clear *(right).* The difference in target settings is the cylindrical power of the lens. **B,** Upward displacement of the target pattern indicates the presence of base-up prism. *(Modified from Gutmark R, Guyton DL, Irsch K. Prescribing prisms.* Focal Points: Clinical Modules for Ophthalmologists. *American Academy of Ophthalmology; 2011, module 10:4.)*

the measurement of cylindrical power, as illustrated in Figure 9-2A, the cross-line target is first rotated, as well as moved forward or backward, until 1 set of lines is sharp. Then, it is moved forward or backward until the perpendicular set of lines is sharp. The difference in target settings is the cylindrical power. The cylinder axis is read from a scale that indicates the orientation of the cross-line target in degrees.

Prism in spectacles can also be detected by means of a lensmeter. If there is no prism present in the lens, the center of the cross-line target will appear in the center of the lensmeter reticule. If, however, the intersection of the target lines is off-center (Fig 9-2B), and the lens must be shifted away from the patient's normal viewing position to recenter it in the reticule, prism is present in the spectacle lens. If the intersection of the target lines is decentered horizontally, horizontal prismatic power is present, whereas a vertical shift indicates the presence of vertical prism power, with the shift in the direction of the prism base. In Figure 9-2B, the target lines are vertically displaced upward from the center, as is the case when vertical prism power, base-up, is present.

When determining a patient's reading add, the examiner places the spectacles on the nose cone with the temples turned around, toward the examiner, so that the front of the glasses rests on the nose cone. The front vertex power of the distance portion is measured; this will be significantly different from the back vertex power for high-plus lenses (in cases other than a distance lens with strong plus power, there is usually little or no clinically significant difference in the measurements), and the front vertex power of the near portion is measured. The difference in power between the distance and near portions of the lens specifies the reading-add power.

Automatic lensmeter

The principles underlying automatic lensmeters differ from those of manual ones. Automated lensmeters do not neutralize the unknown lens but rather measure the deflection of light rays (similar to automated refractors) as they pass through various parts of the lens to calculate lens power and prismatic effect.

Autorefractors

Autorefractors project near-infrared or infrared light into the eye via a beam splitter and employ various optical principles to reveal the eye's refractive characteristics from the measured light reflected from the ocular fundus.

The foundation for most of the optical principles employed in modern autorefractors (including automated lensmeters) and aberrometers was laid by Christopher Scheiner nearly 400 years ago. Using an opaque disk perforated with 2 pinhole apertures (known as the *Scheiner disk*), he demonstrated that an eye's spherical error could be measured. This *Scheiner principle* relies on the fact that a double-pinhole aperture placed before the eye evokes different responses in an ametropic eye than in an emmetropic eye (Fig 9-3). When looking at a small, distant light source, a normal (emmetropic) eye will see a single spot of light with or without the double-pinhole aperture up front. In case of either myopia or hyperopia, on the other hand, 2 separate spots are seen when the double-pinhole aperture is in place. This is because in a myopic eye (for example), the 2 bundles of light that have been created by the double-pinhole aperture

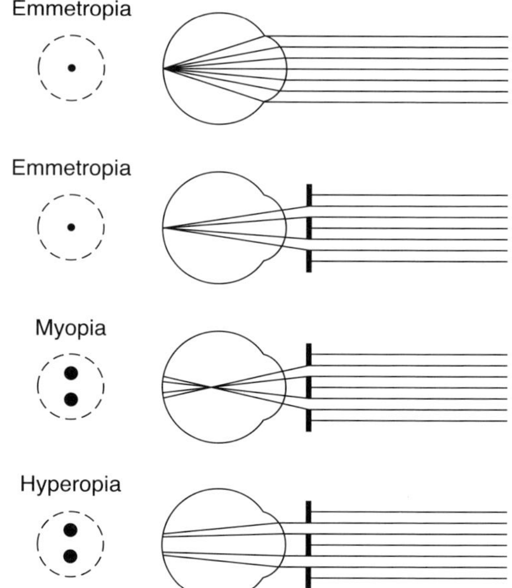

Figure 9-3 The Scheiner principle. Double pinhole apertures placed before the pupil isolate 2 small bundles of light. An object not conjugate to the retina appears doubled. *(Reproduced with permission from Duane TD, ed.* Clinical Ophthalmology, *Vol 1, Revised Edition 1983, Harper & Row.)*

come to focus in the vitreous, crossing over and creating 2 separate spots on the retina; in a hyperopic eye, the 2 bundles of light come to focus beyond the retina, which also leaves 2 separate spots on the retina. One can refract an eye by placing diverse lenses in front of the eye, or by moving the point source axially, until a single spot of light is achieved on the retina.

A modified, objective form of this principle is still used today in most autorefractors. For example, in some instruments, the pinhole apertures are effectively replaced by 2 light-emitting diodes (LEDs) imaged in the pupillary plane. From the axial position of the LEDs required to achieve a single image on a camera, the patient's refractive error is determined. This may be repeated in various meridians to determine any astigmatic component of the refractive error.

Many recent instruments use a stationary source of light to "flood" the eye and then isolate the light emerging from the eye into multiple beams (eg, via a Hartmann screen—essentially a Scheiner disk with multiple holes, or a multilenslet array, as described by Shack). They then measure the deflection or deviation of the emerging light rays from their ideal reference positions to infer the eye's refractive error. This method is commonly referred to as the *ray-deflection principle.* It enables not just the measurement of spherocylindrical errors but also the measurement of higher-order aberrations if multiple parts of the pupil are analyzed, as is done with aberrometers.

The main difficulties with autorefractors are the result of human factors, such as poor fixation and accommodative fluctuation, including so-called *instrument myopia,* that is, the tendency to accommodate when one looks into instruments. Various methods of fogging and automatic tracking have been developed to overcome accommodative fluctuation, with some success.

Keratometer

The keratometer is used to approximate the refracting power of the cornea by determining the curvature of the central anterior corneal surface. It does this by measuring the image size of a reflected mire in each of the principal meridians, accomplished by lining up prism-doubled images at a distance regulated by sharpness of focus. Note that doubling of the image (ie, creating two images that are offset) is performed to avoid problems and inaccuracies from involuntary eye motion. There are 2 basic methods by which the doubled mire images are aligned with one another. For example, in the Javal-Schiøtz keratometer (Haag-Streit USA), the mire separation is adjusted while the image doubling is constant (Fig 9-4A). In the Bausch + Lomb

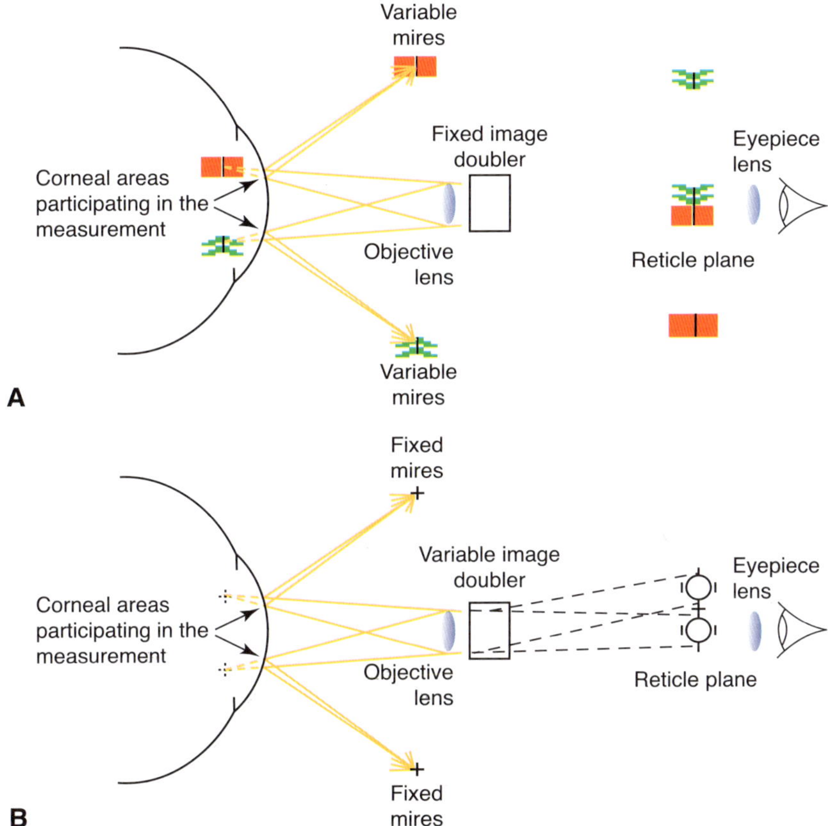

Figure 9-4 Keratometer principle. The curvature of an annulus of the cornea about 3 mm in diameter is determined by measuring the image size of reflected mires in each of the principal meridians. This is accomplished by the examiner lining up the prism-doubled images. Corneal refractive power is inferred from the obtained radius of curvature using the formula for surface power, $D = (n - 1)/r$, where D is the corneal power in diopters; n is the keratometric refractive index at 1.3375, an empirically derived "standardized" refractive index for the cornea that takes the minus power of the corneal back surface into account; and r is the radius of the corneal curvature (in meters). **A,** The Javal-Schiøtz style keratometer employs a fixed-image doubling device, and the mire separation is variable. **B,** The Bausch + Lomb style of keratometer employs a variable-image doubling device, and the mire dimensions are constant. *(Reproduced from Guyton DL, et al.* Ophthalmic Optics and Clinical Refraction. *Prism Press; 1999. Illustration modified by Kristina Irsch, PhD.)*

keratometer, on the other hand, the mire location is fixed and the image doubling is variable (Fig 9-4B). Corneal refractive power is inferred from the calculated radius of curvature using the formula for surface power $D = (n - 1)/r$. In practice, a correction for the small refractive effect (minus power) of the corneal back surface is incorporated in the value for the refractive index of the cornea (yielding a "keratometric" refractive index of $n = 1.3375$).

Corneal Topography

Unlike keratometry instruments, corneal topography instruments produce a detailed map of the entire corneal surface. Originally, corneal topography was limited to analysis of the anterior corneal surface, with the predominant technique being based on the Placido-disk principle (Fig 9-5). Computerized Placido disk–based topographers assess the reflection of a circular mire of concentric lighted rings (Fig 9-6). Note that an ideal, spherical cornea would produce a Placido-disk image with equally spaced rings, while a steeper or flatter

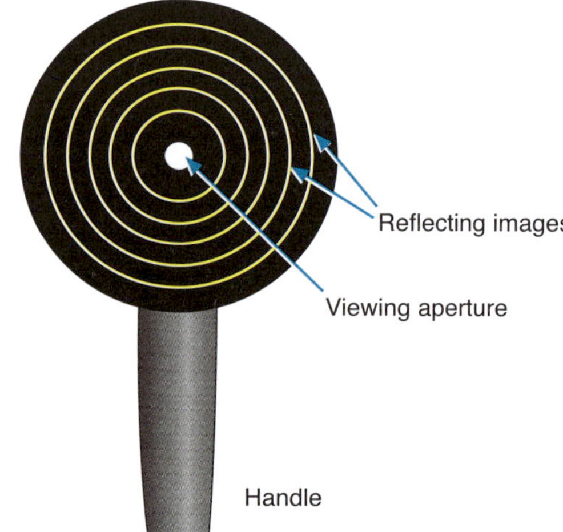

Figure 9-5 A Placido disk. *(Courtesy of Neal H. Atebara, MD. Redrawn by C. H. Wooley.)*

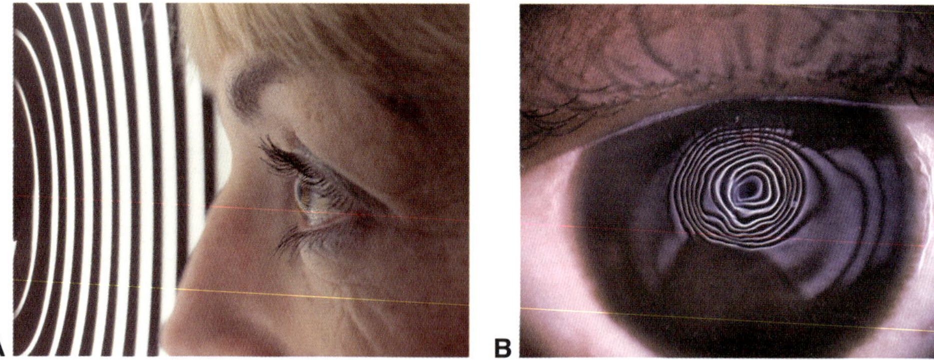

Figure 9-6 Computerized Placido disk–based topography of the cornea. **A,** The ring reflections of the Placido disk–based topographer can be seen on this patient's cornea. This image is then captured and analyzed. **B,** Image of distorted mires on a cornea with keratoconus. *(Courtesy of M. Bowes Hamill, MD.)*

cornea will produce rings that are spaced closer together or farther apart, respectively. Hence, by measuring the distance between the rings, computerized topographers estimate the height of the cornea and display the result in a variety of corneal surface maps that provide quantitative information (eg, on axial curvature, tangential curvature, and elevation; see BCSC Section 13, *Refractive Surgery*). Note that axial maps provide a global representation of anterior corneal curvature, as they are calculated based on the assumption of all light rays being refracted (by the anterior corneal surface) to a common focal point on the optical axis. Tangential maps are calculated based on the fact that not all refracted rays are focused on a central reference axis; tangential maps thereby provide a local representation of anterior curvature, with less smoothing of data than axial maps.

Technological advances enable the characterization of both the anterior and posterior corneal surfaces. These alternative techniques are actually tomography based (and therefore are also suited for corneal pachymetry) and derive topography information via elevation measurements from cross-sectional images of the cornea obtained photographically. They involve the projection of slit beams of light that scan the cornea and use either a stereo-triangulation method (slit-scanning technique) or a camera that rotates perpendicular to the slit beams to capture the illuminated corneal cross sections. The latter, known as a *Scheimpflug camera*, corrects for the nonplanar shape of the cornea and thus enables distortion-free imaging and greater accuracy in the creation of a 3-dimensional map.

Wavefront Aberrometers

Corneal topography can measure the shape of the surface of an irregular cornea, but it cannot measure the actual refractive topography of the entire lens–cornea optical system.

Wavefront aberrometers are essentially ray-deflection autorefractors, the prototype of which was the Scheiner disk. However, unlike autorefractors that measure the deflection of light rays passing through just a few locations of the pupil, which is sufficient to determine spherocylindrical errors of the eye, aberrometers measure the ray deflection through many pupil locations.

For ophthalmic applications, the most popular method employed for wavefront aberrometry is Hartmann-Shack aberrometry, which was first demonstrated by Josef Bille and colleagues in 1994.

Before getting into the details of the underlying principles, let us first review the nature of a wavefront. Wavefronts represent the wave crests, namely the locations for which a wave is maximum at a given time. This is perhaps best understood in the example of water waves, as illustrated in Figure 9-7. The perfect wavefront shown in Figure 9-7A nicely illustrates that, in general, wavefronts are perpendicular to the ray direction and connect the points (that travel at the same speed, from a common source) in a light ray bundle. The concept of wavefront aberrations is simulated in Figure 9-7B, where a floating twig has caused distortion of the waves, creating an irregular wavefront.

In Hartmann-Shack aberrometry, ocular wavefront distortions are measured by using a Hartmann-Shack wavefront sensor (Fig 9-8), which consists of a microlenslet array and a charge-coupled device (CCD) camera. A microlenslet array is a lattice of tiny lenses that can be thought of as a multifaceted lens, like an insect eye (Fig 9-9). An object imaged through such a lens results in multiple images of the same object arranged in an array.

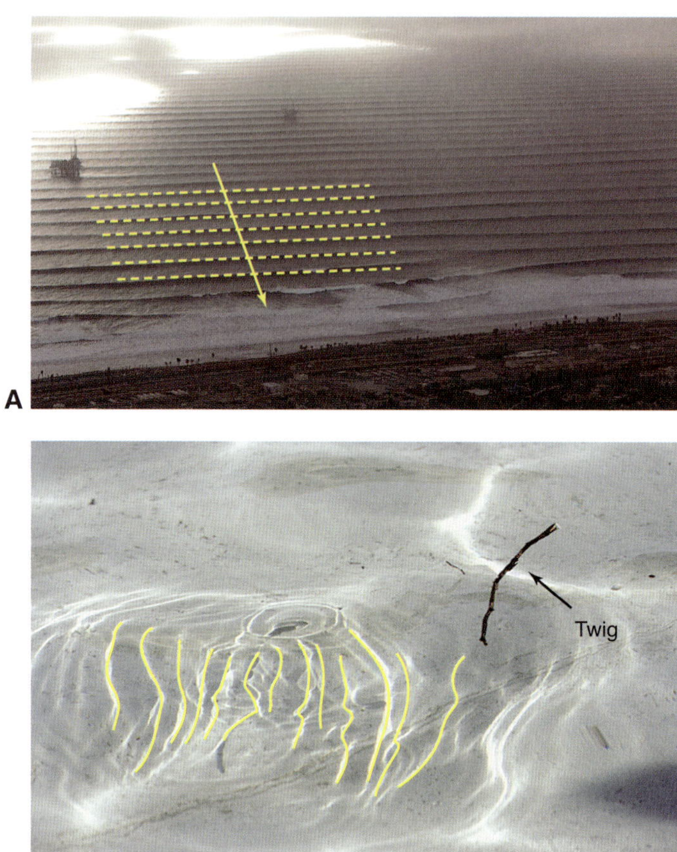

Figure 9-7 Pictorial explanation of wavefront aberrations by means of water waves. **A,** A perfect, regular wavefront. **B,** An irregular wavefront; once a regular wavefront, it has become distorted by a floating twig. *(Part A by Sang Pak, modified by Kristina Irsch, PhD. Part B by Alain Vagner, modified by Kristina Irsch, PhD.)*

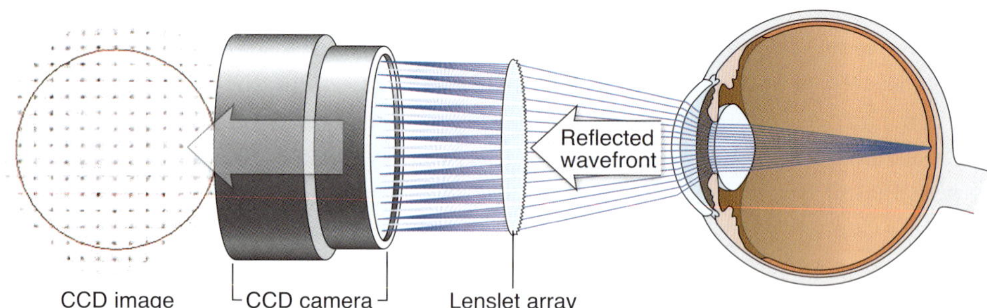

Figure 9-8 Schematic of a Hartmann-Shack wavefront sensor. In Hartmann-Shack aberrometry, wavefront distortions are measured by using a Hartmann-Shack sensor that consists of a microlenslet array and a charge-coupled device (CCD) camera. *(Illustration by Mark Miller.)*

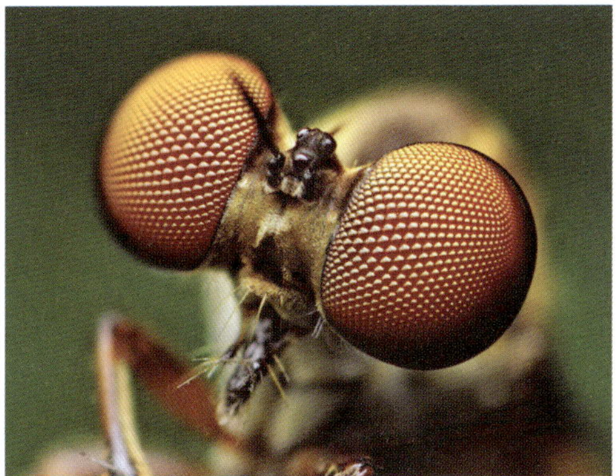

Figure 9-9 Pictorial explanation of a microlenslet array by means of an insect eye. *(Courtesy of Thomas Shahan.)*

For example, in aberrometry, the light reflected from the eye is partitioned into multiple beams by the microlenslet array, forming multiple images of the same retinal spot on the CCD camera. An ideal eye produces a perfect emerging wavefront and thus a regular array of spot images, with each image falling on the grid produced by the optical center of each facet of the multilenslet array (Fig 9-10A). An eye with aberrations, however, produces an irregular wavefront and thus an irregular array of spot images, which are displaced from where they should otherwise fall on the grid (Fig 9-10B). From the displacement of each spot, the shape of the wavefront can be reconstructed and represented in the form of a 2-dimensional wavefront map.

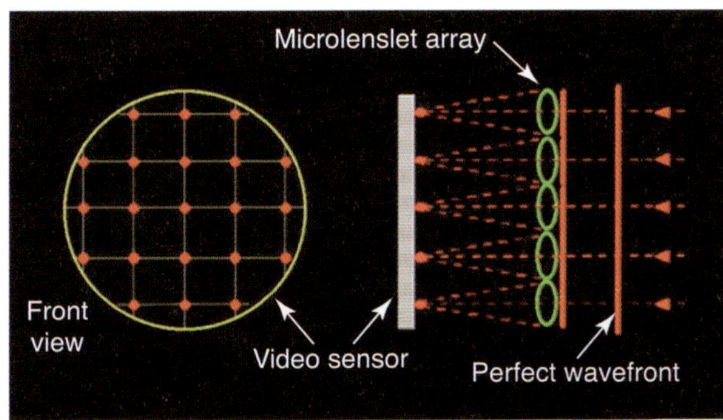

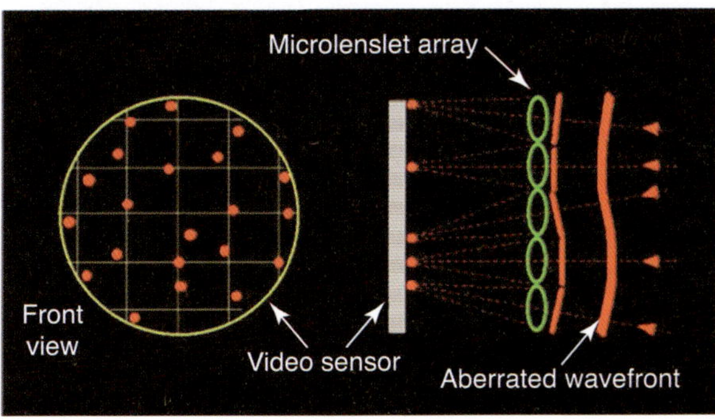

Figure 9-10 An object imaged through a multilenslet array. In aberrometry, the light reflected out of the eye is divided into multiple beams by the microlenslet array, forming multiple images of the same retinal spot on the CCD camera or video sensor. **A,** An ideal eye produces a perfect undistorted emerging wavefront and thus a regular array of spot images, with each image falling on the grid produced by the center of each facet of the multilenslet array. **B,** An aberrated eye produces a distorted wavefront and thus an irregular array of spot images, displaced from where they should otherwise fall on the grid. *(Thibos LN. Principles of Hartmann-Shack Aberrometry.* J Refract Surg. *2000;16(5):S563–S565. doi:10.3928/1081-597X-20000901-14. Reprinted with permission from SLACK Incorporated.)*

Anterior- and Posterior-Segment Imaging

Slit-Lamp Biomicroscope

As with many ophthalmic instruments, it is instructive to consider the illumination and viewing systems of the slit-lamp biomicroscope separately. The illumination system is a light source that is restricted by an adjustable aperture that emits a slit of variable height, width, and orientation, to produce an optical section through the eye. The viewing system is a binocular stereomicroscope with individually focusable eyepieces. To vary the magnification of the viewing system, there may be a Galilean magnification changer (Fig 9-11), a rotating drum of plus and minus lenses. Note that depending on the drum's orientation, a minus–plus lens combination can be oriented either forward (with the minus lens facing the examiner), creating a Galilean telescope to provide higher magnification, or backward (with the plus lens facing the examiner), creating a reverse Galilean telescope to provide lower magnification. Alternatively, there may be 2 sets of eyepieces or objective lenses, or a zoom system in which lenses are moved back and forth to change the magnification.

The illumination system and the viewing system, with its various means of magnification, are mounted on separate arms. In ordinary usage, these rotate about the same vertical axis in a parfocal arrangement, so that they both focus precisely over a common pivot point. This arrangement allows the examiner to study the eye in *direct illumination*. Purposefully separating the illumination and viewing arms from their coupled alignment

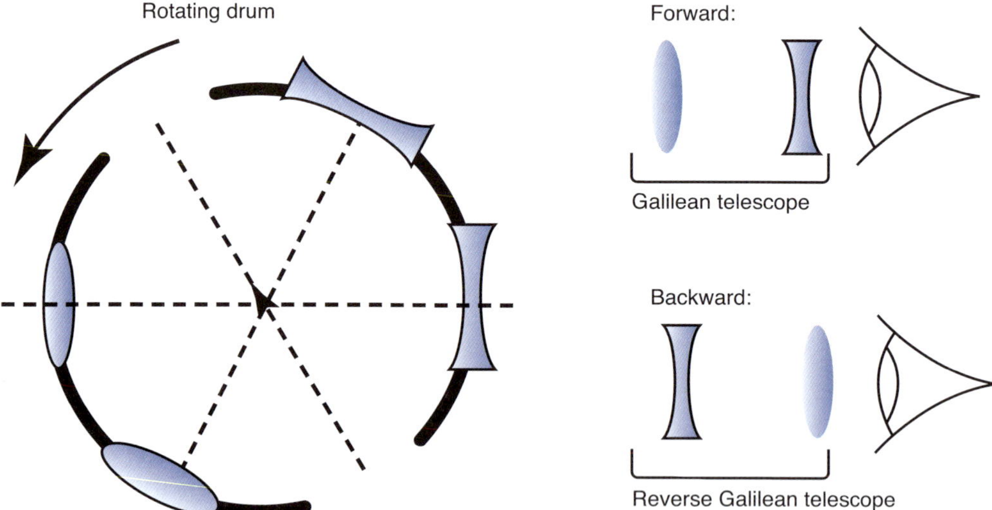

Figure 9-11 Basic concept of Galilean magnification changer, which contains a rotating drum of plus and minus lenses. Depending on the drum's orientation, a minus–plus lens combination may be either orientated forward to create a Galilean telescope and provide higher magnification, or oriented backward to create a reverse Galilean telescope and provide lower magnification. *(Illustration developed by Kristina Irsch, PhD.)*

to horizontally and/or vertically decenter the beam allows for *indirect illumination*. Variations of these illumination techniques allow for examination of the anterior segment in a number of ways, some of which are described next and illustrated in Figure 9-12 (see also BCSC Section 8, *External Disease and Cornea*).

Examination Techniques

- *Direct focal illumination.* This is the most commonly used examination technique, in which the examiner focuses on the area directly illuminated by the slit (Fig 9-12A).
- *Retroillumination.* The beam can be decentered, so that it is striking the iris while the examiner focuses on the cornea, for example. This enables the observer to see corneal opacities illuminated against the black pupil by the reflected light from the iris (iris retroillumination). As another example, by shining the beam through the edge of the pupil, one can observe opacities in the cornea, iris, and lens retroilluminated by the reflected light from the fundus (fundus retroillumination; Fig 9-12B).
- *Sclerotic scatter.* The slit beam is decentered so that it strikes the junction between sclera and cornea, causing light to be totally internally reflected, like a fiber-optic light pipe (Fig 9-12C). In this manner, light follows its longest possible path through the cornea and makes nebular opacities more visible against the background of a dark pupil.
- *Specular reflection.* By looking directly at the bright reflection of the slit beam under high magnification, the examiner can observe irregularities in the corneal surface and see the endothelial cell pattern (Fig 9-12D; this is the principle underlying specular microscopy).

There are several attachments for the slit lamp that extend its use beyond these examination techniques, some of which are described below.

Applanation Tonometry

In tonometry, the intraocular pressure (IOP) of an eye is measured. In Goldmann applanation tonometry specifically, which is performed with an attachment to the slit lamp, IOP is inferred from the amount of force required to flatten a circular region 3.06 mm in diameter on the cornea.

Applanation tonometry is based on Newton's third law of motion, in particular that the pressure (ie, force per unit of surface area) inside the eyeball equals the force applied to its surface divided by the area of contact. This assumes that the eye is infinitely thin walled, perfectly elastic, and dry, none of which is true. Two confounding forces are produced: (1) a force generated by the eye's corneal rigidity (because the eye is not infinitely thin walled or perfectly elastic), which is directed away from the globe; and (2) a force generated by the surface tension of the tear film (because the eye is not dry), which is directed toward the globe. Hans Goldmann determined empirically that if enough force is applied to produce a circular area of flattening 3.06 mm in diameter, the opposing forces caused by corneal rigidity and surface tension cancel each other out, allowing the pressure in the eye to be inferred from the force applied.

The head of the applanation tonometer, which is placed against the patient's cornea, creating a tear film meniscus, contains split-field prisms that split the magnified image

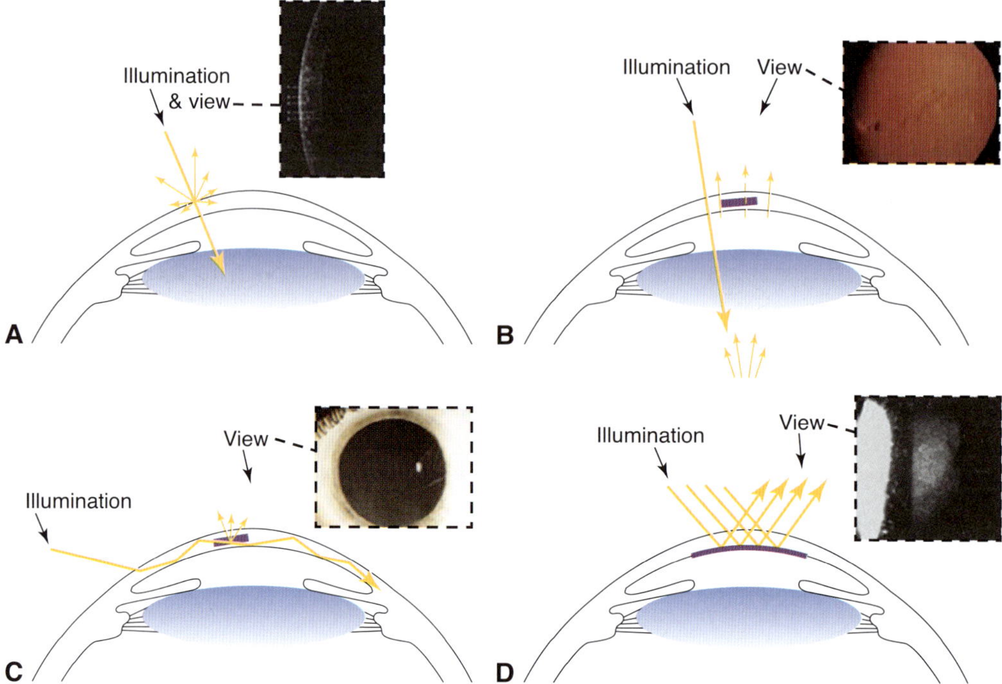

Figure 9-12 Examination techniques with the slit-lamp biomicroscope. **A,** Direct illumination. **B,** Retroillumination. **C,** Sclerotic scatter. **D,** Specular reflection. *(Illustration by Kristina Irsch, PhD. Insets in A–D reproduced with permission from Krachmer JH, Mannis MJ, Holland EJ, eds.* Cornea. *2nd ed. Vol 1. Elsevier/Mosby; 2005:201–217. © CL Mártonyi, WK Kellogg Eye Center, University of Michigan.)*

of tear film meniscus into 2 (like the image doubling associated with keratometry), separated by exactly 3.06 mm. The tear film is often stained with fluorescein dye and viewed under a cobalt blue light to enhance the visibility of the resultant yellow/green circle of tears. The examiner adjusts the applanation pressure until the half-circles are aligned so that their inner margins just touch one another (Fig 9-13). At this point, the circle is exactly 3.06 mm in diameter, and the reading on the tonometer (multiplied by a factor of 10, as it is measured in dynes of force) represents the IOP in millimeters of mercury.

Several factors, especially central corneal thickness, can substantially affect the accuracy of applanation tonometry. Corneas with a smaller or larger central thickness can give artificially low or high IOP readings, respectively.

Surgical Microscope

The operating microscope works on principles similar to those of the slit-lamp biomicroscope. The illumination source of the operating microscope, unlike that of the slit-lamp biomicroscope, is not slit-shaped, and the working distance for the operating microscope is longer to accommodate the specific requirements of ocular surgery. Note that while the illumination is said to be "coaxial," it is technically paraxial (Fig 9-14), as the viewing

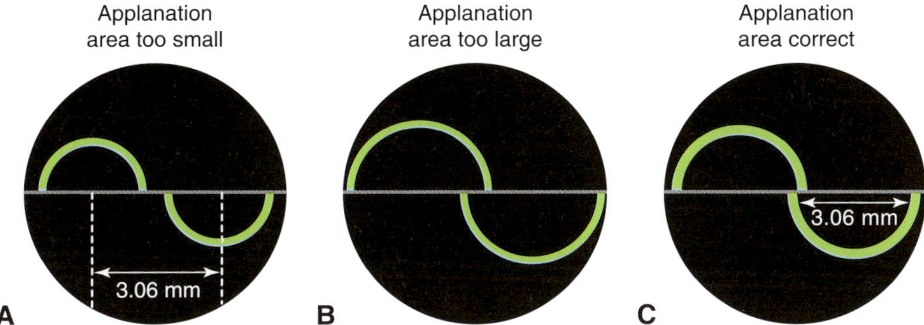

Figure 9-13 The split prism in the applanation head creates 2 offset images. **A,** When the area of applanation is smaller than 3.06 mm, the inner arms of the semicircles remain some distance apart. **B,** When the area of applanation is greater than 3.06 mm, the inner arms of the semicircles overlap. **C,** When the area of applanation is exactly 3.06 mm, the inner arms of the semicircles just touch each other. This is the endpoint for measuring intraocular pressure. The value of 3.06 mm was chosen to approximately balance tear-film surface tension and corneal rigidity. *(Courtesy of Neal H. Atebara, MD. Redrawn by C. H. Wooley.)*

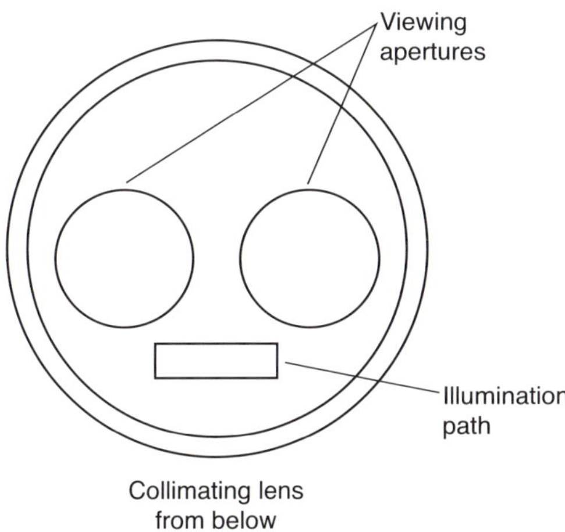

Figure 9-14 Illumination and viewing paths of the surgical microscope as seen from below the collimating lens, demonstrating paraxial rather than coaxial illumination. *(Reproduced from Guyton DL, et al.* Ophthalmic Optics and Clinical Refraction. *Prism Press; 1999. Illustration modified by Kristina Irsch, PhD.)*

apertures and illumination path are separated in modern operating microscopes. The working distance can be selected by the choice of objective lens, though once it is chosen, it is not readily adjustable. In particular for shorter surgeons, for whom the distance from the bottom of the operating table to the eyepieces may exceed the distance from their waists to their eyes, it can be difficult to "get comfortable" at the operating microscope (see Fig 9-15). Sitting up straight at the edge of the stool to allow the thighs to slope downward may be one way to compensate for this difficulty.

Specular Microscopy

Specular microscopy is a modality for examining endothelial cells that uses specular (mirrorlike) reflection from the interface between the endothelial cells and the aqueous humor. The technique can be performed using contact or noncontact methods. In both

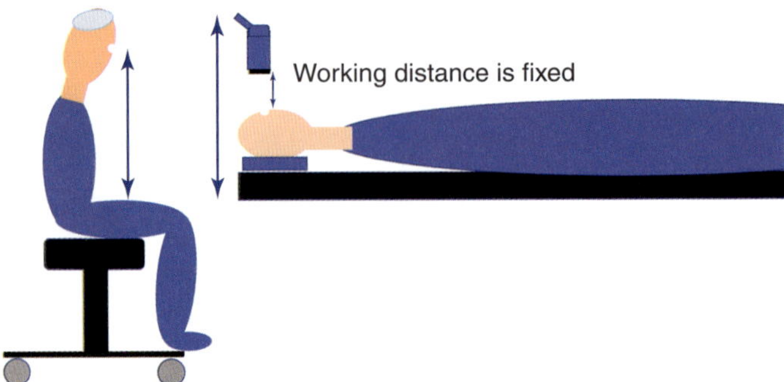

Figure 9-15 Difficulty of "getting comfortable" at the operating microscope. Beware that the distance from the bottom of the operating table to the microscope eyepieces may exceed the distance from the top of the thighs to the surgeon's eyes. To make up for the missing height, a shorter surgeon may have to sit at the edge of the stool to allow their thighs to slope downward. *(Illustration developed by Scott E. Brodie, MD, PhD.)*

methods, the instruments are designed to separate the illumination and viewing paths so that reflections from the anterior corneal surface do not obscure the weak reflection arising from the endothelial cell surface.

As we learned earlier, endothelial cells can also be visualized through a slit-lamp biomicroscope, if the illumination and viewing axes are symmetrically displaced on either side of the normal line to the cornea (see Fig 9-12D). A narrow illumination slit must be used; hence, the field of view is narrow. The use of high-power eyepieces or the maximum magnification setting may facilitate appreciation of the endothelial cell outlines.

Contact specular microscopy allows for higher magnifications than slit-lamp biomicroscopy, making cellular detail and endothelial abnormalities more discernible and allowing for cell counting as well as the study of morphology (see also BCSC Section 8, *External Disease and Cornea*).

Auxiliary Lenses for Slit-Lamp Examination of the Retina

The cornea and lens together provide so much convergence that ordinarily we cannot see the retina using a slit-lamp biomicroscope. At most, the slit lamp can view about half of the way back from the crystalline lens to the retina, and usually no more than one-third of the way. Auxiliary lenses for slit-lamp examination of the retina can be placed in front of the eye to overcome this problem. Table 9-1 lists common auxiliary lenses for slit-lamp examination of the retina.

The Goldmann 3-mirror contact gonioscopy lens is a special viewing lens that is widely used for looking at the eye with the slit lamp. With a power of about –64.00 D, it essentially nullifies the power of the eye (recall that the eye itself has about 60.00 D of plus power) and provides an upright view of the posterior pole. The mirrors inside the contact lens enable views of more and less peripheral portions of the eye, and even of the angle of the anterior chamber (gonioscopy; Fig 9-16). The main disadvantage of the Goldmann lens is its limited field of view, which requires rotation of the lens to visualize more than a small patch of the fundus. Remember that the views in the various mirrors are left-right reversed.

Table 9-1 Auxiliary Lenses for Slit-Lamp Examination of the Retina

Lens	Field of View	Image Magnification	Laser Beam Magnification
Goldmann-style 3-mirror contact lens	60°/66°/76°	1.06×	0.94×
Posterior pole contact lens[a]	70°/84°	1.06×	0.94×
Wide-field contact lens[b]	110°/132°	0.7×	1.4×
Very-wide-field contact lens[c]	120°/144°	0.51×	1.97×
60 D noncontact lens	68°/81°	1.15×	0.87×
78 D noncontact lens	81°/97°	0.93×	1.08×
90 D noncontact lens	74°/89°	0.76×	1.32×

[a] For example, Area Centralis (Volk), Mainster Focal Grid (Ocular Instruments).
[b] For example, TransEquator (Volk), Mainster Wide Field (Ocular Instruments).
[c] For example, QuadrAspheric (Volk), Mainster PRP 165 (Ocular Instruments).

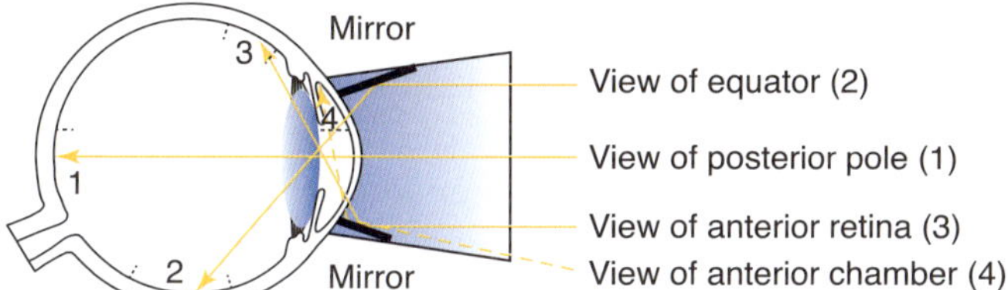

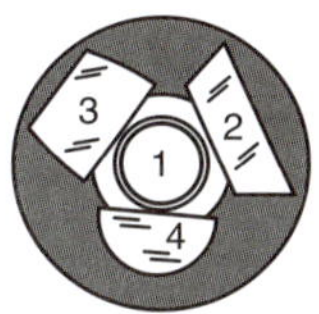

Figure 9-16 Goldmann 3-mirror contact lens. The flat-front contact lens essentially nullifies the power of the eye and provides an upright view of the posterior pole. The mirrors at various angles inside enable alternative (inverted) views of different parts of the retina (2 and 3) and the anterior chamber angle (gonioscopy; 4). *(Image at left reproduced from Guyton DL, et al.* Ophthalmic Optics and Clinical Refraction. *Prism Press; 1999. Illustration modified by Kristina Irsch, PhD.)*

Other examples of contact lenses for the slit-lamp biomicroscope are the fundus contact lenses from manufacturers such as Volk and Ocular Instruments. Examples include the Area Centralis lens (Volk) and Mainster Focal Grid (Ocular Instruments) for viewing the central fundus and the QuadrAspheric and TransEquator lenses (Volk), and the Mainster PRP 165 and Mainster Wide Field lenses (Ocular Instruments), which enable peripheral wide-angle views of the retina.

Holding a high-power plus lens (eg, 60.00 D, 78.00 D, or 90.00 D fundus lenses) in front of the eye produces an inverted aerial image of the retina, which can be viewed with the slit lamp in a manner similar to that of indirect ophthalmoscopy (Fig 9-17).

Ophthalmoscopy

Direct ophthalmoscope

With direct ophthalmoscopy, the examiner uses the optics of the patient's eye as a simple magnifier to look at the retina. If both the examiner and patient have emmetropic vision and are not accommodating, rays of light coming from a point on the patient's retina exit parallel, with zero vergence, and continue through the empty peephole of the direct ophthalmoscope. These parallel rays of light are then focused onto the examiner's retina. Thus, the examiner's retina becomes conjugate to the patient's retina when a direct ophthalmoscope is used.

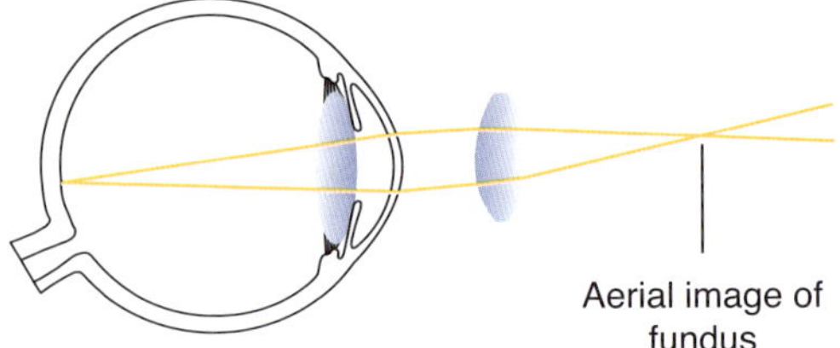

Figure 9-17 High-power plus lenses for slit-lamp indirect ophthalmoscopy (eg, 60.00 D and 90.00 D fundus lenses) held in front of the eye produce an inverted aerial image of the retina within the focal range of a slit-lamp biomicroscope. *(Reproduced from Guyton DL, et al.* Ophthalmic Optics and Clinical Refraction. *Prism Press; 1999. Illustration modified by Kristina Irsch, PhD.)*

When the examiner looks through the peephole of a direct ophthalmoscope, with no lenses in place, just past the edge of (or aperture in) a mirror that reflects light into the patient's eye, almost coaxial to the examiner's view, an upright, virtual, magnified retinal image is seen. The optics of the emmetropic eye are approximately +60.00 D, so using the formula for a simple magnifier (ie, Mag = D/4), the magnification is 60/4, or 15× (Fig 9-18). This means that the patient's retina appears 15 times larger than if the retina were removed from the eye and held at a distance of 25 cm. Only a small field of view is seen with the direct ophthalmoscope (about 7°) because, even when the examiner is as close to the patient as possible, the peripheral rays that come from the peripheral part of the patient's retina cannot be captured, as they do not enter the examiner's pupil (Fig 9-19).

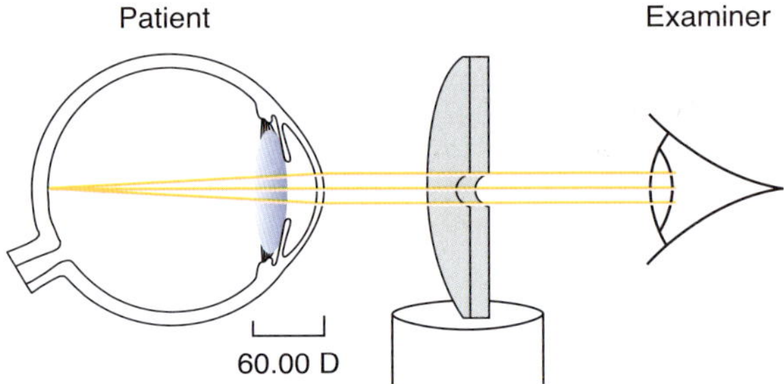

Figure 9-18 Magnification of direct ophthalmoscopy. With direct ophthalmoscopy the examiner uses the optics of the patient's eye as a simple magnifier to look at the retina. The optics of the emmetropic eye are approximately +60.00 D, thus the magnification is 60/4, or 15×, according to the formula for a simple magnifier (Mag = D/4). *(Reproduced from Guyton DL, et al.* Ophthalmic Optics and Clinical Refraction. *Prism Press; 1999. Illustration modified by Kristina Irsch, PhD.)*

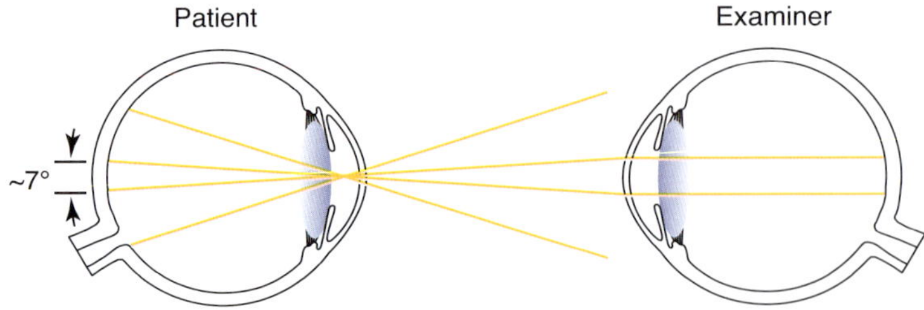

Figure 9-19 Field of view with direct ophthalmoscopy. Even when the examiner is positioned as close to the patient as possible, the peripheral rays that come from the peripheral part of the patient's retina do not enter the examiner's pupil, restricting the field of view to about 7°. *(Reproduced from Guyton DL, et al.* Ophthalmic Optics and Clinical Refraction. *Prism Press; 1999. Illustration modified by Kristina Irsch, PhD.)*

If the patient or examiner has an uncorrected spherical refractive error, a series of auxiliary lenses is available to dial into the path of the direct ophthalmoscope to compensate for it. If the patient's eye is myopic, a minus lens is dialed in to overcome the extra plus power "error lens" inside the patient's eye. These 2 lenses create a Galilean telescope effect, increasing magnification and decreasing the field of view. Similarly, the retina of a hyperopic eye will be magnified less than 15× because of the reverse Galilean telescope created by the minus power error lens inside the patient's eye and the plus lens of the direct ophthalmoscope.

The quality of the view of the fundus through a dilated pupil with the direct ophthalmoscope also has important utility in the preoperative assessment of the optical severity of a cataract.

Indirect ophthalmoscope

In indirect ophthalmoscopy, an ophthalmic "condensing" lens is used to increase the field of view by capturing the peripheral rays (which are lost in direct ophthalmoscopy) and bringing them into the examiner's pupil (Fig 9-20). Thus, a much wider field of view is seen with the indirect ophthalmoscope (eg, about 25° with an ordinary 20.00 D condensing lens).

Assuming that the patient's eye is emmetropic, rays of light coming from a point on the patient's retina leave the eye with zero vergence and are gathered and focused by the condensing lens into what is called an intermediate *aerial image*; that is, an image of the patient's retina in space. In case of a 20.00 D condensing lens, this image is located one-twentieth of a meter from the lens (closer to the examiner). The examiner therefore sees an optically real, inverted image of the patient's retina that appears to be 5 cm closer to the examiner's eye than the 20.00 D lens (Fig 9-21). With the examiner looking at that aerial image, it will be focused on the examiner's retina. Thus, in indirect ophthalmoscopy, the patient's retina, the aerial image, and the examiner's retina are all conjugate to each other.

Equally important conjugate planes in indirect ophthalmoscopy, however, are the cornea and the faceplate of the indirect ophthalmoscope (Fig 9-22). The main purpose of the condensing lens, other than forming the aerial image, is to make the faceplate of the indirect ophthalmoscope conjugate to the patient's cornea, so that the bright illumination light passes at a different place through the cornea, offset from where the examiner's pupils are

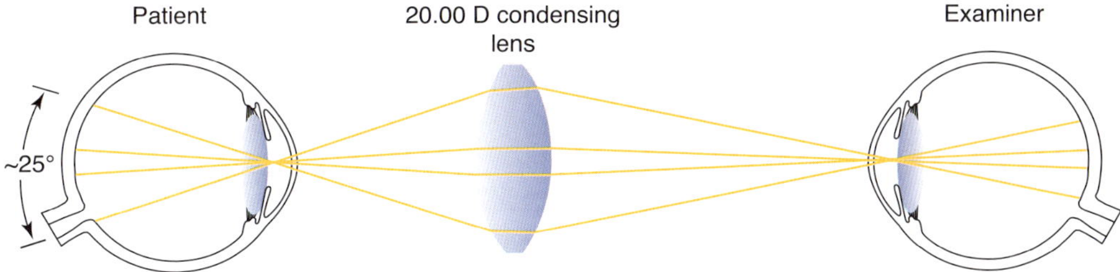

Figure 9-20 Field of view with indirect ophthalmoscopy. Unlike in direct ophthalmoscopy, the condensing lens captures the peripheral rays, enlarging the field of view to about 25° with an ordinary 20.00 D condensing lens. *(Reproduced from Guyton DL, et al.* Ophthalmic Optics and Clinical Refraction. *Prism Press; 1999. Illustration modified by Kristina Irsch, PhD.)*

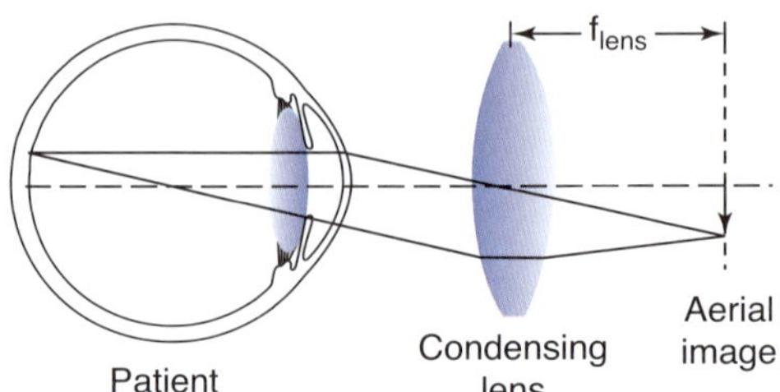

Figure 9-21 Aerial image formation in indirect ophthalmoscopy. The condensing lens held in front of the patient's eye produces an inverted aerial image, that is, a real image of the patient's retina in space. With an emmetropic patient, the light rays coming from a point of the patient's retina exit the eye with zero vergence and the aerial image is formed in the focal plane of the condensing lens. Using an ordinary 20.00 D condensing lens, the image of the patient's retina is thus located 1/20 m = 0.05 m = 5 cm away from the lens. *(Reproduced from Guyton DL, et al.* Ophthalmic Optics and Clinical Refraction. *Prism Press; 1999. Illustration modified by Kristina Irsch, PhD.)*

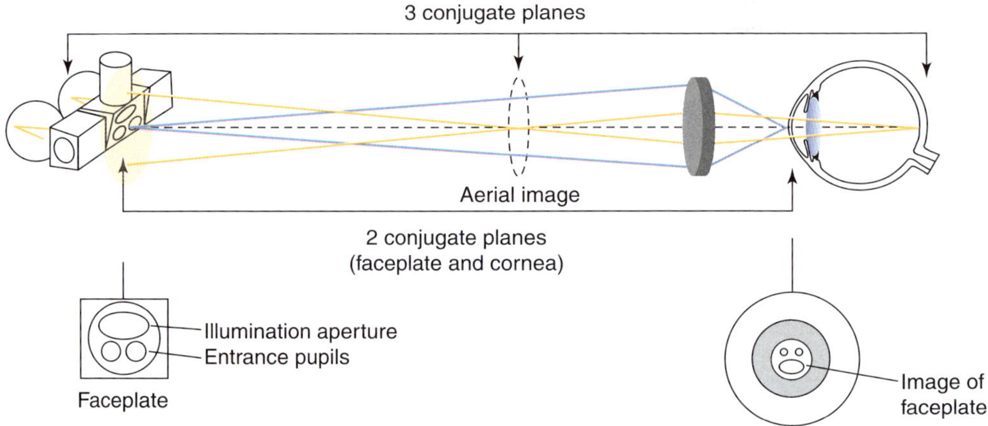

Figure 9-22 Conjugate planes in indirect ophthalmoscopy. The patient's retina, the aerial image, and the examiner's retina, as well as the faceplate of the indirect ophthalmoscope and the patient's cornea, are conjugate to each other when performing indirect ophthalmoscopy. *(Reproduced from Guyton DL, et al.* Ophthalmic Optics and Clinical Refraction. *Prism Press; 1999. Illustration redrawn by Kristina Irsch, PhD.)*

looking, to avoid reflections back from the cornea into the examiner's eyes. This is very important because the cornea reflects about 2% of the light, but the observed retinal image is only 0.1% of the light. Thus, the retina cannot be seen if any light from the cornea is reflected back into the observation pathway. Therefore, in indirect ophthalmoscopy, the light pathway is separated from the observation pathway by imaging the faceplate on the cornea with the condensing lens, so that the aerial image of the retina can be seen. The images of the observer's pupils in the plane of the cornea are very small circles—about 10% of the diameter of the observer's pupil's—and thus form virtual pinholes. These tiny entrance pupils limit the light available for the observer to view the fundus, but also allow very clear images to be appreciated even in the presence of imperfect ocular media, such as cataracts or vitreous debris. This is a mixed blessing—it allows for better views of the fundus than can be obtained in many cases, for example, with the direct ophthalmoscope or slit lamp, but prevents the observer from appreciating the visual impairments caused by the media imperfections.

The binocular eyepieces in the indirect ophthalmoscope, via mirrors and/or prisms, reduce the interpupillary distance from about 60 mm to 15 mm, to fit the images of the examiner's pupils along with the light source into the patient's pupil, allowing for binocular viewing. (If the patient's pupil is small, the illuminating and observation pathways can be brought closer by varying the positions of mirrors or prisms in the eyepieces.) This causes a reduction of the examiner's stereoscopic vision by 60/15, or 4×, which is compensated for by the axial magnification of the aerial image.

This can be appreciated by considering the transverse magnification of the aerial image, which is the power of the eye divided by the power of the condensing lens (see Fig 9-23), that is, 60/20, or 3×, for an emmetropic eye and a 20.00 D condensing lens. The aerial image is thus wider than the actual image on the retina. Recall that the axial magnification is the square of the transverse (lateral or linear) magnification, that is, in our case, 9×. The image that is observed is thus greatly distorted in depth, which helps make up for the loss in stereoacuity due to the reduced interpupillary distance. The eyepieces reduce depth fourfold, so the overall axial magnification is 9/4, or 2.25×. Thus, objects appear to be 3 times wider and 2.25 times increased in depth. Other choices of condensing lens power result in different ratios of transverse and lateral magnification.

However, the threefold transverse magnification of the aerial image is not the overall transverse magnification of indirect ophthalmoscopy. The overall transverse magnification depends upon the distance from which the aerial image is observed. From about 40 cm, from where it is usually observed, the overall transverse magnification is about 3 × 25/40, or 1.87×, with the 20.00 D condensing lens (Fig 9-24), much less than with a direct ophthalmoscope, which provides 15× magnification (see Fig 9-18). Consequently, small details are observed with the direct ophthalmoscope that cannot be seen with the indirect ophthalmoscope.

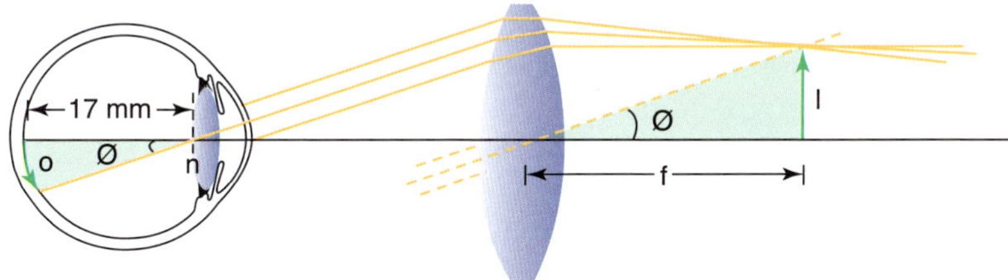

Figure 9-23 Magnification of the aerial image in indirect ophthalmoscopy. For an emmetropic eye, by similar triangles, transverse magnification equals the focal length of the condensing lens divided by the focal length of the eye in air, and therefore the power of the eye divided by the power of the condensing lens. *(Reproduced from Guyton DL, et al.* Ophthalmic Optics and Clinical Refraction. *Prism Press; 1999. Illustration modified by Kristina Irsch, PhD.)*

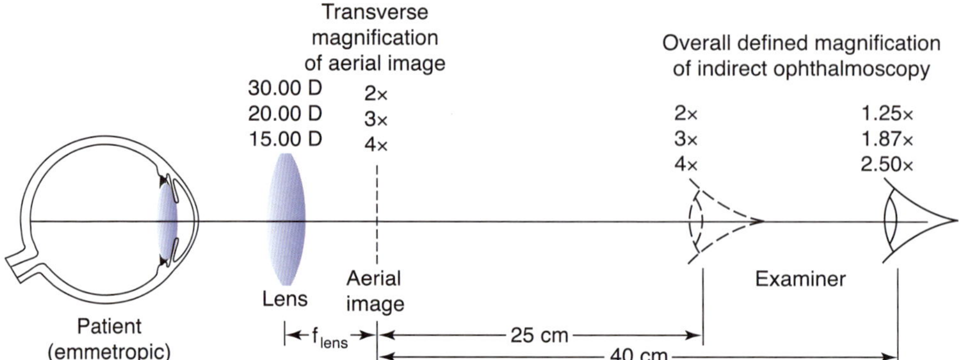

Figure 9-24 Overall magnification of indirect ophthalmoscopy with different condensing lenses depends on the distance from which the aerial image is observed. From about 40 cm, from where it is usually observed, the overall magnification is about 1.87× with the 20.00 D condensing lens. *(Reproduced from Guyton DL, et al.* Ophthalmic Optics and Clinical Refraction. *Prism Press; 1999. Illustration modified by Kristina Irsch, PhD.)*

Fundus Camera

The fundus camera uses the optical principles of indirect ophthalmoscopy. It is essentially an indirect ophthalmoscope with a perforated mirror taking the place of the faceplate of the indirect ophthalmoscope that separates the observation and illumination pathways, and the aerial image is simply reimaged onto the camera's film or sensor array.

With the addition of different filters, *fluorescein angiography* can be performed with the fundus camera. Fluorescein has its absorption maximum at about 490 nm, in the blue part of the spectrum, whereas the emission maximum is at about 530 nm, in the green part of the spectrum. In fluorescein angiography, an "excitation filter" permits blue light to pass and excite the fluorescein; on the return path, a "barrier filter" allows the green light to pass, but blocks the background blue light, allowing the fluorescent image to be recorded with a high-resolution monochrome film or sensor array. Most indirect ophthalmoscopes provide a blue filter to allow "real-time" viewing of the fluorescence pattern.

Scanning Laser Ophthalmoscope

The scanning laser ophthalmoscope (SLO) functions as both an ophthalmoscope and a fundus camera but requires significantly less light than those conventional flood illumination systems. This is because in the SLO, the use of a narrow, highly concentrated (collimated) laser beam of light (eg, from a 670-nm diode laser), which is moved rapidly via scanning mirrors over the retina in a grid (raster) pattern, illuminates only a small spot at a time, hence allowing more of the pupil to be used for viewing than for illumination (Fig 9-25); light returned from each point is detected and synchronously decoded to produce an ocular fundus image. In other words, unlike the ophthalmoscope or fundus camera, in which illumination uses most of the pupillary area, with a separate small area reserved for viewing (Fig 9-25A), the SLO uses the larger area for light collection ("viewing") and the smaller one for illumination (Fig 9-25B).

The following sections describe a few types of SLOs.

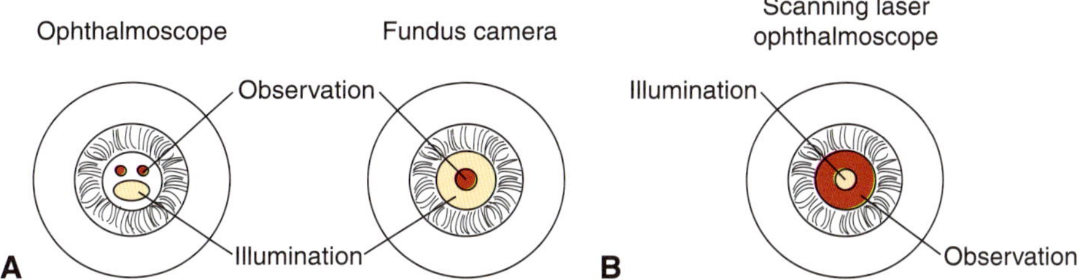

Figure 9-25 Illumination and observation paths in conventional ophthalmoscopy and fundus imaging versus scanning laser ophthalmoscopy. Unlike the ophthalmoscope or fundus camera, in which illumination uses most of the pupillary area and a separate small area is reserved for observation **(A)**, the scanning laser ophthalmoscope uses the larger pupillary area for observation and the smaller one for illumination **(B)**. *(Illustration modified by Kristina Irsch, PhD.)*

Confocal scanning laser ophthalmoscope

In confocal scanning laser ophthalmoscopy (the basis of modern clinical SLOs, eg, from Heidelberg Engineering and Optos), a pinhole is placed in front of the detector to cut off scattered or defocused light coming from outside the point of illumination or interest, which otherwise can blur the image (Fig 9-26). This results in a focused, high-contrast image of a single tissue layer located at the focal plane.

The position of the confocal aperture determines from which layer in the fundus the reflected light is collected, and it enables tomographic information to be extracted. More precisely, by moving the plane of the pinhole, multiple optical sections through the tissue of interest can be acquired.

The series of optical section images forms a layered 3-dimensional image and can be used to construct topography and reflectance images of the fundus. The topography image is constructed by identifying the peak intensity (reflectance) along the z-axis from all optical sections at each pixel location. The reflectance image is constructed as a summation of intensities along the z-axis from all of the optical sections at each pixel location.

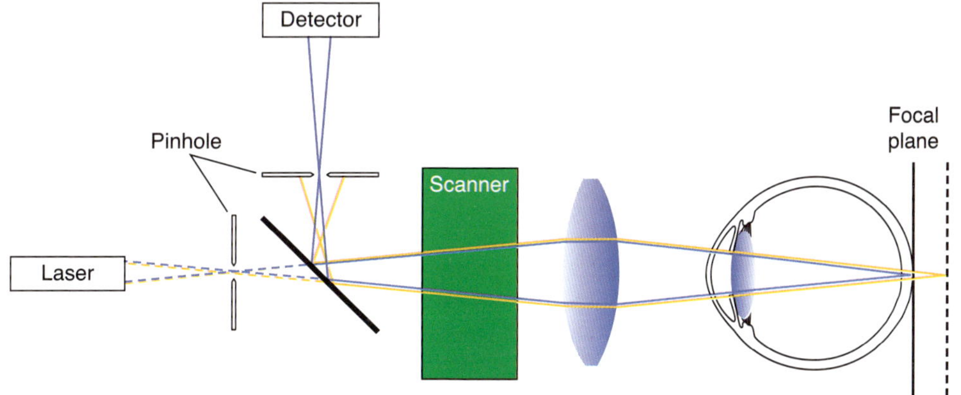

Figure 9-26 Principle of confocal laser scanning ophthalmoscopy. A pinhole aperture prevents defocused or scattered light coming from outside the focal plane, which would blur the image, from entering the detector. *(Illustration modified by Kristina Irsch, PhD.)*

With the use of auxiliary optics, different fields of view can be obtained. Optos, for example, uses a wide ellipsoidal mirror that allows viewing of up to 200° of the ocular fundus in a single image. Two lasers, which emit light at 532 nm (green) and 633 nm (red), are utilized. The light from the 2 lasers, reflected at different depths by the ocular fundus (red wavelengths penetrate deeper), is separated into its green and red components and reassembled into a false-color image (Fig 9-27A). Displaying the images from the red and green channels separately can be of value in visualizing different structures, such as the choroidal vascular pattern (red channel; see Fig 9-27B) and the retinal nerve fiber layer (green channel; see Fig 9-27C).

Confocal scanning laser microscope

With the use of objective lenses, usually put in contact with the patient's corneal surface, the confocal SLO can also be turned into a confocal scanning laser microscope, enabling tomography through different depths of the cornea at cellular resolution (see BCSC Section 8, *External Disease and Cornea*).

Angiography and autofluorescence imaging

The use of various wavelengths allows for additional applications with the confocal SLO, such as fluorescein angiography, indocyanine green angiography, and autofluorescence imaging (see also BCSC Section 12, *Retina and Vitreous*).

For *fluorescein angiography* with the SLO, a blue argon laser at 488 nm is used to excite the dye, while a barrier filter at about 500-nm edge wavelength separates the excitation and fluorescent light.

The same laser uses the natural fluorescence that occurs from the retinal layers (such as lipofuscin, which accumulates in the retinal pigment epithelium) to generate fundus autofluorescence images. It can also create (but without the use of the barrier filter) "red-free" or blue-reflectance images, which can aid in the visualization of pathologies that have low contrast to the red color.

For *indocyanine green angiography*, on the other hand, a diode laser at 790-nm wavelength is used to excite the dye, while a barrier filter at 810-nm edge wavelength separates excitation and fluorescent light.

Optical Coherence Tomography

Optical coherence tomography (OCT) is an optical analogue to ultrasound imaging, capable of generating high-resolution cross-sectional views of the retina and anterior segment. Due to the much higher speed of light compared with sound (eg, lightning can be seen before thunder is heard) the direct electronic measurement of the shorter "echo" times it takes light to travel from different structures at axial distances within the eye is not feasible. Interferometry enables us to overcome this difficulty in the following manner. Light is split into 2 beams, and the beam backscattered from the sample (eg, ocular tissue) is then compared (interfered) with the beam that has traveled a known distance from the reference mirror. Interference patterns are observable when the path–length difference, that is, the optical distances traveled by the 2 beams in the sample and reference arms, is smaller than or equal to the coherence length of the light (see Fig 2-8). In OCT, broadband

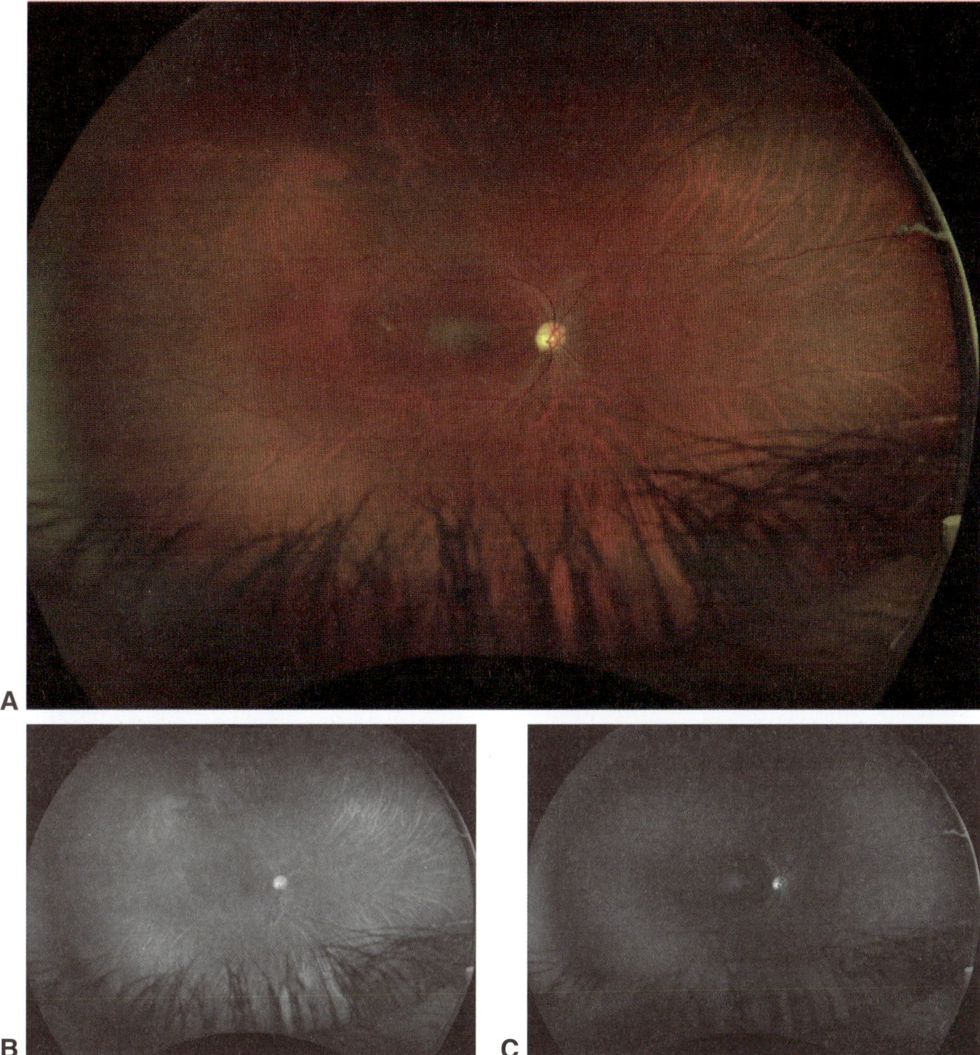

Figure 9-27 Example of wide-field image obtained with Optos' confocal scanning laser ophthalmoscope. A patient with sectoral optic atrophy with loss of papillomacular bundle is depicted. **A,** False-color image representing the superposition of red **(B)** and green **(C)** channels, that is, the reconstructed image from the red and green laser light reflected from the ocular fundus. Because red light penetrates deeper into tissues, monochrome representation of the red channel only aids in the visualization of the underlying choroidal vascular pattern **(B)**. Because green light is more effectively scattered by the nerve fiber layer, the loss of the papillomacular nerve fiber tissue is seen to advantage in the monochrome representation of the green channel only **(C)**. *(Courtesy of Scott E. Brodie, MD, PhD.)*

(ie, low-coherence) light sources are used (eg, a superluminescent diode emitting a beam of light with long [red] wavelengths—reds being chosen because they are scattered in tissue less than is blue light), rather than narrowband (ie, highly coherent) light sources, such as a laser, because they give the instrument greater sensitivity to the differences in path lengths the 2 beams have traveled (see Fig 2-11). In other words, even though the light passes through different structures in the sample, its low coherence aids in separating out the individual reflections originating from each structure at distinct axial distances in the light path. Note that the low-coherence interferometry setup illustrated in Fig 2-11 corresponds to time-domain OCT (TD-OCT) in which the sample may be multilayered corneal or retinal tissue (Fig 9-28).

In TD-OCT (see Fig 9-28), the position of the reference mirror is thus adjusted so that interference patterns show up, as a function of time, whenever the beam reflected from an interface between layers of the tissue has traveled almost the same amount of time as the beam reflected from the reference mirror. In other words, the path-length difference with the sample arm is varied by axially moving the reference mirror, essentially scanning through the depth of the ocular tissue. The mirror position at which interference effects are detected is thus indicative of the depth of the reflecting ocular tissue interface, while the amplitude or "visibility" of the fringes is proportional to its

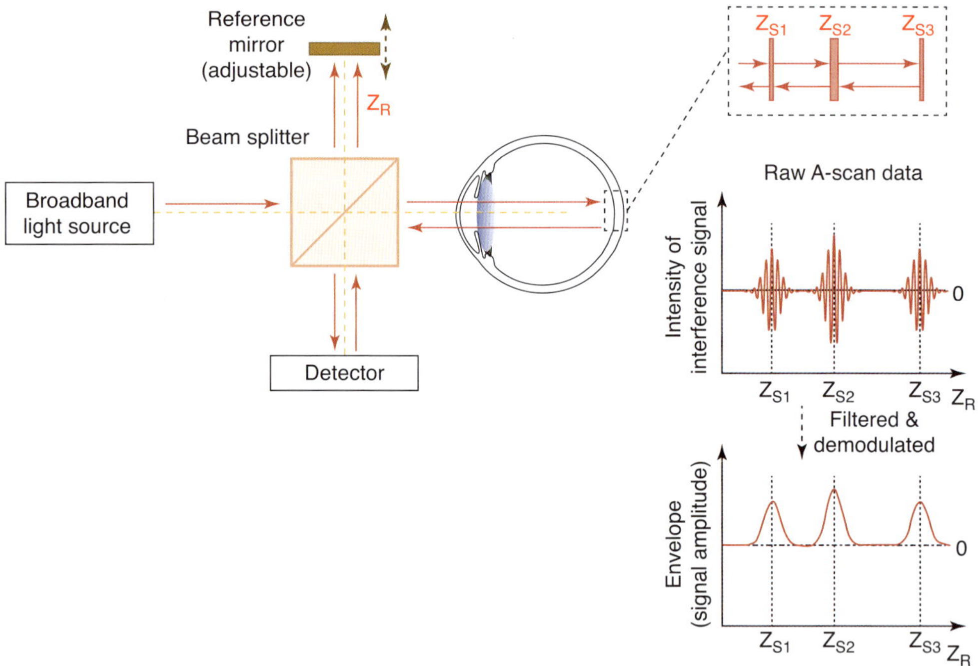

Figure 9-28 Concept of time-domain optical coherence tomography (TD-OCT) based on the principle of low-coherence interferometry. A broadband (ie, low-coherence) light source is used, such as a superluminescent diode that emits a beam of light with long red wavelengths, so that interference effects are registered only when the time traveled by beams in the reference and sample arms is nearly equal. That is, with the reference arm scanned (the reference mirror is altered by a known distance, z_R), fringe patterns are generated as a function of time whenever the position of the reference mirror matches the position of 1 of the reflective interfaces (z_{S1}, z_{S2}, z_{S3}) of the ocular tissue or sample. The detected interference signal is filtered and demodulated, yielding its envelope, from which the ocular tissue's reflectivity profile or 1-dimensional A-scan is derived. *(Illustration developed by Kristina Irsch, PhD.)*

reflectivity. The reflectivity profile of the sample, similar to the ultrasound's A-scan, is derived directly from the envelopes of the interference fringes that are attained, in practice, by filtering and demodulation of the registered interference signal. Cross-sectional images are generated by performing successive A-scans at different transverse positions on the retina or cornea; this yields 2-dimensional results, like an ultrasound's B-scan does (see BCSC Section 12, *Retina and Vitreous* and BCSC Section 8, *External Disease and Cornea*). By acquiring sequential cross-sectional images, 3-dimensional, volumetric results are obtained.

In Fourier-domain OCT (FD-OCT; Fig 9-29), also called *spectral-domain OCT* (SD-OCT) or *frequency-domain OCT*, the reference mirror is fixed at 1 position that approximately corresponds to the location of the sample. In other words, no axial scanning is performed (only lateral scanning across the sample), and the reference arm length remains constant. At a given lateral position, all the light echoes that arise from the various ocular tissue interfaces at different depths are detected simultaneously. Hence, in contrast

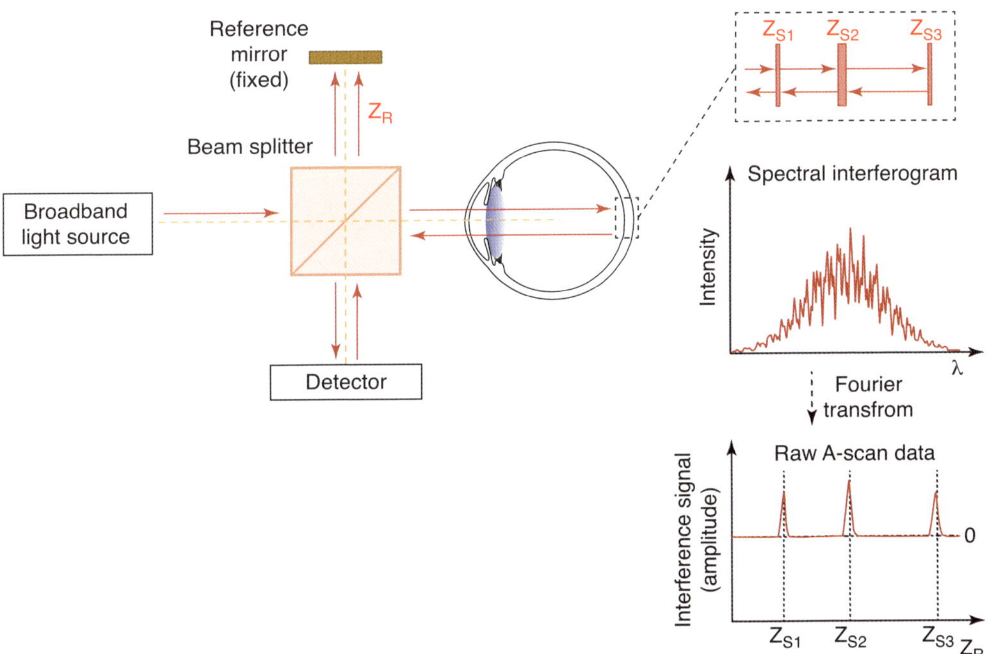

Figure 9-29 Concept of Fourier-domain OCT (FD-OCT). The reference mirror is fixed at a single axial position that approximately corresponds to that of the sample. At a given lateral position, all light echoes arising from the reflecting tissue interfaces at various depths (eg, z_{S1}, z_{S2}, z_{S3}) are detected simultaneously. This detection is performed in the spectral domain, meaning that the composite fringes, all mixed together, are acquired as a function of wavelength, λ. The interferogram is converted from the spectral domain to the spatial or time domain, resulting in the envelope of the familiar interference signal as a function of depth (with fringes occurring at the positions of the ocular tissue's reflectors) by means of spectral-wavelength (ie, Fourier) analysis. *(Illustration developed by Kristina Irsch, PhD.)*

to TD-OCT, the detection of interference-fringe patterns as a function of axial position of the reference mirror and composite fringes, all mixed together, are measured in FD-OCT, but spectral wavelength (or Fourier) analysis enables them to be discerned separately and an A-scan retrieved without the reference mirror being moved.

The key in FD-OCT is the measurement of spectrally resolved interferograms (ie, the composite interference-fringe patterns are acquired as a function of wavelength). In these spectral interferograms, the rate of intensity variation (across wavelengths) is indicative of, and differs from, the axial position of the reflecting interfaces in the sample. In other words, and as explained in Figure 9-30, the light echoes that arise from different ocular tissue depths (ie, different path–length differences with the reference arm) generate differently spaced undulations (so-called frequency modulations) in the spectrally resolved interference signals. For example, when the light echo arises from closer tissue interfaces, there is a slower variation in intensity across different wavelengths in the generated interference-fringe patterns (ie, the fringe patterns' undulations are spaced farther apart,

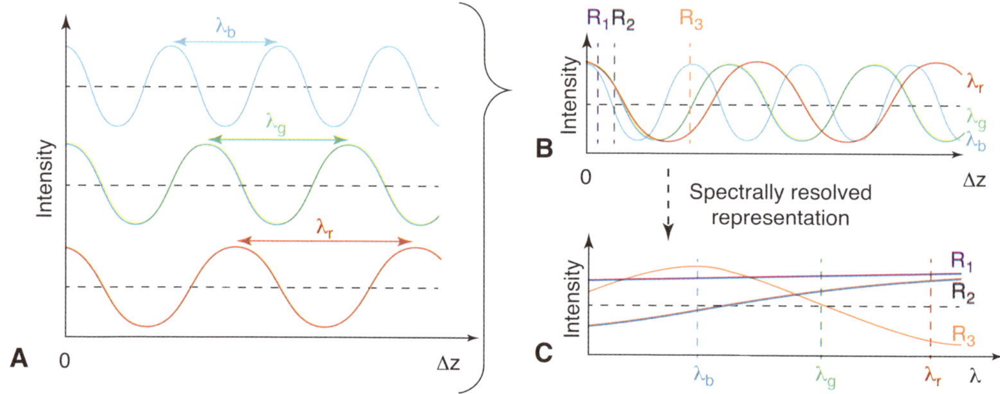

Figure 9-30 Pictorial explanation of encoding of depth information in the rate of intensity variation (frequency modulation) in spectrally resolved interferograms of FD-OCT. **A,** Multiple wavelengths or colors are contained in light from a broadband source. The emitted polychromatic waves (as depicted in the example of 3 distinct colors: blue, green, and red; see also Fig 2-9) are all in-phase only, with all their crests coinciding, for an optical path–length difference of zero ($\Delta z = 0$). **B,** Same as **(A)** but with the polychromatic waves displayed together in a single plot. Consider a sample with 3 reflective tissue interfaces that are located at distances R_1, R_2, and R_3 from the reference mirror (indicated by the purple, gray, and orange dashed lines respectively). Note the waves becoming more and more out of phase. **C,** Spectrally resolved representation of **(B)**: rather than displaying as a function of path–length difference (Δz), or tissue–reflector distance from the reference mirror, the signal (at a given tissue–reflector depth) is plotted as a function of wavelength. As the polychromatic waves became increasingly out of phase with increasing path–length differences or tissue–reflector depths, here, in the spectral representation, this translates to the rate of intensity variation (across wavelengths), which increases with deeper tissue reflectors. In other words, closer reflective tissue interfaces cause slower intensity variations as a function wavelength (ie, lower frequency modulation in the spectral interferogram), whereas deeper reflective tissue interfaces cause faster intensity variations across different wavelengths (ie, faster frequency modulation in the detected spectrally resolved interferogram). *(Illustration developed by Kristina Irsch, PhD.)*

creating a lower frequency modulation) than for those arising from deeper ocular tissue planes, which generate fringes with faster intensity variations as a function of wavelength (ie, the fringe patterns' undulations are spaced more closely together, corresponding to a higher frequency modulation). Consequently, there is frequency encoding of depth: the greater the sample reflector depth, the greater the resultant frequency modulation in the spectrally resolved interferogram. In addition, the amplitude of spectral modulation (or "visibility" of the spectral fringes) is proportional to the amount of reflection from the reflector. In other words, as with TD-OCT, the more highly reflective tissue plane interfaces yield higher-amplitude fringe patterns.

Thus, the spacing of the fringe pattern tells us how deep in the tissue it comes from, and its amplitude tells us how much the light is reflected by that tissue plane interface. This information can be teased out by applying a Fourier transform on the detected spectral interference data (see Fig 9-28). As with TD-OCT, scanning across the retina (or cornea) yields 2- and 3-dimensional images. Thus, FD-OCT is much more efficient than TD-OCT; it results in both greater speed and a higher signal-to-noise ratio, and therefore higher-resolution images.

There are 2 implementations of FD-OCT: spectrometer-based or swept-source implementation. These differ in how they acquire the spectrally resolved interferograms, that is, how they separate light into its spectral components in the detection path or illumination path, respectively. Specifically, a spectrometer-based version of FD-OCT (commonly referred to as SD-OCT) uses a prism or grating in front of the detector to separate light into its spectral components at the output of the spectrometer, whereas a swept-source version of FD-OCT (commonly termed SS-OCT) replaces the superluminescent diode's band of frequencies with a tunable laser. The laser sequentially sweeps through different frequencies, 1 at a time, at the input of the interferometer, and the A-scan is performed for each frequency at each lateral location. Unlike SD-OCT systems, SS-OCT systems are not limited by spectrometer resolutions; they thereby support larger ranges of axial depth measurement. Also, commonly available swept sources have a wavelength centered at about 1 μm (rather than around 800 nm), thus enabling imaging deeper into the tissue. This allows us to see the vitreous, retina, and choroid more easily in a single image. Similarly, the cornea, iris, and crystalline lens can be visualized in a single image with SS-OCT.

Adaptive Optics

Adaptive optics (AO) refers to a technique to compensate for distortions caused by optical aberrations in the media between the camera (or imaging system) and the object being imaged. It was originally developed for use in astronomical telescopes to compensate for optical distortions induced by Earth's inhomogeneous atmosphere. It has since evolved to become a powerful clinical tool in ophthalmology.

In an ophthalmic AO system, a wavefront sensor, such as the Hartmann-Shack wavefront sensor, measures the distorted wavefront emerging from the eye (see Figs 9-8 and 9-10), made irregular by aberrations of the cornea and crystalline lens.

Note that even for a normal eye, as the pupil enlarges, optical aberrations in the peripheral areas of the anterior segment come into play and may result in considerable distortions to the retinal image. For example, under low lighting conditions, the pupil dilates to approximately 5–7 mm in diameter. Higher-order aberrations become significant and lead to broadening of the point spread function (PSF, the image of a point source of light; see Chapter 2).

After measuring the distortion of the retina-reflected light, the AO system "un-distorts" the beam via reflection by a deformable mirror. This is a very special mirror with a flexible surface and multiple electric actuators that can rapidly deform the mirror surface to modify the impinging aberrated wavefront accordingly, thereby effectively removing the distortions, as represented in Figure 9-31.

AO thus enables imaging of the human retina with unprecedented resolution, such as revealing individual photoreceptors or the walls of blood vessels. Note that AO by itself does not provide an image; rather, an AO subsystem is incorporated into an existing imaging device, with the help of a beam splitter, as indicated in Figure 9-32. AO subsystems have thus far been successfully integrated into 3 ophthalmic imaging devices: fundus cameras, SLOs, and OCT devices.

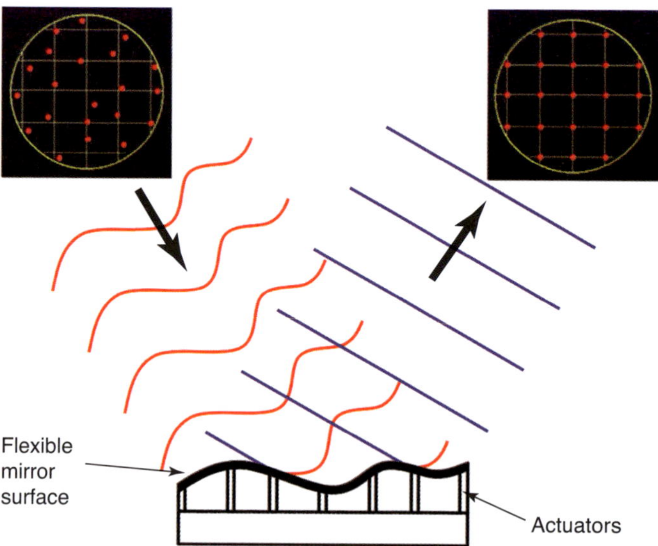

Figure 9-31 Concept of wavefront correction using a deformable mirror. The wavefront sensor reads the displacement of each mini image (produced by the microlenslet array; see Fig 9-10), which allows us to calculate how the flexible-mirror surface should be deformed so that upon reflection, the distorted wavefront is rendered undistorted. *(Illustration modified by Kristina Irsch, PhD; inspired by Austin Roorda, PhD. Inset illustrations reproduced from Thibos LN. Principles of Hartmann-Shack aberrometry.* J Refract Surg. *2000;165(5):S563–S565.)*

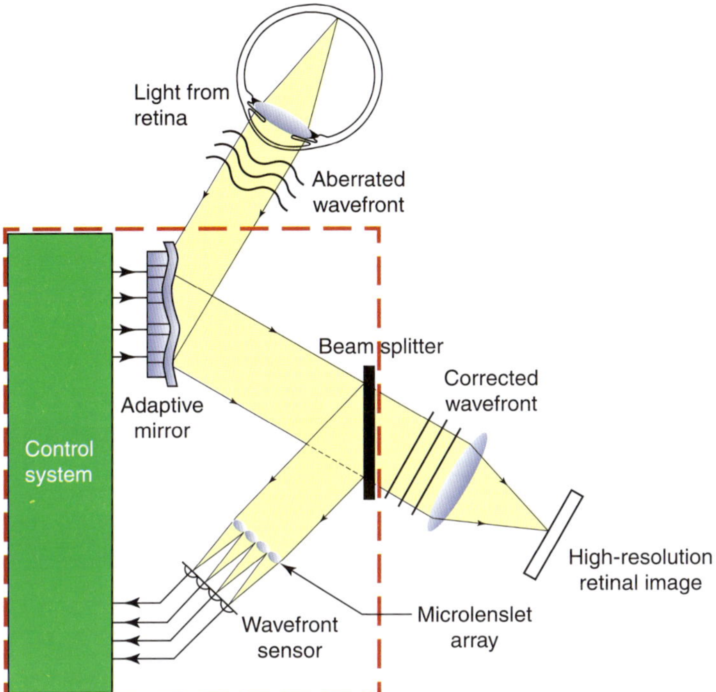

Figure 9-32 Basic principle of adaptive optics (AO). The distorted emerging wavefront from the eye, made irregular by aberrations of the cornea and lens, gives a relatively blurred retinal image at the start. The irregularities in the pattern of multiple images of the object produced by a microlenslet array allow determination of what exactly the distortions produced by the interfering ocular media are; then a deformable mirror can be used to modify the beam accordingly so as to remove the distortions. The result is a high-resolution retinal image. Note that AO by itself does not provide an image; rather, an AO subsystem is incorporated (via a beam splitter) into an existing imaging device, as indicated in red. *(Courtesy of Christopher Dainty, National University of Ireland, Galway.)*

Chapter Exercises

Questions

9.1. Slit-lamp biomicroscopy enables viewing of the corneal endothelium using which technique?
   a. retroillumination
   b. specular reflection
   c. direct focal illumination
   d. sclerotic scatter

9.2. Which statement does *not* characterize how keratometers work?
   a. They measure the radius of curvature of the central cornea.
   b. They assume the cornea to be a convex mirror.
   c. They directly measure the refractive power of the cornea.
   d. They use a mathematical formula to convert radius of curvature to approximate refractive power.

9.3. In what way is the manual keratometer inaccurate for determining corneal power in intraocular lens calculations following myopic laser vision correction?
   a. The keratometry measurement of the posterior surface does not change and is still accurate.
   b. The keratometer mire cannot be imaged at all following laser vision correction.
   c. The assumed relationship between the anterior and posterior surfaces, which is the basis of the assumed index of refraction, is no longer accurate.
   d. Significant irregular astigmatism is present in all corneas that have undergone keratorefractive surgery, and the keratometer is no longer accurate.

9.4. The indirect ophthalmoscope employs one of the brightest light sources used in clinical ophthalmology. Why is such a bright light necessary?

9.5. Which statement is *inaccurate* for fundus examination with the direct ophthalmoscope?
   a. The optic disc will appear larger in a myopic eye than in a normal or hyperopic eye.
   b. The optic disc will appear smaller in a myopic eye than in a normal or hyperopic eye.
   c. The optic disc will appear smaller in a hyperopic eye than in a normal or myopic eye.
   d. Smaller details can be observed than with the indirect ophthalmoscope.

9.6. When a binocular indirect ophthalmoscope is used with a patient with small pupils, binocular visualization can be improved by which technique?
   a. moving the ophthalmoscope's mirrors or prisms closer to the observer
   b. narrowing the observer's effective interpupillary distance
   c. moving the ophthalmoscope's eyepieces farther apart
   d. increasing the distance between the observer's head and the patient
   e. all of the above

Answers

9.1. **b.** With an ordinary slit lamp, the outlines of individual endothelial cells are best seen by viewing the specular reflection of a narrow slit beam at high magnification. A wider field can be viewed using a specular microscope that has a contact optical system to decrease surface reflections.

9.2. **c.** Keratometers approximate the refractive power of the cornea by measuring the radius of curvature of the central cornea and assuming the cornea to be a convex mirror. The formula $D = (n-1)/r$ is then used to convert this radius of curvature into an approximate refractive power, where r is the radius of curvature of the reflective cornea, and n is the keratometric refractive index at 1.3375.

9.3. **c.** The 1.3375 index of refraction is calculated to compensate for the minus-powered posterior corneal surface that cannot be measured with the keratometer. Myopic keratorefractive surgery primarily flattens the anterior surface, and therefore the assumed index of refraction is no longer correct. Another problem following myopic keratorefractive surgery is that the extreme center of the cornea is usually flattened substantially more than the annulus measured by the manual keratometer (approximately 3 mm). Both errors will lead to overestimation of the power of the cornea and a hyperopic postoperative result if not corrected for in the calculation.

9.4. The condensing lens images the observer's entrance pupils as 2 very small discs that fall within the patient's entrance pupil (along with the image of the ophthalmoscope bulb's filament, which must not coincide with the images of the observer's pupils, to avoid obscuring the fundus with reflections from the patient's cornea). Of all the light the ophthalmoscope shines into the patient's eye, only the emergent light that passes through these pupillary images enters the eyes of the observer and is available for viewing the fundus. Because these image discs occupy far less than 1% of the area of the patient's entrance pupil, and only about 0.1% of the light is reflected from the fundus, the ophthalmoscope "wastes" over 99% of the light that enters the patient's eye in forming the image visible to the observer, and so requires a very bright light source.

9.5. **b.** With direct ophthalmoscopy, the examiner uses the optics of the patient's eye as a simple magnifier to look at the retina. The optics of the normal eye are approximately +60.00 D, so using the formula for a simple magnifier (Mag = D/4), the magnification is 60/4, or 15×. If the patient's eye is myopic, a minus lens is dialed in to overcome the extra plus power "error lens" inside the patient's eye. These 2 lenses create a Galilean telescope effect, increasing magnification and decreasing the field of view. Similarly, the retina of a hyperopic eye will be magnified less than 15× because of the reverse Galilean telescope effect created by the minus power error lens inside the patient's eye and the plus lens of the direct ophthalmoscope. Thus, the size of the optic disc will appear larger (and not smaller) in a myopic eye than in a hyperopic or a normal eye.

9.6. **e.** When looking through a small pupil, the observer can improve visualization by narrowing their effective interpupillary distance. This can be accomplished by several means. Moving the ophthalmoscope's mirrors or prisms closer to the observer (the "small-pupil feature" available on some ophthalmoscopes) decreases the distance between the light paths to the observer's left and right eyes, effectively narrowing the observer's interpupillary distance. Moving the ophthalmoscope's eyepieces farther apart also decreases the distance between the light paths to the observer's eyes, similarly narrowing the observer's effective interpupillary distance. Increasing the distance between the observer and the patient decreases the angle formed by the observer's eyes and the patient's eye, thereby allowing the light paths from the observer's eyes to "squeeze through" a smaller pupil.

CHAPTER 10

Vision Rehabilitation

Highlights

- Patients with visual acuities less than 20/40 or scotomata, field loss, or contrast sensitivity loss will benefit from low vision evaluation and multidisciplinary vision rehabilitation to assist them in achieving their goals and maintaining quality of life despite vision loss.
- An evaluation of visual acuity, contrast sensitivity, location and size of scotomata relative to fixation, and extent of mid-peripheral and peripheral field loss allows clinicians to appreciate the impact of vision loss on patients' functioning and informs effective rehabilitation interventions.
- Multidisciplinary vision rehabilitation addresses reading (eg, magnification requirements), daily activities (eg, cell phone accessibility or doing kitchen tasks), safety (eg, fall prevention or ability to take medications), participation (eg, driving), and psychosocial well-being (eg, adjustment to vision loss or depression).
- The range of devices from which patients can benefit includes optical devices, such as reading adds and illuminated magnifiers; electronic devices, such as smartphones, e-readers, video magnifiers, and audio books; and nonoptical devices, such as large-format telephones or television remote controls.
- Patients with any level of vision loss may experience vivid, recurrent visual hallucinations, such as seeing patterns, faces, flowers, or people where there are none. When patients have full insight that these images are not real, and no other neurological symptoms or diagnosis to explain the hallucinations, this is attributed to Charles Bonnet syndrome.

Glossary

Bioptic telescope A spectacle-mounted telescope that is typically placed above the visual axis for spotting distance targets, such as traffic lights, in jurisdictions where bioptic driving is allowed.

Charles Bonnet syndrome A condition in individuals who have some degree of vision loss that is characterized by vivid, recurrent hallucinations and insight that what is being seen is not real. Individuals may see patterns or images, such as people, faces, or landscapes. The degree of vision loss may be moderate or severe, and the vision loss can be acuity loss or visual field loss due to ocular or neurologic disease.

Eccentric fixation Use of nonfoveal fixation to view the object of regard.

Legal blindness A level of vision loss at which patients are entitled to certain concessions or services in various jurisdictions. Legal blindness is defined in the United States as best-corrected visual acuity less than or equal to 20/200 (if measured using a chart such as an ETDRS chart, one cannot read any letters on the 20/100 line) or a central visual field of equal to or less than 20° in diameter.

Low vision Vision loss that cannot be corrected by standard eyeglasses or by medical or surgical treatment. The cause may be ocular or neurologic disease.

Macular microperimeter A perimetry device that images the retina during visual field testing. Eyetracking facilitates reliable perimetry evaluation of patients with unstable fixation or eccentric fixation. The retina can be imaged with a camera or scanning laser ophthalmoscopy. Macular microperimetry is also called *fundus-related perimetry* or *macular perimetry.*

Preferred retinal locus The area of nonfoveal retina that a patient repeatedly uses for fixation when the foveal area is impaired.

Scanning training Training to enhance compensatory visual searching into nonseeing areas of the visual field, such as with hemianopic field loss. Methods of training include performance of search tasks on devices that can be programmed with displays of lights, computer training programs, and scanning training practice typically implemented by occupational therapists.

Video magnifiers Devices that combine digital cameras with electronic screens in handheld, desk, or head-mounted formats. They have also been referred to as closed-circuit televisions (CCTVs).

Vision rehabilitation A multidisciplinary clinical process aimed at enabling individuals with vision loss to reach their goals for visual tasks and improve quality of life. Comprehensive vision rehabilitation assesses and addresses 5 areas: reading, daily life activities, safety, continued participation despite vision loss, and psychosocial well-being.

Visual prosthesis A device to provide vision substitution for individuals who are blind. Devices currently available or under development stimulate the retina (epiretinal, subretinal, or suprachoroidal implants) or stimulate the visual cortex. A device that places an electrode array on the tongue is also available.

Introduction

Ophthalmologists see patients with vision impairment in their offices every day. Those patients may have difficulty reading appointment notices, finding the clinic, or navigating in the office. Simple measures such as knowing how to assist a patient to the examination room with sighted-guide techniques or offering referral to vision rehabilitation services can be valuable. In this chapter we provide an overview of vision rehabilitation so that ophthalmologists may better appreciate the wide range of vision rehabilitation interventions, from smart speakers to support groups, that can assist their patients.

CLINICAL PEARL

Instructions and videos about sighted-guide techniques and how to offer your arm and verbal instructions to a patient who wishes assistance are available online.

In 2010, 4.2 million Americans older than 40 years were estimated to have visual impairment (with best-corrected visual acuity less than 20/40), and 1.3 million were estimated to have legal blindness. Most of these individuals were elderly, as prevalence of vision loss increases with age. Vision loss impacts patient safety, independence, quality of life, and psychosocial well-being. Seniors with vision loss are at risk for falls, injuries, medication errors, nutritional decline, social isolation, and depression at far higher rates than are reported for sighted individuals.

Ophthalmologists should be aware of societal disparities that may have contributed to their patients' vision loss and that can present challenges to its management. For instance, if language differences prevent clear communication between the ophthalmologist and patient, the ophthalmologist should engage the help of an interpreter. If financial circumstances are a barrier to obtaining the services and technology that would allow the patient to improve their quality of life, the ophthalmologist can be ready with low-cost resources. Agencies, services, and technologies that can aid patients with vision rehabilitation are discussed throughout this chapter.

The ophthalmologist is in a unique position to support patients with vision loss by **"recognizing and responding"**: recognizing that vision loss, even moderate vision loss, impacts patients' ability to successfully accomplish the things they need and want to do, and responding by facilitating access to vision rehabilitation services. Appreciation of the strategies and options in the vision rehabilitation "toolbox" allows you to understand why referring patients to such services is important and beneficial and to provide specific examples to your patients of what vision rehabilitation can offer. In addition, your empathy in recognizing a patient's reaction to vision loss, whether it be fear, anger, or sadness, and conveying that you understand the connection of their emotion to their loss, can be a brief but important step in the continuum of care, from diagnosis to rehabilitation.

Any patient with eye disease that cannot be improved with medical or surgical treatment and who is not able to successfully accomplish necessary visual tasks is a candidate for vision rehabilitation. Rehabilitation can be very important even for patients with good acuity and eye disease that is associated with scotomata or with reduced contrast perception, such as patients receiving injections for exudative macular degeneration.

CLINICAL PEARL

The Academy's *Vision Rehabilitation Preferred Practice Pattern* Guidelines recommend that patients with acuity less than 20/40, contrast sensitivity loss, and peripheral or central field loss be referred for vision rehabilitation.

Patients whose only difficulty is reading fine print can usually be assisted by routine eye-care services; however, when vision impairment impacts activities beyond the ability to read fine print, the many practical options of vision rehabilitation are useful.

Vision rehabilitation begins with a low vision evaluation and is followed, as indicated, by training and referral to resources and specialized services. In contrast to an ophthalmic examination, in which visual function and ocular status are evaluated with the intent to diagnose and treat, vision rehabilitation aims to assess and address the whole person by considering five areas: reading and access to text, valued daily life activities, patient safety, continued participation in activities despite vision loss, and psychosocial well-being.

Low Vision Evaluation: History

Patients' Goals

Patients' goals and values help direct and prioritize rehabilitation efforts. Tasks may still be difficult after rehabilitation, but patients highly value success in accomplishing tasks that are important to them. The examiner should ask patients about difficulties with the following 5 areas and encourage them to describe their rehabilitation priorities.

- *Reading tasks,* such as reading newspapers, mail, books, and handwritten notes.
- *Daily life activities,* such as shopping, cooking, using a cell phone or computer, shaving, and watching television. What does the patient do for fun?
- *Safety,* for instance, falls, difficulty reading medications, and kitchen safety.
- *Barriers to participation,* including driving status, transportation alternatives, and isolation.
- *Well-being,* for instance, anxieties, including worry about visual hallucinations experienced; depressive symptoms; and concerns about responsibilities, such as financial or caregiving responsibilities.

Ocular History

The disease, rate of progression, and previous ocular treatments will typically correlate with the patient's functional concerns. For example, patients with macular degeneration would be anticipated to have reading difficulty, whereas a patient with glaucoma may have difficulty with ambulation, but be able to read.

General History

Current living arrangements, responsibilities, employment, hobbies, illnesses, and use of glasses, devices, cell phones, and computers are all relevant issues in the history. Systemic diseases can impact rehabilitation interventions, such as when arthritis or tremors impair a patient's ability to hold a book or magnifier. As in other areas of health care, social determinants of health such as living situation, education, income, social supports, health literacy, social inclusion, and access to services can impact an individual's ability to access rehabilitation.

Charles Bonnet Syndrome

Patients with Charles Bonnet syndrome see images of objects that are not real. The condition affects up to one-third of visually impaired persons. Patients are often relieved to discuss their hallucinations. They may see vivid, recurrent images of patterns, such as wallpaper or barbed wire, or images of people or landscapes. Many patients are puzzled by this symptom. Some are anxious, as they do not understand what they are experiencing, and a small proportion are very upset. Most patients will not report the hallucinations unless the clinician inquires, for fear of being labeled as mentally unwell.

> **CLINICAL PEARL**
>
> A diagnosis of Charles Bonnet syndrome can be made if the patient has 4 clinical characteristics: (1) vivid recurrent visual hallucinations; (2) some degree of vision loss; (3) insight into the unreality of the images, when it is explained to them; and (4) no other neurologic or psychiatric diagnosis to explain the hallucinations.

Charles Bonnet syndrome is a diagnosis of exclusion, and patients should be referred for neurologic or psychiatric evaluation if they have any other neurologic signs or symptoms (see BCSC Section 5, *Neuro-Ophthalmology*). Strategies such as eye movement, blinking, and increasing lighting or activity can decrease hallucinations for some patients.

Low Vision Evaluation: Assessment of Visual Function

Visual Acuity

Accurate visual acuity measurements can be made to very low levels. Charts can be brought to closer-than-standard viewing distances; for example, the ETDRS chart is commonly used at 1 or 2 m (Fig 10-1). For patients with very poor vision, the Berkeley Rudimentary Vision Assessment, a set of 25–cm^2 cards held at 25 cm, is available for quantifying visual acuity as low as 20/16,000.

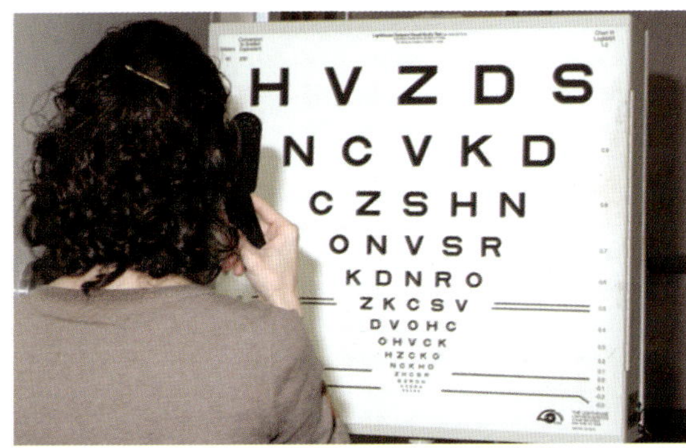

Figure 10-1 Measuring visual acuity with the ETDRS chart at 1 meter. *(Courtesy of Scott E. Brodie, MD, PhD.)*

Refraction

The goal of refraction for patients with low vision is to check for significant uncorrected refractive errors; however, only about 10% of low vision patients will benefit from alternate refractive correction, as the source of their poor vision is typically ocular disease, not refractive error. The vision rehabilitation clinician must temper unreasonable expectations that patients may have, such as the expectation that new glasses can solve vision problems associated with the eye disease, and ensure that patients do not deplete their financial resources on spectacles that offer little benefit, especially when they could put that money toward other devices that significantly improve function. Purchase of new glasses is often best delayed until the patient can compare the benefit of other rehabilitation options and devices to the benefit of spectacles.

Specific strategies can assist low vision refraction, including using a trial frame, performing retinoscopy at a shorter distance with greater working-distance lens power, using a +1.00/−1.00 cross cylinder for patients with poorer acuity to allow them to appreciate the differences between choices, and using an automated refractor. The vision rehabilitation clinician should check for balance lens corrections in an eye that may now be the better-seeing eye. Full corrections, rather than balance lens corrections, are encouraged. Impact-resistant lens material can be considered for ocular safety.

Contrast Sensitivity

The ability to discern contrast is a visual function separate from visual acuity, and these functions are not directly correlated. Patients with poor contrast sensitivity have difficulty seeing the edges of steps, reading light-colored print, driving in foggy or snowy conditions, and recognizing faces. Contrast sensitivity varies with target size (spatial frequency), and the relationship between contrast threshold and spatial frequency may be displayed as a contrast sensitivity curve (see Chapter 3 in this volume). Formal tests of contrast sensitivity include paper charts and computer tests, the latter allowing greater testing range. Paper charts may test a range of spatial frequencies or a single spatial frequency (Fig 10-2).

Patients whose visual impairment includes loss of contrast sensitivity may benefit from illuminated magnifiers or electronic magnification; nonoptical strategies, such as task lighting; or modification of contrast in tasks, such as using a black felt-tip marker rather than a fine-point pen.

Central Visual Field

Traditional field testing with Goldmann or Humphrey perimeters maps the visual field relative to a central fixation point, which is located at the fovea in patients with normal central field. Patients with disease that affects central field, however, may fixate with eccentric areas of the retina, called preferred retinal loci (PRL) (Fig 10-3). Clues to understanding fixation behavior include head and eye movements, the patient's subjective reports, observation of fixation during ophthalmoscopy, and measured fixation with macular microperimetry, also called *fundus-related perimetry.*

The macular microperimeter monitors fundus location and then determines the patient's direction of gaze before each target is presented. Macular microperimetry documents the

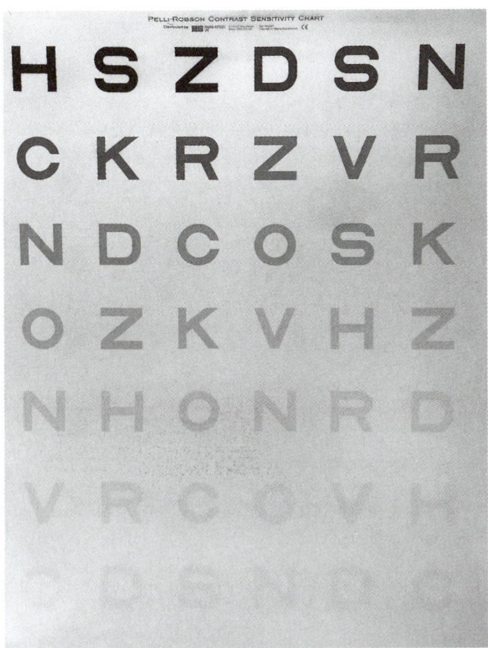

Figure 10-2 Pelli-Robson chart. Contrast of large Sloan letters decreases in groups of 3 from top to bottom and left to right within each line. *(Courtesy of Mary Lou Jackson, MD.)*

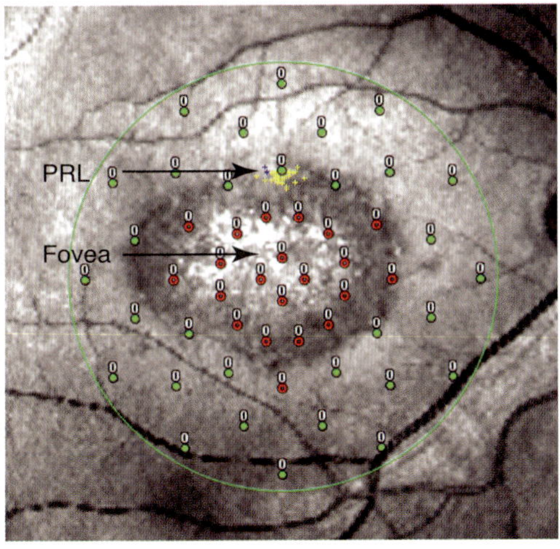

Figure 10-3 The patient has eccentric fixation and uses a preferred retinal locus (PRL) superior to the fovea. *(Courtesy of Mary Lou Jackson, MD.)*

patient's retinal point of fixation, identifies scotomata, and documents the relationship of the fixation to the scotomata. Other nonautomated testing methods, such as Amsler grids, cannot assess fixation and will not detect approximately half of central or paracentral scotomata due to perceptual completion, or "filling in" of visual field defects. Although most patients with central scotomata spontaneously develop eccentric fixation, they may have poor oculomotor control at the eccentric area or PRL. They may use multiple PRLs, change fixation depending on target size or illumination, or develop a sense of "straight ahead" related to their PRL rather than their fovea.

The vision rehabilitation clinician needs to appreciate the nature of the patient's fixation (foveal or eccentric), the presence and nature of scotomata (central or paracentral), and the relationship of fixation and scotoma. Scotomata can vary widely in size, shape, number, and density, and they may not correspond to the fundus appearance of atrophy, scarring, or pigment alteration. For example, a scotoma may be right of fixation and obscure next words, or be left of fixation and make it difficult to carry out an accurate saccade to the beginning of the next line of print. It is not uncommon that patients with macular disease have very small areas of foveal retina surrounded by dense scotomata, called foveal-sparing scotomata (Fig 10-4A). Such scotomata are seen in both dry and treated wet macular degeneration, Stargardt disease, and other macular diseases. Patients with foveal-sparing scotomata may be unable to read the larger letters on a visual acuity chart, causing the examiner to abandon the testing and record very low acuity. More careful testing, or testing at a closer distance, however, may reveal that the patients can in fact discern smaller letters when they are able to align the limited central field with the targets on the eye chart (Fig 10-4B). Scotomata that surround seeing retina may interfere with the recognition of large objects, fluent reading, or using magnification, depending on the size of the central seeing field.

Crossland MD, Culham LE, Kabanarou SA, Rubin GS. Preferred retinal locus development in patients with macular disease. *Ophthalmology*. 2005;112(9):1579–1585.

Crossland MD, Jackson ML, Seiple WH. Microperimetry: a review of fundus related perimetry. *Optom Rep*. 2012;2:11–15.

Peripheral Visual Field

Peripheral visual field defects cause patients to bump into objects or people, trip over objects and curbs, and lose their orientation, particularly in unfamiliar areas. Goldmann fields, automated peripheral fields, and carefully conducted confrontational fields can be informative in the setting of patients with glaucoma, peripheral retinal disease, or optic nerve or neurologic disease that affects visual pathways.

Assessment of Other Visual Functions

Glare, color vision (discussed in BCSC Section 5, *Neuro-Ophthalmology* and in Section 12, *Retina and Vitreous*), binocularity, eye movements, and accommodation (see BCSC Section 6, *Pediatric Ophthalmology and Strabismus*) may be considered in some situations. Patients may describe discomfort from glare or impairment of vision caused by scattered light (mainly Mie-type scattering in the forward direction; see Chapter 2). Patients with reduced contrast sensitivity often require increased illumination, which may, in turn, exacerbate glare, necessitating a balance between lighting recommendations and glare management strategies.

As in ophthalmology in general, visual acuity is an important and common measure of visual function in vision rehabilitation; however, other measures of visual function are also important and in vision rehabilitation can be equally important. As Figures 10-5, 10-6, and 10-7 illustrate, there is a range of visual function not only for visual acuity, but

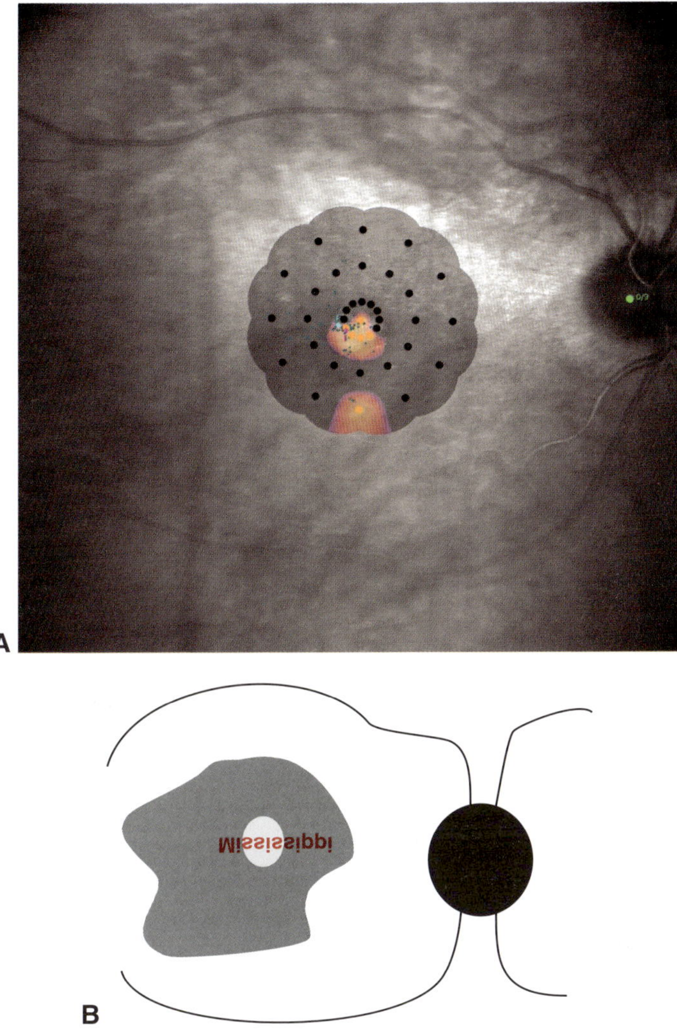

Figure 10-4 Foveal-sparing scotoma. **A,** Fixation is in an area of remaining central field that extends only a few degrees and is surrounded by a dense paracentral scotoma. **B,** Effect of a foveal-sparing scotoma on visualization of text. *(Part A courtesy of Mary Lou Jackson, MD, and part B courtesy of Mary Lou Jackson, MD, and the American Academy of Ophthalmology/Vision Rehabilitation Committee.)*

also for contrast sensitivity and for visual field, both central and peripheral. A composite of visual function, together with patient variables and goals, determines the most effective rehabilitation strategies for that patient.

Performance of Visual Tasks

A practitioner can assess patients' current success with visual tasks by observing them doing such things as reading, using their cell phone or computer, writing, or ambulating. Difficulties, successes, and adaptive strategies may be apparent. Reading tests vary and

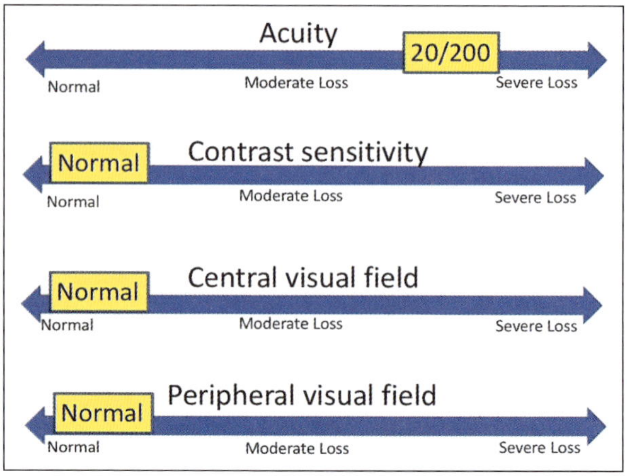

Figure 10-5 Test results of a 65-year-old patient diagnosed to have albinism. This patient has poor visual acuity and will benefit from magnification. Given the excellent contrast sensitivity and central visual field, optical magnification will likely be very successful. The patient is entitled to legal blindness concessions. *(Courtesy of Mary Lou Jackson, MD.)*

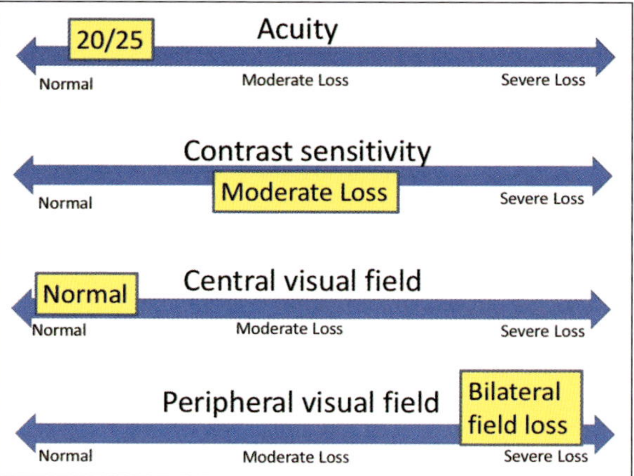

Figure 10-6 Test results of a 65-year-old patient diagnosed to have moderately severe glaucoma. This patient has near-normal visual acuity and moderate loss of contrast sensitivity, but significant loss of bilateral peripheral visual field. He is not legally able to drive and will benefit from orientation and mobility training with a white cane to ambulate safely, particularly in unfamiliar settings. He does not require magnification and can read fluently with a moderate increase in reading add. *(Courtesy of Mary Lou Jackson, MD.)*

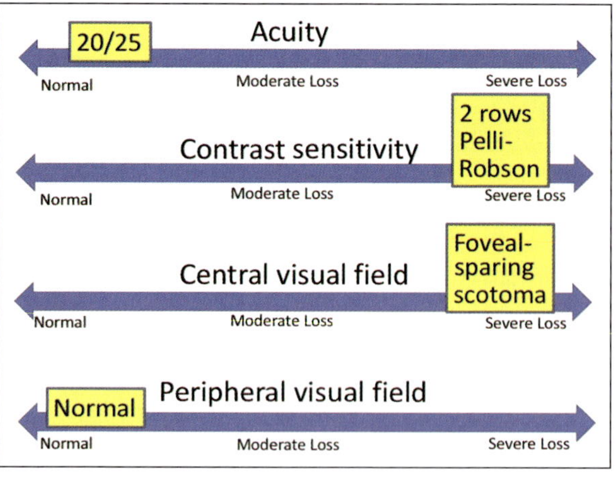

Figure 10-7 Test results of a 65-year-old patient diagnosed to have macular degeneration. This patient has near-normal visual acuity and both significant loss of contrast sensitivity and dense encircling paracentral field loss in the better-seeing eye. He can spot-read and use minimal magnification, but cannot read continuous print fluently due to the limited horizontal span around the fovea. He will benefit from reading with audio books, addressing contrast and lighting in daily tasks such as cooking, and applying fall-prevention strategies. Seeing faces, using a computer, or driving a car may be impacted by the encircling foveal-sparing scotoma. Given the normal peripheral visual field, he does not report difficulty with ambulation. *(Courtesy of Mary Lou Jackson, MD.)*

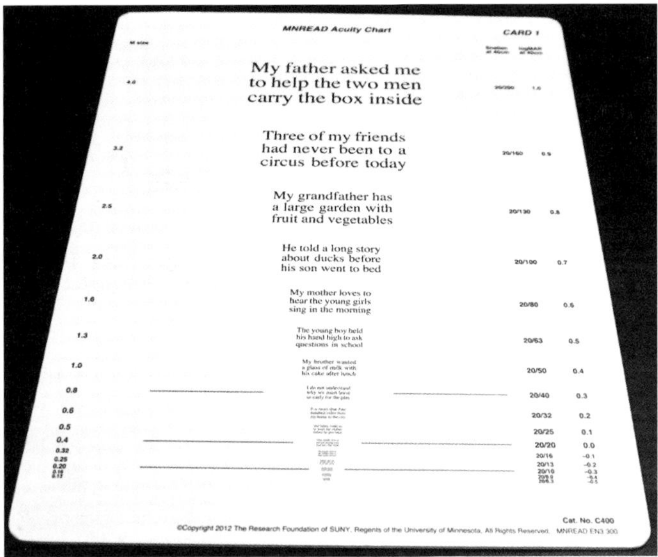

Figure 10-8 The Minnesota Low-Vision Reading Test has a range of text sizes. Patients with a limited area of central seeing retina may have difficulty reading the larger text, yet find it easier to read smaller text. *(Courtesy of Mary Lou Jackson, MD.)*

include tests to assess reading single numbers or words (spot reading), paragraphs (continuous print reading; eg, the International Reading Speed Texts [iReST]), or sentences with decreasing size of text (eg, the Minnesota Low-Vision Reading Test [MNREAD], Fig 10-8). Useful variables include the minimum size of print that can be read with the patient's current glasses or devices (reading acuity), reading errors, and the optimal size text for reading fluency (critical print size). The last variable can inform magnification goals. It is important to note that because different powers of reading add will change reading acuity, reading add power used should always be documented when near vision is measured.

Observing a patient ambulate provides valuable insight into the need for orientation and mobility training, white-cane or support-cane use, or scanning training.

Many different questionnaires have been used to elicit patient reports of difficulties with visual tasks.

Interventions

There is a wide range of vision rehabilitation interventions, including electronic devices, optical devices, nonoptical devices, practical alternate strategies to accomplish tasks, strategies to enhance safety (such as fall prevention strategies), and programs to support adjustment to vision loss, such as peer support groups.

Technology and Electronic Devices

Smartphones and tablets are now increasingly important as devices that allow patients with vision impairment not only to make phone calls, but also magnify text and images and use audio options to send texts, send emails, read books and newspapers, identify colors, read bar codes, navigate in unfamiliar areas, and search the internet. Cell phone cameras can be used to magnify. Smart speakers and virtual assistants also can be very useful for individuals with vision impairment. A variety of applications (Table 10-1) and devices (Table 10-2) are available.

Audio books, most often in Digital Accessible Information System (DAISY) format, are used widely by patients with vision loss and are available free through the Library of Congress in the United States, the Center for Equitable Library Access in Canada, and from online libraries such as Bookshare. These are extensive libraries. The Bookshare accessible library, for example, has more than 1 million titles that can be accessed via audio, by listening while seeing highlighted text, by using digital braille, and by converting standard text to large print or paper braille format.

A variety of video magnifier devices (Fig 10-9) combine cameras and screens to allow not only magnification, but also modification of contrast and color. Both electronic devices that are designed for individuals with low vision (such as video magnifiers) and electronic devices such as computers, tablets, and cell phones that have accessibility features are commonly used by patients with vision impairment. The major difficulties with electronic devices are cost and training requirements; however, in some jurisdictions, and for certain individuals, devices are provided gratis or at reduced cost. For example, devices are provided by some state societies and are also provided to veterans.

Optical Devices

High adds

Ophthalmologists are strongly encouraged to consider +4.00 adds or simple over-the-counter readers, such as +4.00 readers, as long as patients can learn to maintain the closer

Table 10-1 Examples of Smartphone Accessibility Features and Free Applications Used by Individuals With Vision Impairment

iOS operating system
- Siri for phone calls, texts, email, calendars, etc.
- Speak Screen and Speak Selection screen reading options
- VoiceOver screen reader in operating system
- Soundscape app (3D audio cues for navigation)
- Seeing AI app (reads printed text aloud; identifies handwriting, colors, currency, people, landscapes)

Android operating system
- TalkBack (spoken, audible and vibration feedback)
- Select to Speak (screen reading)
- iVision app (optical character recognition [OCR] reader)

Android and iOS operating systems
- Be My Eyes app (connects to volunteers by video call to identify objects and help with other tasks
- TapTapSee app (identifies objects)
- Libby app by Overdrive (plays ebooks and audio books from public libraries)
- Magnifier app with flashlight

Table 10-2 Technology Used by Individuals With Vision Impairment

Electronic Magnification Devices

Advantages
- Greatest range of magnification
- Excellent contrast, reverse contrast, different colors, and brightness
- Allows comfortable position and binocularity
- Can be portable
- Digital devices provide magnification for many tasks (email, internet searching, etc.)

Disadvantages
- Cost
- Must be charged
- Requires some training

Type	*Cost*
Portable video magnifiers	\$400–\$1800
Desk video magnifiers	\$1500–\$4000
Head-worn video magnifiers	\$3000–\$8000
Tablets, eReaders, computers, cell phones	\$500–\$4000

Audio Devices

Advantages
- Allow fluent reading
- Access to more than 1 million books
- Audio books can be played on a device from library, cell phone, eReader, or computer
- Can be portable
- Text-to-speech function is part of many desk video magnifiers
- Audio can be used for texts, phone calls, email, searching the internet, home control, etc.

Disadvantages
- May require practice to become comfortable with synthetic voice
- Devices require training
- May require internet

Type	*Cost*
Audio books	free from public library or subscription
Audio book players	loaned–\$500
Smartphone with apps	variable cost of phones
Text-to-speech in video magnifiers	\$3000–\$4000
Text-to-speech apps	free–\$125
Handheld and head-worn text-to-speech	\$1500–\$7000
Smart speakers (eg, Echo, Google Home)	\$50–\$300

focal distance and use supplemental lighting if beneficial. This can be recommended prior to referral for comprehensive vision rehabilitation. Patients will often use readers in powers from +6.00 D to +12.00 D with appropriate base-in prism and focal distance.

CLINICAL PEARL

A +10.00 D reading add will require a reading distance at the focal point of the lens, which will be 1/10 m (ie, 10 cm, or 4 in).

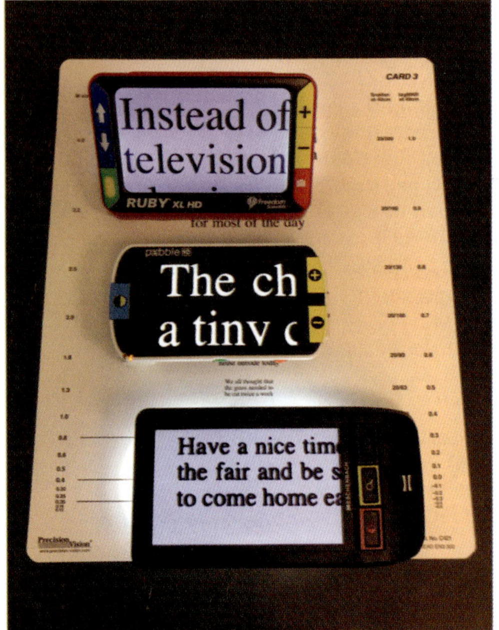

Figure 10-9 Portable handheld video magnifiers. *(Courtesy of Mary Lou Jackson, MD.)*

> **CLINICAL PEARL**
>
> In binocular patients, prism is required to assist convergence and relax accommodation. The recommended prism strength is 2 prism diopters (Δ) more base-in (BI) than the numerical add power, in each eye. For example, if the distance prescription is plano OU and the appropriate add power for reading is +8.00 D, then the prescription should read as follows: OD: +8.00 sphere with 10Δ BI; OS: +8.00 sphere with 10Δ BI. Prism is not required in adds up to +4.00 D.

Historically an add was calculated as the inverse of the visual acuity (Kestenbaum rule: the inverse of the visual acuity fraction is the add power, in diopters, to read 1M type—about 8 points, corresponding to the 20/50 line on a standard near-vision card calibrated for use at 14 inches), and this calculation may provide a general starting point. However, it is now appreciated that many other factors also influence reading fluency, such as fixation location, scotomata, perceptual span, crowding, and contrast sensitivity. The Kestenbaum rule would estimate that a patient with 20/200 acuity would require 200/20, or 10.00 D of add. For fluent reading, patients with 20/200 acuity may actually require a higher add than calculated.

Computer glasses with the intermediate power in the upper segment of the bifocal can be useful.

Magnifiers

A wide range of optical magnifiers are available with and without illumination (Fig 10-10 and Table 10-3). There are 2 methods of calculating the magnification of magnifiers, which can lead to confusion. Simple or nominal magnification is defined as the dioptric power

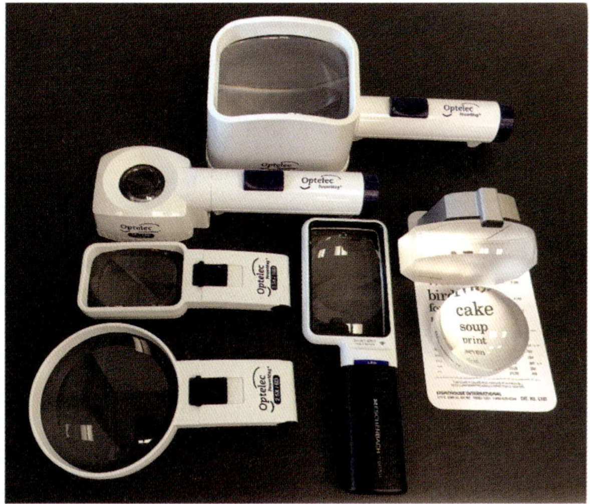

Figure 10-10 Handheld and stand magnifiers. *(Courtesy of Mary Lou Jackson, MD.)*

divided by 4 and assumes that the object is held at the anterior focal point of the magnifier. For example, the power of a +24.00 D magnifier is 6× (24.00 D / 4.00 D). Commercially available magnifiers are often labeled with a "trade magnification" power calculated as (the diopter power of the hand magnifier)/4 + 1, so the trade magnification of +4.00 D handheld lens is 2×. In practical settings, the amount of magnification depends on the dioptric power and how the lens is used. (Magnification is discussed in Chapter 1).

Telescopes

There are 2 types of telescopes: astronomical (also called Keplerian) telescopes and Galilean telescopes. (Optics of telescopes are discussed in Chapter 1). Telescopes are much less commonly used than magnifiers due to their various limitations (Table 10-3) and also because tasks that require magnification for distance viewing are less common than those that require magnification for near viewing (Fig 10-11).

Bioptic telescopes are spectacle-mounted telescopes set to focus at distance; they are mounted in the upper portion of the spectacle lens. In some states drivers can use a bioptic to briefly read signs or look into the distance. The rest of the time, the individual drives while looking through the regular prescription portion of their spectacles. Driving with a bioptic telescope requires prescription of the device as well as device training, driver training, and, in some states, on-road evaluation. Patients with good contrast sensitivity and intact central field are optimal candidates for bioptic driving.

> **CLINICAL PEARL**
>
> State-by-state driving licensing requirements including vision requirements and status for bioptic driving are outlined in the Clinician's Guide to Assessing and Counseling Older Drivers, which can be accessed at: https://www.nhtsa.gov/sites/nhtsa.gov/files/812228_cliniciansguidetoolderdrivers.pdf

Table 10-3 Optical Devices Used by Individuals With Vision Impairment

High-Add Readers

Advantages
- Glasses are a familiar device format
- Allow a wide field of view
- Leave hands free
- Portable

Disadvantage
- Closer focal distance, depending on power

Type	*Cost*
Readers without prism, +4.00 D to +6.00 D	\$20–\$50
Readers with prism, +6.00 D to +14.00 D	\$125–\$200
Monocular aspheric, +6.00 D to +32.00 D (used less often)	\$150–\$200

Handheld Optical Magnifiers

Advantages
- Available with and without illumination
- Low-powered (5.00 D to 12.00 D) version with light-emitting-diode illumination is popular
- Easy to carry
- Ideal for brief spot reading, such as checking prices
- Can be used by some for continuous print reading, ideally with the material on a reading stand

Disadvantages
- Have to be held steady and moved along line of text
- Limited field of view; with power higher than 20.00 D, the field of view is very limited

Type	*Cost*
Handheld, 6.00 D to 32.00 D	\$30–\$150 (LED illuminated frequently used)
Pocket magnifiers, 10.00 D to 20.00 D	\$20–\$100 (frequently used device)

Stand Optical Magnifiers

Advantages
- Magnifier sits on page, eliminating the need to hold it at the proper distance
- Available with and without illumination
- Useful for individuals with a tremor
- Best used with a reading stand and a reading add
- Some types allow writing under the magnifier

Disadvantages
- Higher-power magnifiers are less comfortable for extended print reading, such as reading books
- Larger and less portable
- Often require reading stand to preserve posture

Types	*Cost*
Stand, 8.00 D to 40.00 D	\$40–\$200
Dome, 4.00 D to 20.00 D	\$30–\$250

Table 10-3 *(continued)*

Other Hands-Free Optical Magnifiers

Advantage
- Allow distance from the magnifier to the hands (for writing, sewing, etc.)

Disadvantages
- Distance of object must be maintained
- Easiest to use in lower powers
- Best for stationary tasks

Type	*Cost*
Magnifier on a flexible stand, 3.00 D to 16.00 D	$75–$150
Around-the-neck craft magnifier, 4.00 D to 8.00 D	$50–$75
Head-worn magnifying visor, 3.00 D to 20.00 D	$100–$125

Telescopes

Advantages
- Available for magnification at distance or near focus
- Hands-free
- Close-focus telescopes (loupes) have greater working distance than high-adds
- Astronomical telescopes have a greater focusing range and better image quality
- Galilean telescopes have a wider field of view and are smaller and lighter

Disadvantages
- Reduced field of view
- Decreased contrast
- Narrow depth of field

Type	*Cost*
Handheld monoculars	$40–$350
Handheld binoculars	$50–$500
Spectacle-mounted, bioptic	$400–$3000
Simple telescopic spectacle without casing	$200–$250 (frequently used device)

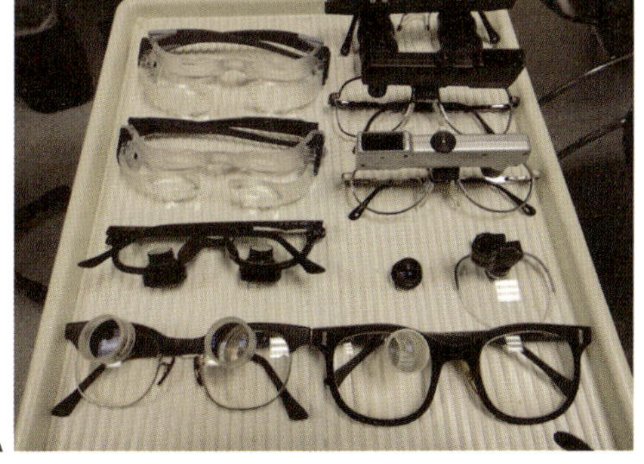
A

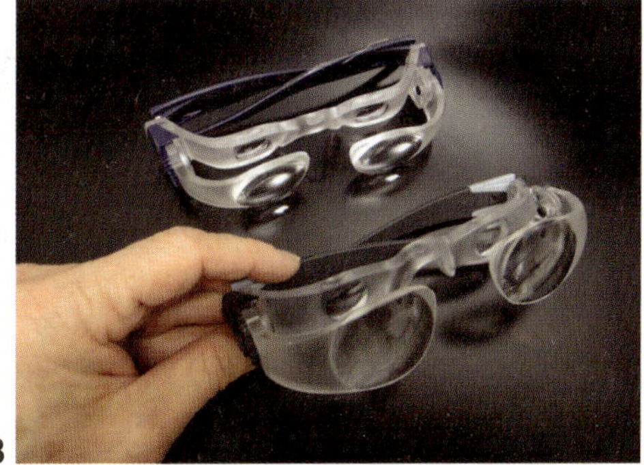
B

Figures 10-11 Telescopic devices. **A,** The range of telescopic devices includes monocular and binocular telescopes. **B,** This binocular spectacle telescope is lightweight and can be used for stationary distance viewing such as watching television. *(Courtesy of Mary Lou Jackson, MD.)*

Nonoptical Aids and Alternative Strategies

An armamentarium of tools is available to assist patients with impaired vision, and it extends beyond electronic, optical, and audio devices. Simple, practical devices include large-format watches, telephones, remote controls, playing cards, and checks. Bold-lettered computer keyboards, needle threaders, dark-lined writing paper, felt-tip pens with black ink, and talking clocks, scales, and timers are a partial list of items that are often useful. Vision rehabilitation often includes learning new ways to address patients' goals with technology, optical devices, nonoptical devices, or new strategies (Table 10-4).

Sight Substitution

Patients with very limited or no vision, particularly those who lose vision quickly, will require blind rehabilitation with sight substitutes that may include electronic text-to-speech or braille. Refreshable braille displays can be connected to computers and tablet devices. They have small, moving pins that rise or lower to create braille patterns that can be read tactilely. Short-term residential blind rehabilitation services, available in some areas, can be of great benefit to patients faced with the daunting task of adjusting to sudden and profound loss of vision. Prosthetic visual devices are being developed, and many groups around the world are developing subretinal, suprachoroidal, and epiretinal devices, in addition to cortical visual prostheses that stimulate the brain directly. Currently, devices allow patients to see direction of motion or contrast.

Training

After the low vision evaluation and creation of a vision rehabilitation plan for interventions, patients should be trained to accomplish tasks with modifications and to use appropriate devices. Medicare and some other health insurers in the US fund occupational therapists to train patients, just as rehabilitation is provided for patients with other disabilities, such as neurological and orthopedic conditions. Occupational therapists, or other state- or privately funded vision rehabilitation therapists or technology specialists, can assess home safety, modify lighting, provide labels for appliances and dials, assist with strategies to manage glare, and instruct patients in accessibility features with computers,

Table 10-4 Examples of How Interventions Can Address Patient Goals

Patient Goals	Technology	Optical	Nonoptical/Strategies
Reading	Audio books played on a smart phone	Hand magnifier for spot reading	Large-print books
Daily Life Tasks	Smartphone Seeing AI app to read prices aloud	Pocket magnifier to read labels	Large-format playing cards
Safety	Audio medication labels	High-plus readers leaving hands free to check insulin dosage	Fall prevention
Participation	Smartphone GPS to independently navigate	Telescope to see numbers	Alternative transportation services
Well-being	Attending support groups virtually		In-person peer support groups

tablets, and cell phones. Physical, cognitive, psychosocial, and environmental factors that may impact performance must be considered. Although eccentric fixation will develop spontaneously in patients with central field loss, training may improve the efficiency of using eccentric fixation. Current research is evaluating perceptual training, oculomotor training, and training a new direction of fixation (trained retinal locus). A large-sample, randomized, placebo-controlled, double-masked trial comparing prisms for assisting eccentric viewing in maculopathy showed no significant benefit.

Gaffney AJ, Margrain TH, Bunce CV, Binns AM. How effective is eccentric viewing training? A systematic literature review. *Ophthalmic Physiol Optics*. 2014;34(4):427–437.

Pijnacker J, Verstraten P, van Damme W, Vandermeulen J, Steenbergen B. Rehabilitation of reading in older individuals with macular degeneration: a review of effective training programs. *Neuropsychol Dev Cogn B Aging Neuropsychol Cogn*. 2011;18(6):708–732.

Smith HJ, Dickinson CM, Cacho I, Reeves BC, Harper RA. A randomized controlled trial to determine the effectiveness of prism spectacles for patients with age-related macular degeneration. *Arch Ophthalmol*. 2005;123(8):1042–1050.

Vision Rehabilitation for Field Loss

Scanning training, sector prisms to displace images to the seeing field, and vision restoration with computer training are rehabilitation strategies proposed for patients with hemianopia. A comparative trial of scanning and prisms showed improvement in vision-related quality of life with scanning training and very common adverse events (typically headaches) with prisms. Scanning training may also be provided for patients with field loss from disease such as retinitis pigmentosa. Orientation and mobility specialists provide training in using white canes and strategies to ambulate safely.

Rowe FJ, Conroy EJ, Bedson E, et al. A pilot randomized controlled trial comparing effectiveness of prism glasses, visual search training and standard care in hemianopia. *Acta Neurol Scand*. 2017;136(4)310–321.

Trauzettel-Klosinski S. Rehabilitation for visual disorders. *J Neuroophthalmol*. 2010;30(1): 73–84.

Discussion With Patients

Often physicians must communicate information to patients with low vision that patients will perceive as "bad news," such as that they are not able to drive or that their vision will not improve. Communication techniques have been conceptualized in different communication models (Fig 10-12); however, keys to delivering bad news include allowing sufficient time for the discussion, acknowledging patient emotions, and conveying that the physician appreciates that the emotions are connected to the negative news. The *Guide to Assessing and Counseling Older Drivers* is an informative resource and includes a chapter about counseling patients who can no longer drive.

American Geriatrics Society. Pomidor A, ed. *Clinician's Guide to Assessing and Counseling Older Drivers*. 3rd ed. (Report No. DOT HS 812 228). National Highway Traffic Safety Administration; 2016.

The SPIKES Health Care Communication Model

S—*Setting:* The clinician is seated, appears comfortable, and does not interrupt when the patient speaks.

P—*Perception:* "What have you been told about your driving up to now?"

I—*Invitation:* "How much detail would you like to know about the licensing requirements?"

K—*Knowledge:* "Today I do need to discuss your driving with you." (Warning shot)

E—*Empathy:* "Hearing that you do not meet the licensing requirements is clearly a major shock to you. I wish the news were better."

(The patient cries, and the clinician pauses and looks away.) "I see that this news upsets you. Let's just take a break now until you're ready to start again."

S—*Strategy and summary:* "So the summary of all this is that your vision does not meet the requirements to maintain a valid driver's license, and, unfortunately, you will now not be able to drive. Is that your understanding?"

A

The Four Es Model of health care communication

Engagement: "Would you like to take your coat off? We talked about your vision and the diagnosis of age-related macular degeneration in your last visit. Is there anything else you were wondering about?"

Empathy: "It is tough to have to think about alternate ways to get around if you cannot drive the way you used to."

Education: "What would you like to know about licensing requirements and vision standards?"

Enlistment: "I believe we have common ground here, since neither of us wants you to be involved in an accident. We both want to keep you driving safely as long as possible and make the decision not to drive at the right time."

B

Figure 10-12 Communication models. **A,** The SPIKES Healthcare Model of Communication was authored by Robert Buchman. **B,** The Four-E Model of Health Care Communication was developed by the Institute for Healthcare Communication. *(Part B from Buchman R. Breaking bad news: the S-P-I-K-E-S strategy.* Community Oncology. *2005;2:138–142.)*

Other Services

Many other agencies and services are involved in multidisciplinary vision rehabilitation, including optometric practices, state services, services for veterans, driving-rehabilitation services, talking-book libraries, transportation services, counseling, and support groups. Orientation and mobility training is offered by some agencies to provide instruction in using visual cues, telescopes, white canes, and GPS devices for safe and independent ambulation. Vision loss also affects the patient's spouse and family. Referral to psychological counseling and support groups may be part of the rehabilitation team's approach to helping patients and their families cope and adapt. The goal of multidisciplinary vision rehabilitation is collaboration among services to best address patients' goals and achieve optimal clinical outcomes.

Binns AM, Bunce C, Dickinson C, et al. How effective is low vision service provision? A systematic review. *Surv Ophthalmol.* 2012;57(1):34–65.

Owsley C, McGwin G Jr, Lee PP, Wasserman N, Searcey K. Characteristics of low-vision rehabilitation services in the United States. *Arch Ophthalmol.* 2009;127(5):681–689.

Pediatric Vision Rehabilitation

Although vision loss is less frequent in the pediatric population, this cohort is an important group that requires the ophthalmologist's attention. Every child with loss of vision needs to be recognized, and the ophthalmologist's response should include recommending vision rehabilitation. Most adults with low vision have lost vision because of an ocular disease incurred later in life. Thus, they have already acquired many of the vision-aided skills (eg, reading, understanding social cues, cooking, self-care tasks) that are important for functioning in society. Children with low vision, however, need to learn these skills despite poor or no vision.

The most prevalent causes of visual impairment in children in the US are cortical visual impairment, retinopathy of prematurity, optic nerve hypoplasia, albinism, optic atrophy, and congenital infections. Many of these children have coexisting physical and/or cognitive disabilities that create further challenges to successful integration into society.

Resources

Materials for Patients

The American Academy of Ophthalmology's vision rehabilitation patient handout is available for download (at www.aao.org/low-vision-and-vision-rehab). It provides essential tips for making the most of remaining vision and offers a list of resources, including a website that allows patients to search for services in their communities.

Materials for Ophthalmologists

- *BCSC Section 6: Pediatric Ophthalmology and Strabismus*
- American Academy of Ophthalmology. Vision Rehabilitation Committee. Preferred Practice Pattern Guidelines. *Vision Rehabilitation.* American Academy of Ophthalmology; 2022. Accessed October 6, 2023. https://www.aao.org/education/preferred-practice-pattern/vision-rehabilitation-ppp-2022
- American Academy of Ophthalmology. Vision rehabilitation web page updated with information about vision rehabilitation initiatives and education. Accessed October 6, 2023. www.aao.org/low-vision-and-vision-rehab
- Mishra A, Jackson ML, Mogk, LG. Comprehensive vision rehabilitation. *Focal Points: Clinical Practice Perspectives.* American Academy of Ophthalmology; 2017, module 4.

Chapter Exercises

Questions

9.1. What level of visual function is considered "legal blindness"?
   a. cannot read any letters on the 20/100 line of an ETDRS acuity chart
   b. best-corrected visual acuity 20/70
   c. visual field extending 30° around fixation
   d. hemianopic visual field

9.2. What is the optimal prescription for a patient who requires +8.00 reading add?
   a. +8.00 OU with 10 prism diopters (Δ) base-in OU
   b. OD +8.00 with 8Δ base in; OS +8.00 with 8Δ base in
   c. +8.00 OU with 8Δ OU
   d. +8.00 OU with 10Δ OD

9.3. The American Academy of Ophthalmology's Preferred Practice Pattern Guidelines regarding vision rehabilitation recommend referral to low vision consultation at what level of visual function?
   a. only when patients become legally blind
   b. when a patient's acuity is less than 20/40 or the patient has reduced contrast sensitivity, field loss, or a scotoma
   c. only if the patient asks for referral to vision rehabilitation
   d. when a patient cannot read fine print

Answers

9.1. **a.** Legal blindness is defined in the United States as visual acuity less than or equal to best-corrected visual acuity of 20/200 (ie, if evaluated with a chart such as an ETDRS chart, a person cannot read any of the letters on the 20/100 line) or a visual field of equal to or less than 20 degrees around central fixation. (See https://www.ssa.gov/disability/professionals/bluebook/2.00-SpecialSensesandSpeech-Adult.htm)

9.2. **a.** A guideline for adding prism to high-add spectacles over 4.00 D is to incorporate base-in prism for each eye at a correction that is 2.00 D greater than the required add power.

9.3. **b.** The American Academy of Ophthalmology's Preferred Practice Pattern Guidelines regarding vision rehabilitation recommend that patients with acuity less than 20/40, contrast sensitivity loss, peripheral field loss, or central field loss be referred for low vision evaluation.

Epilogue

A 15-year-old girl was referred from a major teaching hospital to a retina specialist for evaluation of unexplained visual impairment, including electroretinography testing. Her vision had been poor from infancy, and she was attending a school for the visually impaired. Visual acuity was 20/300 in both eyes. Her pupils reacted normally and symmetrically, without afferent defect. Ocular rotations were normal; there was no nystagmus.

Slit-lamp examination and dilated fundus examination were unremarkable. ERG testing was normal under photopic and scotopic conditions.

A fluorescein angiogram was obtained. There were no abnormalities of the retinal vasculature.

Study of the angiogram revealed myopic fundus markings, with easily visible choroidal vessels, which suggested a large myopic refractive error. Retinoscopy initially revealed the dim, immobile pseudoneutralization reflex that indicates high myopia. With a final manifest refraction of −5.50 sp OU, acuity promptly improved to 20/30 + 2 in each eye.

There was no other ocular pathology.

This child had grown up with a severe visual impairment—effectively legally blind—because no one had ever gone to the trouble to perform a competent refraction.

Additional Materials and Resources

Related Academy Materials

The American Academy of Ophthalmology is dedicated to providing a wealth of high-quality clinical education resources for ophthalmologists.

Print Publications and Electronic Products

For a complete listing of Academy clinical education products, including the BCSC Self-Assessment Program, visit our online store at aao.org/store. Or call Customer Service at 866.561.8558 (toll free, US only) or +1 415.561.8540, Monday through Friday, between 8:00 AM and 5:00 PM (PST).

Online Resources

Visit the **Ophthalmic News and Education (ONE®) Network** at aao.org/comprehensive-ophthalmology to find relevant videos, podcasts, webinars, online courses, journal articles, practice guidelines, self-assessment quizzes, images, and more. The ONE Network is a free Academy-member benefit.

Access free, trusted articles and content with the Academy's collaborative online encyclopedia, **EyeWiki,** at aao.org/eyewiki.

Get mobile access to *The Wills Eye Manual*, watch the latest 1-minute videos, and set up alerts for clinical updates relevant to you with the free **AAO Ophthalmic Education App.** Download today: Search for "AAO Ophthalmic Education" in the Apple app store or in Google Play.

Basic Texts and Additional Resources

Albert DM, Miller JW, Azar DT, Young LH, eds. *Albert & Jakobiec's Principles and Practice of Ophthalmology.* 4th ed. Springer International Publishing; 2022.

Corboy JM. *The Retinoscopy Book: An Introductory Manual for Eye Care Professionals.* 5th ed. Slack; 2003.

Guyton DL, West CE, Miller JM, Wisnicki HJ. *Ophthalmic Optics and Clinical Refraction.* Prism Press; 1999.

Hunter DG, West CE. *Last-Minute Optics.* 2nd ed. Slack; 2010.

Lipson A, Lipson SG, Lipson H. *Optical Physics.* 4th ed. Cambridge University Press; 2011.

Milder B, Rubin ML. *The Fine Art of Prescribing Glasses Without Making a Spectacle of Yourself.* 3rd ed. Triad Publishing Co; 2004.

Rubin ML. *Optics for Clinicians.* Triad Publishing Co; 1993.

Stein HA, Slatt BJ, Stein RM, Freeman MI. *Fitting Guide for Rigid and Soft Contact Lenses: A Practical Approach.* 4th ed. Mosby; 2002.

Yanoff M, Duker JS. *Ophthalmology.* 5th ed. Elsevier; 2018.

Requesting Continuing Medical Education Credit

The American Academy of Ophthalmology is accredited by the Accreditation Council for Continuing Medical Education (ACCME) to provide continuing medical education for physicians.

The American Academy of Ophthalmology designates this enduring material for a maximum of 15 *AMA PRA Category 1 Credits*™. Physicians should claim only the credit commensurate with the extent of their participation in the activity.

To claim *AMA PRA Category 1 Credits*™ upon completion of this activity, learners must demonstrate appropriate knowledge and participation in the activity by taking the posttest for Section 3 and achieving a score of 80% or higher.

To take the posttest and request CME credit online:

1. Go to aao.org/education/cme-central and log in.
2. Click on "Claim CME Credit and View My CME Transcript" and then "Report AAO Credits."
3. Select the appropriate media type and then the Academy activity. You will be directed to the posttest.
4. Once you have passed the test with a score of 80% or higher, you will be directed to your transcript. *If you are not an Academy member, you will be able to print out a certificate of participation once you have passed the test.*

CME expiration date: June 1, 2025. *AMA PRA Category 1 Credits*™ may be claimed only once between June 1, 2022 (original release date), and the expiration date.

For assistance, contact the Academy's Customer Service department at 866-561-8558 (US only) or 415-561-8540 between 8:00 AM and 5:00 PM (PST), Monday through Friday, or send an e-mail to customer_service@aao.org.

Study Questions

Please note that these questions are not part of your CME reporting process. They are provided here for your own educational use and identification of any professional practice gaps. The required CME posttest is available online (see "Requesting Continuing Medical Education Credit"). Following the questions are answers with discussions. Although a concerted effort has been made to avoid ambiguity and redundancy in these questions, the authors recognize that differences of opinion may occur regarding the "best" answers. The discussions are provided to demonstrate the rationale used to derive the answers. They may also be helpful in confirming that your approach to a problem was correct or, if necessary, in fixing a principle in your memory. The Section 3 faculty thanks the Resident Self-Assessment Committee for developing these self-assessment questions and the discussions that follow.

1. The simplest imaging system is a pinhole camera. What is a characteristic feature of this device?
   a. high magnification
   b. superb depth of field
   c. upright image formed at the image plane
   d. rapid exposure times

2. As it is unsafe to view a partial eclipse of the sun directly, observers are often advised to use a simple pinhole camera viewer to form an image of the eclipse. Of course, these pinhole images are small and dim. A better alternative is to use a +1.00 lens to project an image of the sun on the ground (see figure). How far should the lens be held from the ground to obtain a sharp image?

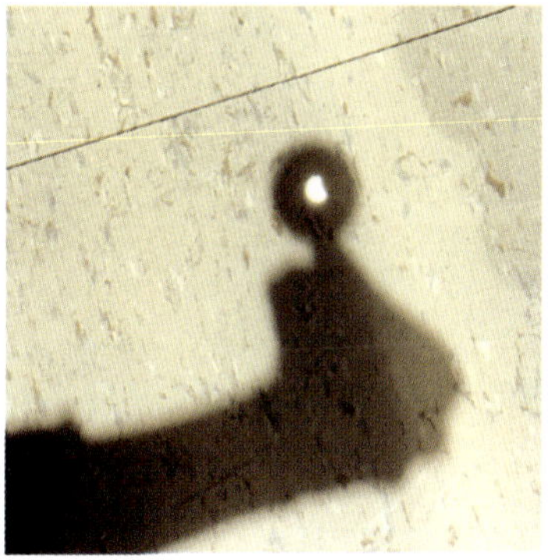

   a. 0.5 m
   b. 1.0 m
   c. 2.0 m
   d. It doesn't matter—any distance works well, just as in a pinhole camera.

3. Suppose a distant object is located to the left of a lens system, which focuses light from this object at 1.0 m to the right of the lens system. If a +3.00 D lens is added adjacent to the lens system, where is the new image located?
   a. 25 cm to the right of the lenses
   b. 50 cm to the right of the lenses
   c. 1.5 m to the right of the lenses
   d. 4.0 m to the right of the lenses

4. Where does the image of a distant object form for an eye with an uncorrected myopic refractive error?
   a. in front of the retina
   b. on the retina
   c. behind the retina
   d. This depends on whether the patient is accommodating.

5. The power-cross description of a toric lens is +1.00 @ 25°, −2.00 @ 115°. What is the spherocylindrical specification of this lens, expressed in minus cylinder form?
   a. $+1.00 \subset -2.00 \times 115°$
   b. $-2.00 \subset +1.00 \times 025°$
   c. $+1.00 \subset -3.00 \times 025°$
   d. $-2.00 \subset +3.00 \times 025°$

6. When cross cylinder refinement of an astigmatic correction is performed, it is necessary to adjust the spherical component of the correction to keep the circle of least confusion on the retina as cylinder power is varied. What is the proper rule for this compensation with a plus cylinder phoropter?
   a. Increase the plus sphere power by 1 click (0.25 D) for each 0.25 D increase in plus cylinder power.
   b. Increase the plus sphere power by 1 click (0.25 D) for each 0.25 D decrease in plus cylinder power.
   c. Increase the plus sphere power by 1 click (0.25 D) for each 0.50 D increase in plus cylinder power.
   d. Increase the plus sphere power by 1 click (0.25 D) for each 0.50 D decrease in plus cylinder power.

7. What is the spherocylindrical specification of the most commonly used Jackson cross cylinder (JCC)?
   a. $+0.25 \subset -0.25 \times 090$
   b. $-0.25 \subset -0.50 \times 180$
   c. $-0.25 \subset +0.50 \times 170$
   d. $+0.50 \subset -0.25 \times 080$

8. A cycloplegic streak retinoscopy is performed at a testing distance of 67 cm. What is the correct refraction, if the results are as follows:

   +3.00 D sphere neutralizes the reflex when the streak is horizontal (180°);

   +4.00 D sphere neutralizes the reflex when the streak is vertical (90°).

   a. +1.50 sphere +1.00 × 090
   b. +1.50 sphere −1.00 × 090
   c. +3.00 sphere +1.00 × 090
   d. +3.00 sphere −1.00 × 090

9. While surfing, a person spots a shark nearby in the water. Where is the shark, in reality, compared with where the person sees its image from the surfboard?
   a. closer to the person
   b. further from the person
   c. precisely where it appears
   d. the same distance, but to the opposite side

10. What part of the conoid of Sturm is on the retina if only a spherical lens is used to give the clearest image?
    a. circle of least confusion
    b. elliptical meridian
    c. horizontal focal line
    d. vertical focal line

11. When a beam of white light passes through a prism, it is dispersed into a spectrum of colors. Which color of visible light is deflected the most?
    a. red
    b. yellow
    c. green
    d. violet

12. The radius of curvature of a convex passenger-side automobile rear-view mirror is typically about 1.0 m. Where does such a mirror form an image of an object 10.0 m behind the car?
    a. 0.91 m in front of the mirror (ie, on the opposite side of the mirror from the source object)
    b. 0.47 m in front of the mirror (ie, on the opposite side of the mirror from the source object)
    c. 0.47 m behind the mirror (ie, on the same side of the mirror as the source object)
    d. 0.91 m behind the mirror (ie, on the same side of the mirror as the source object)

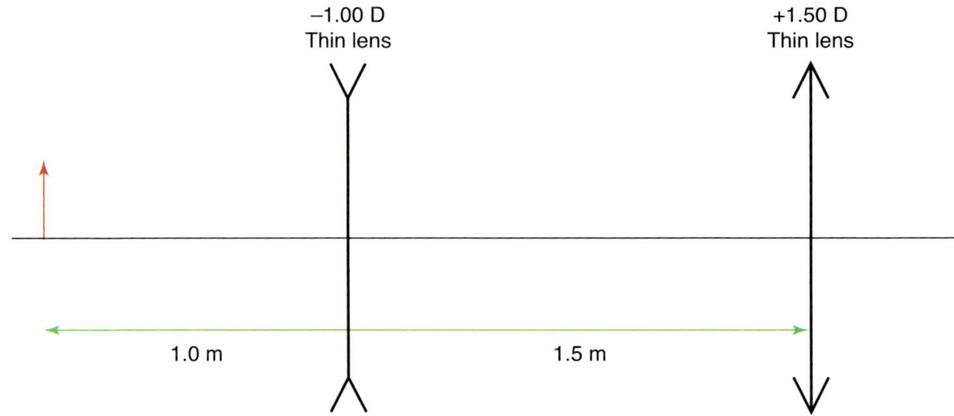

13. In the figure above, an object is 1.0 m to the left of a −1.00 D thin lens. The −1.00 D lens is, in turn, 1.5 m to the left of a 1.50 D thin lens. What is the size of the final image compared with the original object?,
    a. one-fourth the size
    b. one-half the size
    c. same size
    d. twice the size

14. A decrease in the size of the Airy disc image on the retina will result from what change, as light rays are entering the eye?
    a. smaller pupil
    b. longer wavelength of light
    c. decreased focal length of the eye
    d. temporally shifted macula

15. What type of astigmatism is found in a patient with a refraction of $-0.25 + 0.25 \times 090$?
    a. compound astigmatism
    b. simple myopic astigmatism
    c. simple hyperopic astigmatism
    d. mixed astigmatism

16. The radius of the bowl of the Goldmann perimeter is 333 mm. The diameter of the largest available target ("V4") is 9 mm. What is the diameter of the image of this target on the retina?
    a. 0.23 mm
    b. 0.46 mm
    c. 0.90 mm
    d. 3.60 mm

17. LogMAR notation (base-10 logarithm of the minimum angle of resolution) is frequently used to record visual acuity in clinical trials. What is the difference in logMAR scores associated with a doubling of the minimum angle of resolution (such as the difference between visual acuity of 20/40 and 20/80 or between 6/12 and 6/24)?
    a. 0.01 logMAR
    b. 0.20 logMAR
    c. 0.30 logMAR
    d. 0.50 logMAR

18. While refracting a patient, the ophthalmologist uses the duochrome test. The patient states that the green letters are much clearer than the red letters. What does this signify about the patient's visual acuity?
    a. The patient is overminused.
    b. The patient is overplussed.
    c. The patient is presbyopic.
    d. The patient is anisometropic.

19. The clinician is given a small examination room and will refract a patient. If the visual acuity screen is mounted on the wall 3 m from the patient, which step will ensure that the refraction is correct?
    a. Add –0.33 D to the final prescription.
    b. Take no additional step. The refraction should be correct as measured.
    c. Perform a duochrome test.
    d. Refine the final sphere with a trial frame in a longer hallway (6 m).

20. Which bifocal type results in the least amount of image jump?
    a. executive bifocal
    b. flat-top bifocal
    c. round-top bifocal
    d. transition-zone bifocal

21. A patient wears glasses with the following prescription: OD –1.00 sphere and OS +2.00 sphere. When he reads, his eyes move 8 mm below the optic center. What is the induced phoria (in prism diopters [Δ])?
    a. 0.8Δ
    b. 1.6Δ
    c. 2.4Δ
    d. 3.2Δ

22. A patient sees well with contact lenses of −10.00 sph in both eyes. If glasses are made with a vertex distance of 13 mm, which prescription is required to correct the refractive error?
    a. −8.70 D
    b. −10.90 D
    c. −11.50 D
    d. −12.80 D

23. A 46-year-old patient with myopia has blurred distance vision wearing his 5-year-old pair of glasses, which have −4.00 D lenses for both eyes. He has no problem reading. The new distance spectacle power is found to be −5.50 D in both eyes. He expresses an interest in contact lenses. What is the likely effect on the patient's vision of changing the distance correction?
    a. He will be able to see well, far and near, with single-vision spectacles, −5.50 D OU.
    b. He will be able to see well, far and near, with contact lenses −4.00 D for each eye.
    c. He will be able to see well, far and near, with contact lenses −5.50 D for each eye.
    d. He will find it difficult to read with single-vision spectacles, −5.50 OU, and even more difficult to read with contact lenses.

24. A patient has a refractive error of −4.50 D and a *K* measurement of 45.00 D (7.50 mm). What is the residual refractive error if a plano rigid contact lens with a base curve of 7.67 mm (44.00 D) is placed on the eye?
    a. −3.50 D
    b. −4.00 D
    c. −5.00 D
    d. −5.50 D

25. What is the purpose of a square-edge design for an intraocular lens implant?
    a. minimization of positive dysphotopsias
    b. reduced rotation of toric lenses
    c. diminished incidence of iris chafing
    d. decreased posterior migration of lens epithelial cells

26. On postoperative examination, an appropriately powered toric intraocular lens (IOL) is found to be misoriented by 30°. What is the result of this misalignment?
    a. This misalignment will reduce the patient's preoperative astigmatism by one-third.
    b. This misalignment will reduce the patient's preoperative astigmatism by one-half.
    c. This misalignment will neither improve nor worsen the patient's preoperative astigmatism.
    d. This misalignment will double the patient's preoperative astigmatism.

27. How does silicone oil affect the power of a biconvex intraocular lens (IOL)?
    a. Because the refractive index of oil is greater than that of vitreous, the lens power will be increased.
    b. Because the refractive index of oil is less than that of vitreous, the lens power will be increased.
    c. Because the refractive index of oil is greater than that of vitreous, the lens power will be reduced.
    d. Because the refractive index of oil is less than that of vitreous, the lens power will be reduced.

28. A patient presents for laser in situ keratomileusis (LASIK) evaluation to eliminate the need for a distance contact lens correction of −10.00 D. What is the lowest (flattest) treatable keratometric reading that will still avoid excessive corneal flattening?
    a. 40.00 D
    b. 41.00 D
    c. 42.00 D
    d. 43.00 D

29. A 25-year-old hyperopic patient presents to you for refractive surgery evaluation. You measure a large angle kappa. Otherwise, they are a good candidate for photorefractive keratectomy (PRK). What is your plan?
    a. Center the ablation based on the optical axis.
    b. Center the ablation based on the pupillary axis.
    c. Center the ablation based on the visual axis.
    d. Recommend that they continue to use contact lenses rather than undergo refractive surgery.

30. What method can be employed to reduce the risk of night vision difficulties such as glare, starbursts, and haloes in patients who will undergo keratorefractive surgery?
    a. decreasing the size of optical zone
    b. creating a transition zone larger than the pupil
    c. treating preoperatively with miotics
    d. increasing the ablation depth

31. What light phenomenon is the underlying basis of optical coherence tomography (OCT)?
    a. reflection
    b. interference
    c. fluorescence
    d. polarization

32. Considering that the eye acts as a simple magnifier, what is the magnification experienced when one uses a direct ophthalmoscope?
    a. 2×
    b. 4×
    c. 15×
    d. 20×

33. What level of visual field loss qualifies a patient for legal blindness concessions in the United States?
    a. hemianopic field loss
    b. foveal-sparing scotoma
    c. constriction to 20°
    d. severe glaucoma field loss with a mean defect of −19.00 D on 30° field testing

34. A patient with macular degeneration reports blurred vision at near. Their visual acuity is 20/160 in each eye with no refractive error in either eye. What is the most appropriate prescription for low-vision reading glasses?
    a. OD: +4.00 sphere 4Δ BI, OS: +4.00 sphere 4Δ BI
    b. OD: +4.00 sphere 8Δ BI, OS: +4.00 sphere 8Δ BI
    c. OD: +8.00 sphere 8Δ BI, OS: +8.00 sphere 8Δ BI
    d. OD: +8.00 sphere 10Δ BI, OS: +8.00 sphere 10Δ BI

35. What findings reflect the expected effects of a foveal-sparing scotoma from age-related macular degeneration (AMD) on vision and contrast sensitivity?
    a. 20/200 visual acuity, 7 rows on Pelli-Robson chart, normal confrontation visual field
    b. 20/25 visual acuity, 2 rows on Pelli-Robson chart, normal confrontation visual field
    c. 20/25 visual acuity, 4 rows on Pelli-Robson chart, bilaterally constricted confrontation visual field
    d. 20/25 visual acuity, 7 rows on Pelli-Robson chart, normal confrontation visual field

Answers

1. **b.** The magnification of a pinhole camera is limited by the distance from the pinhole to the image plane. The image formed by a pinhole camera is inverted, not upright. The small aperture limits the light available for image formation, and so lengthy exposure times are required and sensitivity is poor in dim light. The depth of field is nearly unlimited.
2. **b.** By definition, a lens with +1.00 D of refractive power forms an image of a distant object 1 m from the lens. The sun is certainly a "distant object"! The formula for the power of a lens $P = 1/f$ is helpful, where P is the power of the lens in diopters and f is the focal length of the lens. A +1.00 D lens forms images of a distant object 1.0 m from the lens, on the opposite side of the lens from the object. Similarly, a +2.00 D lens could be used and would be held 0.5 m from the ground.
3. **a.** The power of the original lens system is given by the vergence equation: $U + P = V$, where P is the power of the lens in diopters, U *is* the object vergence, and V is the image vergence. It is worth noting that $U = 1/u$ and $V = 1/v$, where u is the distance from the lens to the object and v is the distance from the lens to the image. Here, the distant object can be considered to be located at infinity, so $U = 1/\infty = 0$. Thus, $0 + P = 1/1.00$, so $P = +1.00$ D. The net power of the new lens system is the sum of the original power plus the power of the added lens: $P_{new} = P_{old} + 3.00\text{ D} = 4.00\text{ D}$. This new lens system forms an image according to the vergence equation: $0 + 4.00\text{ D} = 1/v$, so $v = +0.25$ m.
4. **a.** For an eye with uncorrected myopia, the refractive power is stronger than necessary to focus the light rays on the retina, and the image of a distant object will form in front of the retina. This is true whether or not the eye is accommodating. For an eye with uncorrected hyperopia, the image of a distant object will form behind the retina. For a younger patient with hyperopia or an older patient with a low hyperopic refractive error, accommodation may be used to bring a near object into focus on the retina.
5. **c.** The key to converting a power-cross description to a spherocylindrical specification is to determine the *difference* between the power in the 2 principal meridians. Here, the difference is 3.00 diopters (D). For a spherocylindrical lens, the power of cylindrical correction is oriented 90° away from its power. As we are asked for the answer in minus cylinder form, the spherical component is the power in the more positive meridian, here +1.00. The cylindrical component is thus −3.00 D. This power is observed along the 115° meridian and is created by a minus cylinder lens component with axis 90° away; that is, axis 25°. When expressed in plus cylinder form, the spherocylindrical specification of this lens is −2.00 ⊂ +3.00 × 115°.
6. **d.** The compensation of the sphere power is always in the opposite direction from the change in cylinder power, in the ratio of a change in the sphere of one-half the change in cylinder. This is because the spherical equivalent power of a given refraction equals the spherical power plus one-half of the cylindrical power. When transposing a glasses prescription between minus and plus cylinder notation, one adds the spherical and cylindrical powers to obtain the new spherical power, reverses the sign of the cylindrical power, and rotates the axis 90°.
7. **c.** The Jackson cross cylinder (JCC) lens is a single lens that combines 2 cylindrical lenses whose powers are numerically equal and of opposite signs, with axes perpendicular to each other. This combination makes the spherical equivalent always equal to 0. The primary

use of a JCC is to subjectively refine the axis and magnitude of cylinder after placing the best available estimate of the spherical equivalent of the refraction in front of the eye. In a phoropter, the most common JCC powers are +0.25 D and −0.25 D, with the axes determined by the orientation of the lens, or +0.25 ⊃ − 0.50 × __ = −0.25 ⊃ +0.50 × __. Red dots identify the axis of the minus cylinder power, and white dots identify the axis of the plus cylinder power.

8. **a.** If the retinoscopy streak is horizontal, the axis of the cylindrical lens is also horizontal (180°). So the spherocylindrical lens combination for this patient, before the working distance adjustment is subtracted, is +3.00 + 1.00 × 090. The working distance (67 cm, or 0.67 m) must be subtracted from the final refraction. Thus, subtracting 1/0.67 m, or 1.50 D, yields the correct answer: +1.50 + 1.00 × 090. Note that the cylindrical power acts 90° from the axis. If the retinoscopy streak is horizontal, the axis of the cylindrical lens is 180°, but the actual power is at 90°. Accordingly, the powers, after subtracting the working distance, are +1.50 D at 90° and +2.50 D at 180°.
9. **a.** If light travels from a denser medium (in this case, water; refractive index 1.33) to a less dense medium (in this case, air; refractive index 1.00), then light rays bend away from the surface normal, according to Snell's law. This redirection of light produces image displacement, thus causing the shark to appear further away than it actually is. Thus, the shark is closer than it appears to the surfer. However, for a shark (in the water) looking up at a surfer (in the air), the surfer would actually be further from the shark than the surfer appears. See Chapter 1, Figure 1-2.
10. **a.** Unlike light that passes through a spherical lens and is focused to a single point, light that passes through a spherocylindrical lens is focused to a 3-dimensional image termed the conoid of Sturm. The images at the ends of the conoid are lines, and the image at the center of the conoid is a circle. Images between the ends and center of the conoid are elliptical in shape. The circle of least confusion is the circular cross section of the conoid of Sturm that is halfway between the 2 focal lines; it occurs at the spherical equivalent value of a spherocylindrical lens and provides the best visual acuity.
11. **d.** A prism disperses white light into a spectrum of wavelengths, creating a rainbow. While each of the various colors of light is deflected toward the base of the prism, shorter wavelengths of light, such as violet, are bent more than longer wavelengths of light, such as red. This effect—referred to as chromatic aberration—is caused by dispersion, in which the index of refraction of a medium may vary with the wavelength of the light passing through it. This phenomenon is the basis for the duochrome test for accommodative control, in which green light rays are bent more and come into focus more anteriorly than do red light rays.
12. **b.** Mirrors have reflecting power but no refracting power. The reflecting power of a mirror is calculated as $P = -1/f = -2/r$, where the focal length (f) equals half of the radius of curvature (r). For this mirror, $P = -2/r = -2.0$ D. Thus the vergence equation $U + P = V$ reads $-1/10.0 + (-2.0) = 1/v$, so $v = 1/(-2.1) = -0.47$ m; that is, 0.47 m away from the mirror on the side opposite the source object. This will be an erect, virtual image, minified by a factor of 0.47/10.0 = 0.047. Such a small image is interpreted by the driver as an object farther away than the original source object—as the reminder printed on the mirror states: "OBJECTS IN MIRROR ARE CLOSER THAN THEY APPEAR."
13. **a.** The vergence equation ($U + P = V$, or $1/u + P = 1/v$) can be used to determine the location of the intermediate and final images, and the formula for transverse magnification ($M_T = U/V$)

can be used to calculate the image size. Application of the vergence equation determines that the intermediate image is located 0.5 m to the left of the first lens (applying $U + P = V$, $-1 - 1 = -2$; applying $v = 1/V$, $1/-2 = -0.5$). Based on $M_T = U/V$ ($M_T = -1/-2 = +0.5x$), the intermediate image is half the height of the original image and upright, given the positive sign. Now, $U + P = V$ is represented by $-0.5 + 1.5 = +1$, and the final image is located 1 m to the right of the second lens. Again, by $M_T = U/V$ ($M_T = -0.5/+1 = -0.5x$), the final image is half the height of the intermediate image and inverted. The magnification of the final image can be calculated as $(0.5)(-0.5) = -0.25$, which means that the final image is one-fourth the size of the original object and inverted. Of note, transverse magnification describes the image height, while axial (longitudinal) magnification describes the length, or depth, of the image (measured along the optical axis) and can be calculated as $M_L = (M_T)^2$.

14. **c.** Eyes with shorter focal lengths have smaller Airy discs than eyes with longer focal lengths and therefore diffract light rays less. The Airy disc is the central portion of a pattern of light and dark rings formed when light from a point source passes through a circular aperture and is diffracted. Diffraction describes the divergence of light as it traverses through an aperture. The smaller the aperture is relative to the wavelength of light, the more pronounced the diffraction. The formula for the diameter of the Airy disc is diameter = $2.44\lambda f/D$, where λ is the wavelength of the light, f is the focal length of the eye, and D is the diameter of the pupil. Diffraction increases as the focal length of the eye increases, the wavelength of light increases, or the pupil size decreases. Retinal conditions have no effect on the size of the Airy disc.
15. **b.** The prescription in the question stem can be written in plus cylinder notation as −0.25 + 0.25 × 090 or in minus cylinder notation as plano −0.25 × 180. This is an example of simple myopic astigmatism, with 1 focal line on the retina. A patient with simple hyperopic astigmatism has a hyperopic refraction with 1 focal line on the retina; an example is plano +0.50 × 090 (same as +0.50 −0.50 × 180). Compound myopic astigmatism involves 2 focal lines in front of the retina (sph and cyl negative in both plus and minus cyl notation), while compound hyperopic astigmatism involves 2 focal lines behind the retina (sph and cyl positive in plus and minus cyl notation). Mixed astigmatism involves 1 focal line behind the retina and 1 in front (sph and cyl with opposite signs in both plus and minus cyl notation).
16. **b.** The nodal point in the Gullstrand schematic eye is located 17 mm in front of the retina. Using the geometric principle of similar triangles, the diameter of the retinal image of an object located 333 mm from the eye, with a diameter of 9 mm, is 9 mm × (17/333) = 0.46 mm. The corresponding retinal image is about 20 times smaller than its target light in a Goldmann perimeter. This is because the perimeter's radius (333 mm) is approximately 20 times larger than the distance from the eye's nodal point to the retina (17 mm). Similarly, the retinal image size of a Snellen letter on an eye chart can be calculated as follows: retinal image height / Snellen letter height = 17 mm / distance from chart to eye.
17. **c.** A change in acuity by a factor of 10 (such as a change from 20/20 to 20/200) corresponds to a difference of 1.0 logMAR, since 1.0 is the common logarithm of 10. The common logarithm of 2 is 0.301, which we round to 0.30 for clinical purposes. This is "built-in" to the common ETDRS eye charts, which feature proportional steps of 0.10 logMAR between lines, so that a 3-line change in acuity corresponds to a change of 0.30 logMAR (ie, a doubling [or halving] of the visual angle). The logMAR is calculated as the logarithm of the reciprocal of the Snellen fraction (eg, 20/200 –> reciprocal is 200/20 = 10 –> logarithm of 10 = 1).

18. **a.** This patient is overminused. Shorter wavelengths of light, such as green, are bent more than longer wavelengths, such as red. When the patient sees the green letters more clearly than the red letters, the shorter (more bent) green wavelength is more in focus and closer to the retina than the longer red wavelength of light. Therefore, more plus would need to be added to the refraction to bring the red wavelength closer to the retina. A balanced refraction is achieved when the green and red letters are equidistant from the retina and each one appears equally clear. RAM-GAP is a mnemonic device to help learners remember to "*r*ed *a*dd *m*inus, *g*reen *a*dd *p*lus."

19. **d.** Refracting in a short room will produce results that are inherently inaccurate because normal fogging techniques to relax accommodation will not be effective. One method to relax the accommodation would be to move the patient to a longer hallway to complete the refraction in a trial frame. Another option would be to install mirrors to optically extend the room length to 6m.

20. **a.** Prism is induced when one looks through a lens at any point other than its optical center. Therefore, when the eye is looking down and encounters the top of a bifocal add, the image jumps, unless the optical center of that bifocal add is at the top of the segment. Executive-style segments have their optical centers at the top of the segment; therefore, they induce no image jump. The optical center of a flat-top segment is typically 3 mm from the top of the segment, whereas the optical center of a round-top segment is much lower. Therefore, flat-top segments cause some image jump, but less than that caused by round-top segments. The "transition zone" is the name for the area of progressive change in lens power in a progressive addition lens (PAL). While PALs do not induce image jump, they are (by definition) not bifocals.

21. **c.** Prentice's rule states that the prism power of a lens at any point on its surface, in prism diopters (Δ), is equal to the distance away from the optic center *(h)* in centimeters times the power of the lens in diopters (D), or $\Delta = hD$. Minus-power lenses can be drawn as 2 prisms with the bases directed outward, while plus-power lenses can be drawn as 2 prisms with the bases directed inward. For the right eye, $\Delta = 0.8 \times 1 = 0.8\Delta$. Based on the diagram on the left, below, we know that this is 0.8Δ base down. For the left eye, $\Delta = 0.8 \times 2 = 1.6\Delta$. Based on the diagram on the right, below, we know that this is 1.6Δ base up. Given that the prisms are opposite each other vertically, the prism diopters are added together, and the induced phoria is calculated to be 2.4Δ.

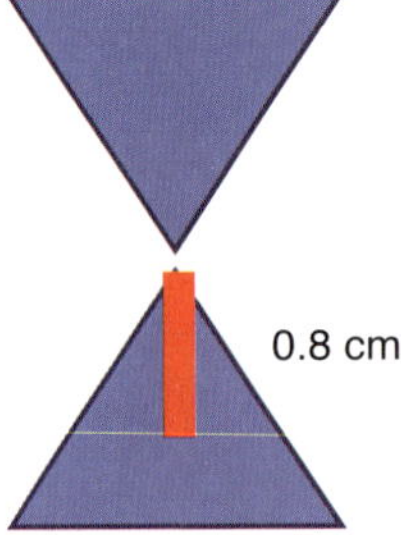

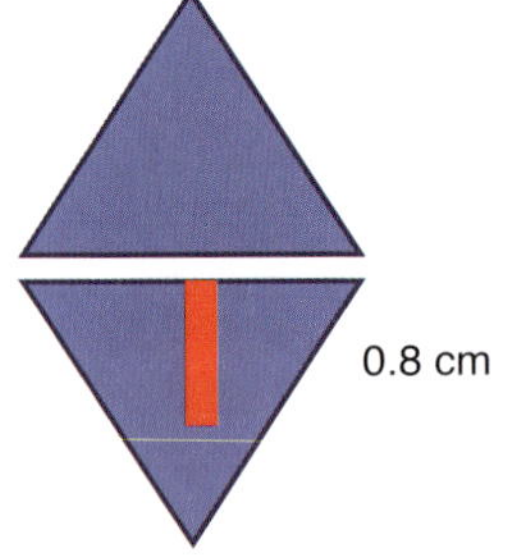

22. **c.** Ametropia is corrected with a lens whose focal point coincides with the eye's far point. First, locate the far point of the eye. Because the patient is myopic, we know that the far point is in front of the eye; by convention, this is represented as a negative number. The distance from the patient's eye to the far point is 10 cm, and the vertex distance is 1.3 cm.

Thus, the far point of the eye and the focal point of the contact lenses coincide at this location: –0.100 m – (–0.013 m) = –0.087 m (in front of the eye). Therefore, the required lenses have a power of 1/(–0.087) = –11.50 D.

23. **d.** The old glasses do not give clear vision for distance, and they now function almost as reading glasses. New spectacles, fully correcting the distance vision about 12 mm from the eye, have the advantage of "near effectivity," which reduces accommodative demand, compared to an emmetropic eye or one corrected by a contact lens. People with myopia who are in the patient's age range and who are still able to read with their correct distance glasses are likely to find it more difficult to read with contact lenses. The presbyopic myopic patient who wears glasses can read more easily by pushing the glasses farther away from the eyes.

24. **a.** The curvature of the contact lens (44.00 D) is flatter than the cornea (45.00 D) by 1 D. This means that the tear film creates a negative lens power: –1.00 D. To counteract this tear film, +1.00 D must be added to the refraction: –4.50 D + 1.00 D = –3.50 D. This can be remembered with the SAM-FAP rule: *s*teeper *a*dd *m*inus, *f*latter *a*dd *p*lus. Since the contact lens is flatter by 1.00 D, add +1.00 D to the refraction of –4.50 D for a power of –3.50 D.

25. **d.** Lenses with a square edge produce increased pressure of the lens edge against the posterior capsule, resulting in decreased posterior migration of lens epithelial cells and a diminished rate of posterior capsular opacification (PCO). Many modern lens implants are created with a rounded anterior edge and square posterior edge to maintain a decreased risk of PCO while reducing the risk of iris chafing, which can be especially high with sulcus placement of a lens with a square anterior edge. A square-edge lens design has been associated with positive dysphotopsias, with smooth edges found to minimize dysphotopsias. A frosted-edge haptic design has been shown to reduce rotation of toric lenses.

26. **c.** Misalignment of a toric intraocular lens by as little as 10° will result in a substantial reduction in the efficacy of the astigmatism correction. Misalignment by 30° will have a neutral effect, negating the benefit of the toric lens. Misalignment by 90° will double the patient's resultant astigmatism. Any misalignment of a toric intraocular lens (other than a misalignment of exactly 90°) will also rotate the patient's postoperative astigmatic axis.

27. **c.** Because the refractive index of silicone oil is greater than that of vitreous, the oil filling the vitreous cavity reduces the optical power of the posterior surface of the intraocular lens (IOL) in the eye when a biconvex IOL is implanted. This problem must be counteracted by an increase in IOL power of 3 to 5 diopters.

28. **b.** For myopic laser in situ keratomileusis (LASIK), a change of approximately 0.80 D in the average keratometry value *(K)* results from each 1.00 D of refractive change. The following equation is used to predict corneal curvature after keratorefractive surgery: $K_{postop} = K_{preop} + (0.8 \times RE)$, where K_{preop} and K_{postop} are the preoperative and postoperative K readings, respectively, and RE is the refractive error to be corrected at the corneal plane. When myopic corrections are performed, the minimum corneal power tolerable is 33.00 D. Therefore, the formula becomes $33.00 = K_{preop} + (0.8 \times -10.00)$, where K_{preop} equals 41.00. Both excessively flat (<33.00 D) and excessively steep (>50.00 D) corneal powers should be avoided postoperatively, as these can result in decreased visual quality and increased higher-order aberrations. For hyperopic LASIK, approximately 1.00 D of corneal steepening occurs per 1.00 D of corneal ablation.

29. **c.** Corneal refractive ablations should be centered on the visual axis in a patient with a high angle kappa, in order to avoid a decentered ablation. Angle kappa is the angle between the pupillary axis (line perpendicular to the corneal surface, passing through the pupillary midpoint) and the visual axis (line connecting point of fixation to fovea); see Chapter 3, Figure 3-3. High angle kappa may result from hyperopia, exotropia, or macular dragging. When identified preoperatively, the ablation can be shifted more nasally to center on the visual axis, rather than the pupillary axis. Patients with decentered ablations may develop coma, which occurs when rays at one edge of the pupil converge before rays at the opposite edge of the pupil do. This higher-order aberration can result in an image resembling a comet with a tail. Decentered ablations are particularly problematic in a hyperopic correction. Large angle kappa is not a contraindication to refractive surgery.

30. **b.** Postoperative night-vision problems are well described and are often associated with large pupil sizes (>8 mm). These symptoms, which include the appearance of glare, starbursts, and haloes, decreased contrast sensitivity, and decreased quality of vision at night, tend to occur in patients with both large pupils and small treatment zones (≤6 mm). In appropriate candidates, third-generation lasers utilize larger optical and transition zones to help reduce the incidence and severity of night-vision problems. The accepted standard transition zone between ablated and unablated cornea is 0.5–1.0 mm larger than the pupil to help reduce night-vision problems, but in order to conserve corneal tissue, smaller optical zones are used in the correction of high myopia. The incidence of night-vision problems in these patients increases in part because of the mismatch between the size of the pupil and that of the optical zone. In this patient, increasing the optical zone may not be feasible without significantly thinning the cornea and increasing the risk of postsurgical corneal ectasia. Preoperative treatment with miotics does not reduce the risk of night-vision problems. In some of the patients, postoperative miotics such as brimonidine 0.2% or pilocarpine 0.5% or 1% may help reduce the postoperative night-vision problems.

31. **b.** Optical coherence tomography (OCT) is an optical analogue to ultrasound imaging and uses infrared light instead of sound. The much higher speed of light compared with sound allows for finer resolution, but direct electronic measurement of the shorter "echo" times it takes light to travel from different structures at axial distances within the eye is not feasible. Interferometry makes it possible to overcome this difficulty. More precisely, OCT uses interference of tunable broadband coherent light to generate optical sections of the retina and cornea.

32. **c.** With direct ophthalmoscopy, the examiner uses the optics of the patient's eye as a simple magnifier to look at the retina. The optics of the emmetropic eye are approximately +60.00 D, thus the magnification is approximately 60/4, or 15×, according to the formula for a simple magnifier (Mag = D/4). Interestingly, this magnification varies. The optic disc will appear larger in a myopic patient and smaller in a hyperopic patient when the dial on the direct ophthalmoscope is rotated to correct the patient's refractive error. For a myopic patient, a minus lens is dialed in to overcome the extra plus power "error lens" inside the patient's eye. The 2 lenses create a Galilean telescope, increasing magnification and decreasing the field of view. Similarly, a reverse Galilean telescope is formed during examination of a hyperopic patient, which decreases magnification.

33. **c.** The definition of legal blindness in the United States requires the better-seeing eye to exhibit best-corrected visual acuity (BCVA) of 20/200 or worse, or a visual field with 20° or less around central fixation, measured with a Goldmann III 4e target. A point seen at 10 dB or higher on a static automated threshold field test is considered to be seen with a

4e stimulus. A mean defect of 22 dB or greater on an automated 30° static threshold perimetry test is also considered legal blindness by the Social Security Administration in the United States. Referral to visual rehabilitation services should occur before the patient is legally blind; the AAO Preferred Practice Pattern guideline says to refer a patient when visual acuity is <20/40, contrast sensitivity has declined, or significant peripheral or central visual field loss is present.

34. **d.** In patients with low visual acuity, high-plus reading glasses may be helpful reading aids. The Kestenbaum rule provides the dioptric power of the reading lens, which is defined by the following equation: [lens dioptric power] = 1 / [visual acuity fraction]. In this case, the lens dioptric power would be 160/20, which is +8.00 D. Because of the high power of the lens (greater than 4.00 D), prisms are added to help reduce convergence. As a general rule, the amount of prism added to the glasses is 2Δ base-in more than the dioptric power of the lens, or in this case, 10Δ base-in (BI) in each eye.

35. **b.** This patient with age-related macular degeneration (AMD) has preserved central visual acuity with reduced-vision near fixation, resulting in severely decreased contrast sensitivity, as reflected by the ability to read only 2 rows on the Pelli-Robson chart. This patient may have difficulty reading larger text (eg, headlines), despite having excellent visual acuity when reading the Snellen chart. The patient described in answer a has decreased central visual acuity from foveal hypoplasia due to albinism, with preserved contrast sensitivity reflected in the ability to read all 7 lines on the Pelli-Robson chart. The patient described in answer c has peripheral vision loss with moderately reduced contrast sensitivity due to glaucoma. The patient described in answer d has normal vision.

Index

(*f* = figure; *t* = table)

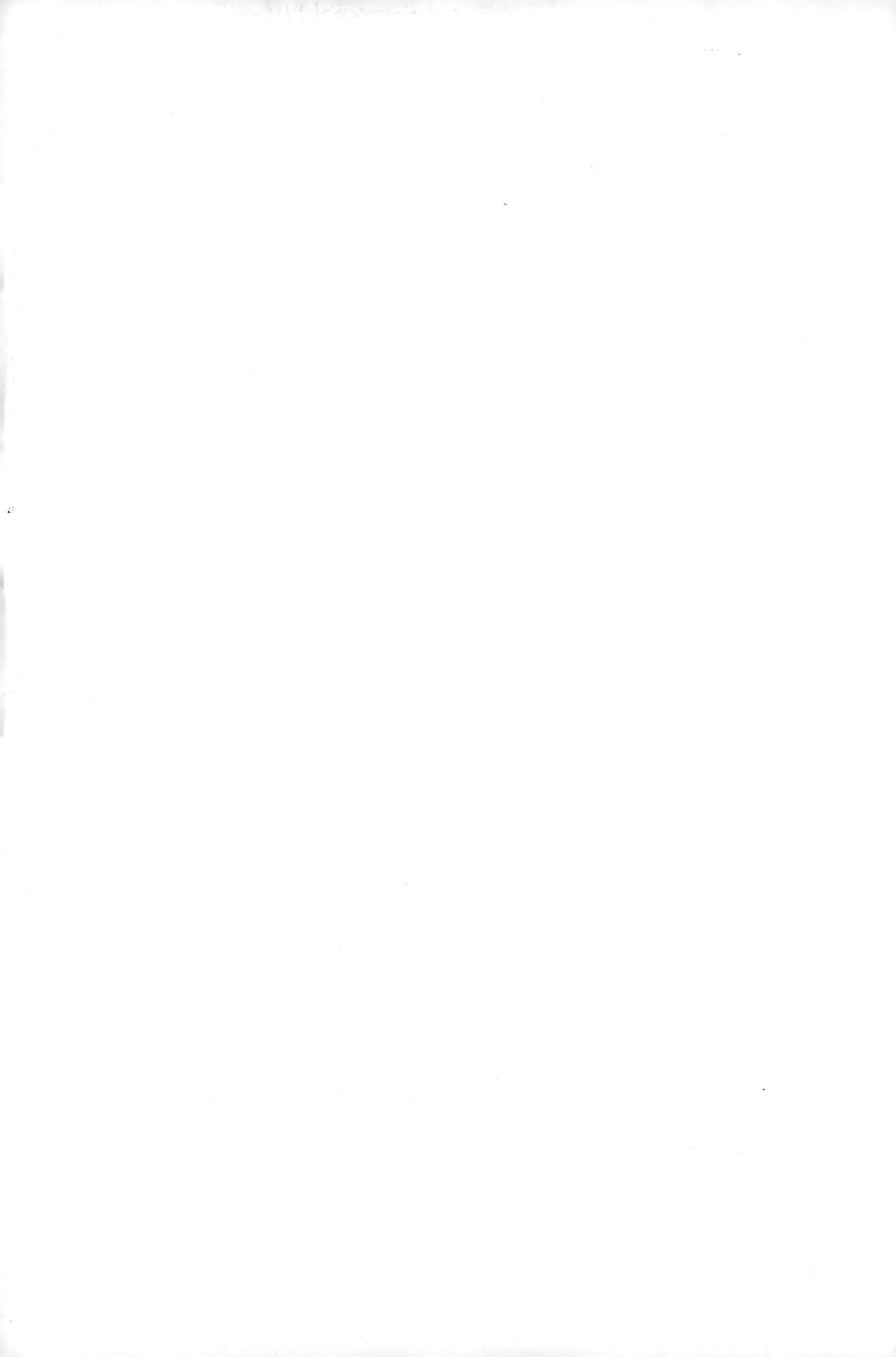